Renal and Urologic Issues

Editors

MICHELLE N. RHEAULT
LARRY A. GREENBAUM

CLINICS IN PERINATOLOGY

www.perinatology.theclinics.com

Consulting Editor
LUCKY JAIN

September 2014 • Volume 41 • Number 3

ELSEVIER

1600 John F. Kennedy Boulevard • Suite 1800 • Philadelphia, Pennsylvania, 19103-2899

http://www.theclinics.com

CLINICS IN PERINATOLOGY Volume 41, Number 3
September 2014 ISSN 0095-5108, ISBN-13: 978-0-323-32337-6

Editor: Kerry Holland
Developmental Editor: Casey Jackson

Clinics in Perinatology (ISSN 0095-5108) is published quarterly by Elsevier Inc., 360 Park Avenue South, New York, NY 10010-1710. Months of issue are March, June, September, and December. Business and Editorial Offices: 1600 John F. Kennedy Blvd., Ste. 1800, Philadelphia, PA 19103-2899. Customer Service Office: 3251 Riverport Lane, Maryland Heights, MO 63043. Periodicals postage paid at New York, NY and additional mailing offices. Subscription prices are $285.00 per year (US individuals), $445.00 per year (US institutions), $340.00 per year (Canadian individuals), $545.00 per year (Canadian institutions), $420.00 per year (foreign individuals), $545.00 per year (foreign institutions), $135.00 per year (US students), and $195.00 per year (Canadian and foreign students). Foreign air speed delivery is included in all Clinics subscription prices. All prices are subject to change without notice. **POSTMASTER:** Send address changes to *Clinics in Perinatology*, Elsevier Health Sciences Division, Subscription Customer Service, 3251 Riverport Lane, Maryland Heights, MO 63043. **Customer Service: Telephone: 1-800-654-2452** (U.S. and Canada); **1-314-447-8871** (outside U.S. and Canada). **Fax: 1-314-447-8029. E-mail: journalscustomerservice-usa@elsevier.com** (for print support); **journalsonlinesupport-usa@elsevier.com** (for online support).

Reprints. For copies of 100 or more, of articles in this publication, please contact the Commercial Reprints Department, Elsevier Inc., 360 Park Avenue South, New York, NY 10010-1710. Tel. 212-633-3874; Fax: 212-633-3820; E-mail: reprints@elsevier.com.

Clinics in Perinatology is also pubilshed in Spanish by McGraw-Hill Interamericana Editores S.A., P.O. Box 5-237, 06500 Mexico D.F., Mexico.

Clinics in Perinatology is covered in *MEDLINE/PubMed (Index Medicus) Current Contents, Excepta Medica, BIOSIS* and *ISI/BIOMED.*

Printed in the United States of America.

Contributors

CONSULTING EDITOR

LUCKY JAIN, MD, MBA
Richard W. Blumberg Professor and Executive Vice Chairman, Department of Pediatrics, Emory University School of Medicine; Executive Medical Director, Children's Physician Group, Emory Children's Center, Children's Healthcare of Atlanta, Atlanta, Georgia

EDITORS

MICHELLE N. RHEAULT, MD
Assistant Professor, Division of Pediatric Nephrology; Medical Director of Dialysis, Department of Pediatrics, University of Minnesota Children's Hospital, Minneapolis, Minnesota

LARRY A. GREENBAUM, MD, PhD
Marcus Professor of Pediatrics, Division Director, Pediatric Nephrology, Children's Healthcare of Atlanta and Emory University School of Medicine, Atlanta, Georgia

AUTHORS

ANGELA M. ARLEN, MD
Fellow in Pediatric Urology, Children's Healthcare of Atlanta, Emory University School of Medicine, Atlanta, Georgia

WILLIAM R. ARMSTRONG III, MD
Department of Urology, Urology Resident, University of Illinois Chicago College of Medicine, Chicago, Illinois

DAVID J. ASKENAZI, MD, MSPH
Associate Professor of Pediatrics, Division of Pediatric Nephrology, University of Alabama at Birmingham, Birmingham, Alabama

LAUREN BALDINGER, DO, MS
Division of Pediatric Urology, The Children's Hospital of Philadelphia, Perelman School of Medicine, University of Pennsylvania, Philadelphia, Pennsylvania

ROSSANA BARACCO, MD
Assistant Professor of Pediatrics, Division of Pediatric Nephrology, Children's Hospital of Michigan, Wayne State University, Detroit, Michigan

DONALD L. BATISKY, MD
Director, Pediatric Hypertension Program, Children's Healthcare of Atlanta, Emory – Children's Center; Associate Professor of Pediatrics, Emory University School of Medicine, Atlanta, Georgia

M. JANE BLACK, BSc (Hons), PhD
Associate Professor, Department of Anatomy and Developmental Biology, Monash University, Clayton, Victoria, Australia

DETLEF BOCKENHAUER, MD, PhD
Nephrology Unit, UCL Institute of Child Health, Great Ormond Street Hospital for Children NHS Foundation Trust, London, United Kingdom

JOHN W. BROCK III, MD
Chief, Division of Pediatric Urologic Surgery; Professor, Department of Urologic Surgery, Monroe Carrel Jr. Children's Hospital, Nashville, Tennessee

MICHAEL C. CARR, MD, PhD
Associate Professor, Pediatric Urology; Attending Physician, Division of Urology, The Children's Hospital of Philadelphia, Philadelphia, Pennsylvania

DOUGLASS B. CLAYTON, MD
Division of Pediatric Urologic Surgery, Assistant Professor, Department of Urologic Surgery, Monroe Carrel Jr. Children's Hospital, Nashville, Tennessee

WILLIAM O. COOPER, MD, MPH
Division of General Pediatrics, Department of Pediatrics, Vanderbilt University School of Medicine, Nashville, Tennessee

STUART L. GOLDSTEIN, MD
Professor of Pediatrics, University of Cincinnati; Center for Acute Care Nephrology, Cincinnati Children's Hospital Medical Center (CCHMC), Cincinnati, Ohio

STEPHANIE M. JERNIGAN, MD
Assistant Professor of Pediatrics, Division of Pediatric Nephrology, Emory University School of Medicine and Children's Healthcare of Atlanta, Atlanta, Georgia

JENNIFER G. JETTON, MD
Clinical Assistant Professor of Pediatrics, Division of Nephrology, Dialysis and Transplantation, University of Iowa Children's Hospital, Iowa City, Iowa

DEBORAH P. JONES, MD, MS
Division of Pediatric Nephrology, Department of Pediatrics, Vanderbilt University School of Medicine, Nashville, Tennessee

AHMAD KADDOURAH, MD, MS
Clinical Fellow of Pediatric Acute Care Nephrology, Center for Acute Care Nephrology, Cincinnati Children's Hospital Medical Center (CCHMC), Cincinnati, Ohio

ALISON L. KENT, BMBS, FRACP, MD
Professor, Department of Neonatology, Centenary Hospital for Women and Children, Canberra Hospital; Australian National University Medical School, Canberra, Australian Capital Territory, Australia

DENNIS B. LIU, MD, FAAP, FACS
Clinical Instructor of Urology, Ann and Robert H. Lurie Children's Hospital of Chicago, Department of Urology, Northwestern University Feinberg School of Medicine, Chicago, Illinois

MAX MAIZELS, MD
Professor of Urology, Ann and Robert H. Lurie Children's Hospital of Chicago,
Department of Urology, Northwestern University Feinberg School of Medicine,
Chicago, Illinois

TEJ K. MATTOO, MD, DCH, FRCP
Professor of Pediatrics, Division of Pediatric Nephrology, Children's Hospital of Michigan,
Wayne State University, Detroit, Michigan

YOSUKE MIYASHITA, MD, MPH
Assistant Professor, Division of Pediatric Nephrology, Department of Pediatrics,
Children's Hospital of Pittsburgh of UPMC, University of Pittsburgh School of Medicine,
Pittsburgh, Pennsylvania

THOMAS M. MORGAN, MD
Division of Medical Genetics, Department of Pediatrics, Vanderbilt University School of
Medicine, Nashville, Tennessee

ABHIJITH MUDEGOWDAR, MD
Division of Pediatric Urology, The Children's Hospital of Philadelphia, Perelman School of
Medicine, University of Pennsylvania, Philadelphia, Pennsylvania

MICHELLE N. RHEAULT, MD
Assistant Professor, Division of Pediatric Nephrology; Medical Director of Dialysis,
Department of Pediatrics, University of Minnesota Children's Hospital, Minneapolis,
Minnesota

DANA RYAN, BSc (Hons)
Department of Anatomy and Developmental Biology, Monash University, Clayton,
Victoria, Australia

ELLEN SHAPIRO, MD
Department of Urology, Director of Pediatric Urology, New York University School of
Medicine, New York, New York

ASEEM R. SHUKLA, MD, FAAP
Division of Pediatric Urology, Director of Minimally Invasive Surgery, The Children's
Hospital of Philadelphia; Associate Professor of Surgery (in Urology), Perelman School of
Medicine, University of Pennsylvania, Philadelphia, Pennsylvania

EDWIN A. SMITH, MD, FAAP, FACS
Clinical Associate Professor of Urology, Children's Healthcare of Atlanta, Emory
University School of Medicine; Georgia Urology, PA, Atlanta, Georgia

MEGAN SUTHERLAND, BBiomedSci (Hons), PhD
Department of Anatomy and Developmental Biology, Monash University, Clayton,
Victoria, Australia

PRIYA VERGHESE, MD, MPH
Assistant Professor, Division of Pediatric Nephrology, Department of Pediatrics; Medical
Director of Pediatric Kidney Transplantation, Amplatz Children's Hospital, University of
Minnesota, Minneapolis, Minnesota

BRADLEY A. WARADY, MD
Professor of Pediatrics, University of Missouri — Kansas City School of Medicine; Senior
Associate Chairman, Department of Pediatrics; Director, Division of Pediatric Nephrology;
Director, Dialysis and Transplantation, Children's Mercy Hospital, Kansas City, Missouri

JOSHUA J. ZARITSKY, MD, PhD
Chief, Division of Nephrology; Associate Professor of Pediatrics, Thomas Jefferson University Medical College; Nemours/A.I. duPont Hospital for Children, Wilmington, Delaware

JAKUB ZIEG, MD, PhD
Department of Pediatrics, 2nd Faculty of Medicine, Charles University in Prague and Motol University Hospital, Praha, Czech Republic

Contents

Critically ill neonates are at risk for acute kidney injury (AKI). AKI has been associated with increased risk of morbidity and mortality in adult and pediatric patients, and increasing evidence suggests a similar association in the neonatal population. This article describes the current AKI definitions (including their limitations), work on novel biomarkers to define AKI, diagnosis and management strategies, long-term outcomes after AKI, and future directions for much-needed research in this important area.

An increased emphasis has been placed on the early identification of chronic kidney disease (CKD) in the neonatal population, given the long-term health consequences that can accompany this diagnosis. The definition of CKD in neonates and young infants differs from that of children older than 2 years and, if severe, treatment may mandate dialysis with appropriate ethical considerations. Special attention must also be directed to optimal nutrition because of its impact on height, weight, and brain development in the young child experiencing impaired kidney function. There has been steady improvement in patient survival over the last decade.

 Video of PD catheter accompanies this article

The incidence of acute kidney injury (AKI) has steadily increased in the last decade in neonates and infants. Despite the extensive proposed pharmacologic approaches to treat or prevent AKI, renal replacement therapy is the only available therapeutic approach to manage the consequences of significant AKI and maintain electrolyte homeostasis and fluid balance in infants with AKI. The objective of this article is to summarize the different approaches and modalities of renal replacement therapy in neonatal intensive care units.

The incidence of neonatal hypertension (HTN) remains low, at less than 2%, and its etiology is varied. Strict definitions of HTN in neonates are unavailable, and the decision to treat is based on opinion rather than evidence. More studies are needed to define normal blood pressure in neonates and to refine current reference values, thus permitting a better definition of HTN. Most causes of neonatal HTN, the most common of which seems to be renovascular disease, are determined by history and basic clinical investigations. Treatment is guided by clinical judgment and expert opinion, given the limited number of clinical trials.

This article provides an up-to-date comprehensive review and summary on neonatal polycystic kidney disease (PKD) with emphasis on the differential diagnosis, clinical manifestations, diagnostic techniques, and potential therapeutic approaches for the major causes of neonatal PKD, namely hereditary disease, including autosomal recessive and autosomal dominant PKD and nonhereditary PKD, with particular emphasis on multicystic dysplastic kidney. A brief overview of obstructive cystic dysplasia and simple and complex cysts is also included.

The normal development of the kidney may be affected by several factors, including abnormalities in placental function, resulting in fetal growth restriction, exposure to maternal disease states, including hypertension and diabetes, antenatal steroids, chorioamnionitis, and preterm delivery. After preterm birth, several further insults may occur that may influence nephrogenesis and renal health, including exposure to nephrotoxic medications, postnatal growth failure, and obesity after growth restriction. In this review article, common clinical neonatal scenarios are used to highlight these renal risk factors, and the animal and human evidence on which these risk factors are based are discussed.

Electrolyte disorders can result in life-threatening complications. The kidneys are tasked with maintaining electrolyte homoeostasis, yet the low glomerular filtration rate of neonatal kidneys, tubular immaturity, and high extrarenal fluid losses contribute to increased occurrence of electrolyte disorders in neonates. Understanding the physiologic basis of renal electrolyte handling is crucial in identifying underlying causes and initiation of proper treatment. This article reviews key aspects of renal physiology, the diagnostic workup of disorders of plasma sodium and potassium, and the appropriate treatment, in addition to inherited disorders associated with neonatal electrolyte disturbances that illuminate the physiology of renal electrolyte handling.

Microscopic and gross hematuria, while rare in healthy newborns, is more common in premature infants, particularly those cared for in the neonatal intensive care unit. Hematuria may be transient, but may require evaluation, investigation, and intervention in a timely manner. This article discusses the causes, workup, and treatment of the more common forms of newborn hematuria.

Glomerular disorders in infancy can include nephrotic and nephritic syndromes. Congenital nephrotic syndrome (CNS) is most commonly caused by single gene mutations in kidney proteins, but may also be due to congenital infections or passive transfer of maternal antibodies that target kidney proteins. Prenatal findings of increased maternal serum α-fetoprotein and enlarged placenta suggest CNS. Neonatal nephritis is rare; its causes may overlap with those of CNS and include primary glomerulonephritis, systemic disease, infections, and transplacental transfer of maternal antibodies. These syndromes in the neonate can cause significant morbidity and mortality, making urgent diagnosis and treatment necessary.

In utero exposure to certain drugs early in pregnancy may adversely affect nephrogenesis. Exposure to drugs later in pregnancy may affect the renin-angiotensin system, which could have an impact on fetal or neonatal renal function. Reduction in nephron number and renal function could have adverse consequences for the child several years later. Data are limited on the information needed to guide decisions for patients and providers regarding the use of certain drugs in pregnancy. The study of drug nephroteratogenicity has not been systematized, a large, standardized, global approach is needed to evaluate the renal risks of in utero drug exposures.

Urinary tract infection (UTI) is the most common bacterial infection in febrile newborns, particularly those born prematurely and with a low birth weight. Vesicoureteral reflux (VUR) predisposes to UTI and renal scarring. Half of neonates with UTI may have only low-grade fever or no fever. Jaundice in the absence of any other symptoms or signs may be the only clinical manifestation of UTI in neonates. The urinalysis may be negative in a significant number of neonates with UTI. Newborns with UTI have a high incidence of congenital anomalies of kidney and urinary tract anomalies, and hence should undergo renal imaging.

Lauren Baldinger, Abhijith Mudegowdar, and Aseem R. Shukla

Abnormalities of the external genitalia span the spectrum from subtle find-ings of limited clinical significance to profound anomalies that call into ques-tion such essential questions as sex determination. In addition, missing a diagnosis of congenital adrenal hyperplasia in a newborn female child with virilized external genitalia can result in near-term mortality, whereas a large inguinal hernia could present rapidly with incarceration if undetected. To that end, this article seeks to present a survey of commonly encountered genital abnormalities while highlighting those scenarios that require multi-disciplinary interventions.

Michael C. Carr

The management of infants born with myelomeningocele depends on understanding how their bladder stores and empties urine. Storage at low pressure with effective emptying periodically throughout the day is the goal. Intervention is designed to impact on one or both of these pro-cesses so that infants can remain infection-free and at the same time allow for appropriate renal growth over time. Urodynamic evaluation plays an important role, so that neonates can be stratified according to their risk. Most patients require intermittent catheterization and pharmacotherapy to achieve these goals at some point in their lives.

PROGRAM OBJECTIVE
The goal of *Clinics in Perinatology* is to keep practicing perinatologists, neonatologists, obstetricians, practicing physicians and residents up to date with current clinical practice in perinatology by providing timely articles reviewing the state of the art in patient care.

TARGET AUDIENCE
Perinatologists, neonatologists, obstetricians, practicing physicians, residents and healthcare professionals who provide patient care utilizing findings from *Clinics in Perinatology.*

LEARNING OBJECTIVES
Upon completion of this activity, participants will be able to:
1. Review acute and chronic kidney conditions in the neonate.
2. Discuss prenatal and postnatal evaluation and management of hydronephrosis.
3. Recognize long term renal consequences of preterm birth.

ACCREDITATION
The Elsevier Office of Continuing Medical Education (EOCME) is accredited by the Accreditation Council for Continuing Medical Education (ACCME) to provide continuing medical education for physicians.

The EOCME designates this enduring material for a maximum of 15 *AMA PRA Category 1 Credit*(s) ™. Physicians should claim only the credit commensurate with the extent of their participation in the activity.

All other health care professionals requesting continuing education credit for this enduring material will be issued a certificate of participation.

DISCLOSURE OF CONFLICTS OF INTEREST
The EOCME assesses conflict of interest with its instructors, faculty, planners, and other individuals who are in a position to control the content of CME activities. All relevant conflicts of interest that are identified are thoroughly vetted by EOCME for fair balance, scientific objectivity, and patient care recommendations. EOCME is committed to providing its learners with CME activities that promote improvements or quality in healthcare and not a specific proprietary business or a commercial interest.

The planning committee, staff, authors and editors listed below have identified no financial relationships or relationships to products or devices they or their spouse/life partner have with commercial interest related to the content of this CME activity:
Angela M. Arlen, MD; William R. Armstrong III, MD; Lauren Baldinger, DO, MS; Rossana Baracco, MD; Donald L. Batisky, MD; M. Jane Black, BSc (Hons), PhD; Detlef Bockenhauer, MD, PhD; John W. Brock, III, MD; Michael C. Carr, MD, PhD; Douglass Brooks Clayton, MD; William O. Cooper, MD, MPH; Stuart L. Goldstein, MD; Larry A. Greenbaum, MD, PhD; Kerry Holland; Brynne Hunter; Lucky Jain, MD, MBA; Stephanie M. Jernigan, MD; Jennifer G. Jetton, MD; Deborah P. Jones, MD, MS; Ahmad Kaddourah, MD, MS; Alison L. Kent, BMBS, FRACP, MD; Sandy Lavery; Dennis B. Liu, MD, FAAP, FACS; Max Maizels, MD; Tej K. Mattoo, MD, DCH, FRCP; Jill McNair; Yosuke Miyashita, MD, MPH; Thomas M. Morgan, MD; Abhijith Mudegowdar, MD; Palani Murugesan; Lindsay Parnell; Michelle N. Rheault, MD; Dana Ryan, BSc (Hons); Ellen Shapiro, MD; Aseem R. Shukla, MD, FAAP; Edwin A. Smith, MD, FAAP, FACS; Megan Sutherland, BBiomedSci (Hons), PhD; Priya Verghese, MD, MPH; Joshua J. Zaritsky, MD, PhD; Jakub Zieg, MD, PhD.

The planning committee, staff, authors and editors listed below have identified financial relationships or relationships to products or devices they or their spouse/life partner have with commercial interest related to the content of this CME activity:
David J. Askenazi, MD, MSPH is on speakers bureau for Baxter Renal.
Bradley A. Warady, MD is a consultant/advisor and has a research grant from Baxter Healthcare.

UNAPPROVED/OFF-LABEL USE DISCLOSURE
The EOCME requires CME faculty to disclose to the participants:
1. When products or procedures being discussed are off-label, unlabelled, experimental, and/or investigational (not US Food and Drug Administration (FDA) approved); and
2. Any limitations on the information presented, such as data that are preliminary or that represent ongoing research, interim analyses, and/or unsupported opinions. Faculty may discuss information about pharmaceutical agents that is outside of FDA-approved labelling. This information is intended solely for CME and is not intended to promote off-label use of these medications. If you have any questions, contact the medical affairs department of the manufacturer for the most recent prescribing information.

TO ENROLL

To enroll in the *Clinics in Perinatology* Continuing Medical Education program, call customer service at 1-800-654-2452 or sign up online at http://www.theclinics.com/home/cme. The CME program is available to subscribers for an additional annual fee of $212 USD.

METHOD OF PARTICIPATION

In order to claim credit, participants must complete the following:

1. Complete enrolment as indicated above.
2. Read the activity.
3. Complete the CME Test and Evaluation. Participants must achieve a score of 70% on the test. All CME Tests and Evaluations must be completed online.

CME INQUIRIES/SPECIAL NEEDS

For all CME inquiries or special needss, please contact elsevierCME@elsevier.com.

CLINICS IN PERINATOLOGY

NOW AVAILABLE FOR YOUR iPhone and iPad

Foreword

Our Kidneys: A Lot Is Riding on Their Shoulders

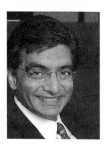

Lucky Jain, MD, MBA
Consulting Editor

Let us admit it: they don't get the respect they deserve! At least not until they start to fail, which is when all sorts of alarm bells go off, and the renal squad gets called! Up until then, other needy organs overshadow the need to protect precious renal tissue. From blood pressure management to clearing infections, many of the most potent agents available to us are not very kind to the kidneys.[1] We are just now beginning to understand the long-term effects on the kidneys of early neonatal disorders and the agents deployed to treat them.[2]

The kidneys are still developing when many preterm babies begin getting exposed to fairly nephrotoxic agents. Animal data and autopsy findings in preterm infants reveal morphologically abnormal glomeruli primarily in the outer renal cortex, suggesting nephrons impacted by the hostile environment after birth.[2,3] Abnormalities observed in these studies include diminished capillarization, cystic Bowman's space, and relatively immature form.[3] Indeed, the majority of nephrons are still being formed in the third trimester. The loss and abnormal function of nephrons have far-reaching consequences with residual effects detected in adult life (**Fig. 1**). Observational studies in humans and studies in animal models point to the association between low birth weight and chronic renal disease in adulthood. These effects are not as readily seen in children and young animals. The precise reason for this finding is unclear; however, it may be related to the decreased final number of nephrons with the remaining (fewer) glomeruli compensating by hyperfiltrating, thus accelerating the normal age-related decline in nephron number and function.[4] This follows Brenner's hyperfiltration hypothesis connecting low nephron number with hypertension, glomerular injury, and proteinuria.[5] Additional factors that may impair nephrogenesis in fetal life include maternal diet, stress, infections, diabetes, chronic utero-placental insufficiency, and medications.

This story sounds very similar to what we already know about premature lungs and brain in that much growth of these organs is yet to occur and that injury can have

Clin Perinatol 41 (2014) xv–xvii
http://dx.doi.org/10.1016/j.clp.2014.06.002
0095-5108/14/$ – see front matter **perinatology.theclinics.com**

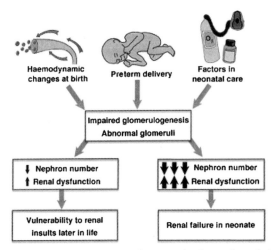

Fig. 1. Overview of the factors that may contribute to the formation of abnormal glomeruli in kidneys from preterm infants and the health consequences of reduced nephron endowment at birth. (*From* Black MJ, Sutherland MR, Gubhaju L, et al. When birth comes early: effects on nephrogenesis. Nephrology (Carlton) 2013;18:181; with permission.)

delayed and permanent consequences. In the case of the kidneys, we are lulled into complacence because of the large natural reserve in renal function, which masks manifestations until the damage is severe. It is for this same reason that our overall knowledge of the pathophysiology of renal disorders lags behind that of the lung and brain. Drs Greenbaum and Rheault are to be congratulated for pulling together a superb series of articles related to renal and urologic issues in the perinatal period with contributions from leaders in the fields of nephrology, urology, neonatology, and other related disciplines. I am confident that this issue of the *Clinics in Perinatology* will serve as a ready source of up-to-date information for our colleagues in neonatal perinatal medicine and restore (hopefully) a healthy level of respect for this vital organ system.

Lucky Jain, MD, MBA
Emory University School of Medicine &
Children's Healthcare of Atlanta
2015 Uppergate Drive
Atlanta, GA 30322, USA

E-mail address:
ljain@emory.edu

REFERENCES

1. Ligi I, Boubred F, Grandvuillemin I, et al. The neonatal kidney: implications for drug metabolism and elimination. Curr Drug Metab 2013;14:174–7.
2. Black MJ, Sutherland MR, Gubhaju L, et al. When birth comes early: effects on nephrogenesis. Nephrology (Carlton) 2013;18:180–2.
3. Maringhini S, Corrado C, Maringhini G, et al. Early origin of adult disease. J Matern Fetal Neonatal Med 2010;23:84–6.

4. Vehaskari VM. Prenatal programming of kidney disease. Curr Opin Pediatr 2010; 22:176–82.
5. Brenner BM, Lawler EV, Mackenzie HS. The hyperfiltration theory: a paradigm shift in nephrology. Kidney Int 1996;49:1774–7.

Preface

Renal and Urologic Abnormalities in the Perinatal Period

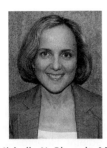 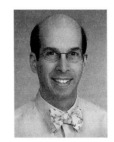

Michelle N. Rheault, MD   Larry A. Greenbaum, MD, PhD
Editors

Kidney and urologic abnormalities are very common in the perinatal period and can have long-term implications for a child's health. This issue of *Clinics in Perinatology* provides an in-depth overview of perinatal kidney and urologic problems, with a special focus on differential diagnosis, initial management, and long-term outcomes of these often challenging conditions. As in much of perinatology, a multidisciplinary team approach is required to diagnose and treat these complex disorders; therefore, leaders in the fields of nephrology, urology, neonatology, and pharmacoepidemiology have contributed their expertise and written comprehensive up-to-date reviews of each topic.

Congenital anomalies of the kidney and urinary tract are the most frequent findings on prenatal ultrasounds and are responsible for 20% to 30% of all prenatally detected anomalies. These anomalies are the most common cause of chronic kidney disease in childhood. This issue of *Clinics in Perinatology* provides the reader with a comprehensive review of these disorders, including hydronephrosis, bladder outlet obstruction, abnormalities of the external genitalia, neurogenic bladder, and cloacal anomalies as well as a review of the management of the resultant chronic kidney disease. Articles covering the diagnosis and management of primary renal disorders, including cystic kidney disease and the rare nephrotic and nephritic syndromes in the newborn, are also included. In the past several years, clinicians have recognized that acute kidney injury is a major problem in the neonatal intensive care unit and there is a great deal of new information in the literature. This issue of *Clinics in Perinatology* includes comprehensive reviews of acute kidney injury and renal replacement therapy in this unique population. Of special interest for all physicians is an excellent review of the long-term renal consequences of preterm birth. With the rise in premature births

Clin Perinatol 41 (2014) xix–xx
http://dx.doi.org/10.1016/j.clp.2014.06.001
perinatology.theclinics.com

over the past decades, this may become a major contributor to adult chronic renal and cardiovascular disease risk. Finally, the very common problems of neonatal hypertension and electrolyte disorders in the neonate are examined in detail.

We would like to thank each of the authors for their contributions to this collection. We would also like to thank Dr Lucky Jain for the opportunity to highlight the important problem of renal and urologic abnormalities in the perinatal period. Finally, we would like to thank the editorial team at Elsevier for guiding us through this process and their assistance in putting together a first-class collection of articles.

Michelle N. Rheault, MD
Assistant Professor, Medical Director of Dialysis
Department of Pediatrics
University of Minnesota Children's Hospital
2450 Riverside Avenue, MB680
Minneapolis, MN 55454, USA

Larry A. Greenbaum, MD, PhD
Marcus Professor of Pediatrics
Division Director, Pediatric Nephrology
Emory University School of Medicine
and Children's Healthcare of Atlanta
2015 Uppergate Drive, NE
Atlanta, GA 31322, USA

E-mail addresses:
rheau002@umn.edu (M.N. Rheault)
lgreen6@emory.edu (L.A. Greenbaum)

Acute Kidney Injury in the Neonate

Jennifer G. Jetton, MD[a], David J. Askenazi, MD, MSPH[b],*

KEYWORDS

- Acute kidney injury • Neonate • Critical illness • Biomarkers
- Chronic kidney disease • Acute renal failure

KEY POINTS

- Acute kidney injury (AKI) is common in neonatal intensive care units and seems to affect patient outcomes.
- AKI is a heterogeneous disorder with many mechanisms and management strategies. Current AKI biomarkers are limited and often late indicators that injury has occurred. Development of new, more precise biomarkers is a major focus of current research.
- Care of the neonate with AKI remains supportive. Maintenance of adequate renal perfusion, prevention of fluid overload, avoidance of nephrotoxic medications, and consideration for early initiation of renal supportive therapy are strategies which should improve outcomes.

INTRODUCTION

Neonates who are critically ill are at high risk for acute kidney injury (AKI) as the result of several potential exposures (eg, nephrotoxic medications, sepsis, hypotension, adverse perinatal events such as asphyxia). Recent data suggest an association between AKI and morbidity and mortality in these patients,[1–6] such that AKI can no longer be viewed as an incidental finding; it is an independent risk factor for poor outcomes. Close attention to at-risk patients and early recognition of changes in kidney function are keys to ameliorating this process.

Funding Sources: Dr D. Askenazi is funded by the American Society of Nephrology Norman Siegel Career Development Grant and by the Pediatric and Infant Center for Acute Nephrology (PICAN) at the University of Alabama at Birmingham and Children's of Alabama. Dr J.G. Jetton has no funding to declare.
Conflicts of Interest: Consultant for Baxter-Gambro Renal (Dr D. Askenazi). Nil (Dr J.G. Jetton).
[a] Division of Nephrology, Dialysis and Transplantation, University of Iowa Children's Hospital, 200 Hawkins Drive, 4023 BT, Iowa City, IA 52242, USA; [b] Division of Pediatric Nephrology, University of Alabama at Birmingham, 1600 7th Avenue South, Lowder Building 516, Birmingham, AL 35233, USA
* Corresponding author.
E-mail address: daskenazi@peds.uab.edu

AKI INCIDENCE AND AT-RISK POPULATIONS IN THE NEONATAL INTENSIVE CARE UNIT

The reported incidence of AKI in the neonatal intensive care unit (NICU) varies widely depending on the patient sample and AKI definition used (see Askenazi and colleagues[7] and Jetton and Askenazi[8] for epidemiology overviews). Groups of newborns recognized as being at increased risk for AKI include infants with perinatal hypoxia;[9–12] premature and very low birth weight (VLBW) infants;[1,4] infants with congenital heart disease, especially those requiring cardiopulmonary bypass;[3,5,13–16] infants requiring extracorporeal membrane oxygenation;[17–23] sick near-term/term infants;[24] and infants with sepsis.[25] In addition, neonates with congenital anomalies of the kidney and urinary tract are at high risk for AKI overlying their underlying chronic kidney disease (CKD). All of these infants should be identified as at risk and undergo close monitoring of kidney function with attention to modifiable risk factors during their NICU stay.

AKI DEFINITIONS AND DIAGNOSIS

AKI is a sudden impairment in kidney function that results in the inability to maintain adequate fluid, electrolyte, and waste product homeostasis. It is a complex and clinically heterogeneous disorder with multiple causes, pathophysiologic pathways, and clinical manifestations. Moreover, there are graded levels of severity that portend different outcomes. To highlight the dynamic and evolving nature of this syndrome, the old description acute renal failure has now been supplanted by the new term AKI. This change in terminology emphasizes the importance of early recognition and intervention at the time of injury rather than waiting until complete organ failure has occurred.[26]

At the bedside, AKI traditionally has been defined as either an increase in serum creatinine (SCr) or decrease in urine output (oliguria; ie, <0.5 mL/kg/h). These traditional biomarkers have several important limitations that are described later. Current focus in AKI research is on the development of more informative and timely biomarkers that will allow earlier detection of AKI, as well as help elucidate the nature of the injury (functional change vs structural damage).[27] Among the most well-studied functional biomarkers are SCr and serum cystatin C, an endogenous proteinase inhibitor that is produced at a constant rate by the body, freely filtered by the glomerulus, and neither secreted nor reabsorbed by the renal tubules.[28] Since 2005, there has been a growing effort to incorporate markers of kidney injury/repair into the definition of AKI. For example, urine neutrophil gelatinase associated lipocalin (NGAL), a small protein that is readily excreted and detectable in the urine following ischemic injury,[29] has been shown to be upregulated hours after renal injury in animal, pediatric, and adult populations (reviewed in Refs.[30–32]). This and other AKI biomarkers show great promise, but are not yet ready for routine use at the bedside.

For now, SCr and urine output remain the standard for identifying AKI events in critically ill infants, although both have limitations. For example, after birth SCr in the newborn reflects maternal creatinine levels. Rather than maintaining a steady state, SCr then declines at varying rates over days to weeks depending on gestational age. Moreover, newborns, especially preterm infants, may have higher SCr levels than their mothers;[33] the creatinine values for these babies may even increase after birth as the result of reabsorption of creatinine in the renal tubules[34–36] and decreased total body fluid. Thus, the natural physiology and immature handling of SCr by the newborn kidney render changes (or lack of change) in SCr difficult to interpret when assessing for AKI. Bruel and colleagues[37] reported critical serum creatinine levels based on gestational age that predicted increased risk of mortality and worse neurodevelopmental outcome at age 2 years: greater than 1.6 mg/dL for preterm infants

24 to 27 weeks, 1.1 mg/dL at 28 to 29 weeks, and 1 mg/dL at 30 to 32 weeks. Further validation of the ability of this and other proposed definitions to predict hard clinical short-term and long-term outcomes is critical for developing a reliable definition of neonatal AKI (**Box 1**).

Other important limitations of SCr-based AKI definitions not unique to the neonatal population have been described in detail elsewhere.[7] Most importantly, SCr is a surrogate for kidney function, not injury. SCr increases late, as much as 24 to 48 hours after the initial injury and not until at least 25% to 50% of renal function is lost. In addition, SCr does not differentiate the nature (eg, prerenal, nephrotoxic medication exposure, or ischemic acute tubular necrosis [ATN]) or timing of the kidney insult (eg, 2 hours, 6 hours, or 24 hours ago). SCr is also readily cleared by dialysis and can no longer be used as a marker for either renal injury or recovery once a patient is receiving renal replacement therapy.

Until recently, the lack of standardized AKI definitions hampered progress in AKI research. Several standardized, categorical definitions of AKI have been proposed to allow consensus across research studies, stratification of levels of severity, and earlier recognition of AKI in clinical practice. The first such definition, the RIFLE (risk, injury, failure, loss, and end-stage renal disease) classification,[38] was adapted for children as the pRIFLE (pediatric RIFLE) definition.[39] These definitions evolved into the AKIN (Acute Kidney Injury Network) definition.[26] In 2013, the Kidney Diseases: Improving Global Outcomes (KDIGO) clinical practice guidelines workgroup published a definition that combines aspects of both RIFLE and AKIN to provide a single tool for use in both research and clinical practice.[40] All of these definitions are based on changes in SCr and/or urine output, with particular emphasis on the way even small changes in SCr (eg, >0.3 mg/dL increase) are significant[41] and that different levels of severity may portend different outcomes.

Although there has been great progress in the diagnosis and classification systems for AKI in the adult and older pediatric populations, the utility of the KDIGO or any of the other AKI definitions for the neonatal population remains uncertain because of factors unique to neonatal renal physiology, as described earlier. At this time, there is general acceptance that an SCr increase of 0.3 mg/dL or more (KDIGO AKI stage 1) is sufficient to trigger concern for AKI in neonatal patients in the appropriate clinical context.[42] Thus, modifications to the KDIGO definition have been made in a proposed neonatal AKI definition as follows.[8] Because SCr normally declines over the first week of life,[43] each SCr is compared with the lowest previous value. In addition, because

---

Box 1
Proposed neonatal AKI classification

Stage	SCr	Urine Output
0	No change in SCr or increase <0.3 mg/dL	≥0.5 mL/kg/h
1	SCr increase ≥0.3 mg/dL within 48 h or	<0.5 mL/kg/h for 6–12 h
	SCr increase ≥1.5–1.9 × reference SCr[a] within 7 d	
2	SCr increase ≥2 to 2.9 × reference SCr[a]	<0.5 mL/kg/h for ≥12 h
3	SCr increase ≥3 × reference SCr[a] or	<0.3 mL/kg/h for ≥24 h or
	SCr ≥2.5 mg/dL or	anuria for ≥12 h
	Receipt of dialysis	

[a] Baseline SCr is defined as the lowest previous SCr value.
Modified from Jetton JG, Askenazi DJ. Update on acute kidney injury in the neonate. Curr Opin Pediatr 2012;24(2):191–6.

SCr of 2.5 mg/dL represents glomerular filtration rate of less than 10 mL/min/1.73 m², this SCr cutoff defines AKI stage 3. Although this definition has not been tested in large cohorts to determine its ability to predict hard clinical outcomes, members of the National Institutes of Health Neonatal Workshop in April 2013 (including both neo-natologists and nephrologists) agreed that this was currently the best definition and encouraged its use until further studies are conducted.

IDENTIFYING THE CAUSE OF AKI IN THE CRITICALLY ILL NEONATE

The traditional anatomic classification of AKI causes as prerenal, intrinsic AKI, and postrenal/obstruction is simple and widely used. Although useful for bedside evalua-tion, it is important to remember that this system is imprecise in terms of clarifying the underlying pathophysiology and appropriate therapeutic interventions.[27] In addition, AKI in a critically ill neonate is often multifactorial (eg, hypotension, nephrotoxic medi-cation exposure), and the risk of AKI increases as the number of prevalent risk factors increases.[9,44,45]

Renal Hypoperfusion (Prerenal Injury)

An increase in blood urea nitrogen (BUN) concentration with little or no change in SCr may represent an appropriate physiologic response to decreased renal blood flow. Renal hypoperfusion leads to increased sodium and water reabsorption (along with active BUN reabsorption) in the renal tubules, stimulated by both angiotensin II and aldosterone.[46] Newborns, especially premature infants, have immature tubular func-tion and are not able to conserve sodium and water to the same extent as older chil-dren and adults, so they may not manifest the expected degree of oliguria.[36] Common causes of renal hypoperfusion in the NICU include increased insensible losses (radiant warmers, phototherapy, and fever), fluid losses from other sources (chest tubes, ven-tricular drains, nasogastric suction, abdominal drains), excessive diuretic use, con-genital kidney disease with inability to concentrate urine appropriately (eg, dysplasia or polyuria following relief of urinary tract obstruction), congestive heart failure, high mean airway pressures from ventilator requirements in patients with severe lung dis-ease, blood loss for any reason (including perinatal events such placental abruption, twin-twin transfusion), and medications such as angiotensin-converting enzyme in-hibitors and nonsteroidal inflammatory drugs that cause reduction in renal blood flow via inhibition of prostaglandin-dependent renal perfusion.[47]

Correction of the underlying problem with restoration of adequate renal blood flow is critical for normalization of renal function and improvement in urine output, but this does not always mean correction with fluid rehydration because patients with conges-tive heart failure may require improved cardiac contractility, and some patients with hypotension may benefit from blood pressure support with dopamine. If renal hy-poperfusion is severe or prolonged, kidney parenchymal damage may ensue, which delays the time to recovery.

Parenchymal (Intrinsic) Kidney Injury

Neonates are at risk for parenchymal injury from a variety of exposures. Many of these have distinct mechanisms of injury and clinical courses. Infants, more than older chil-dren and adults, are prone to renal vein and artery thrombosis. Newborns are also more susceptible to cortical necrosis and irreversible kidney injury, which may in the most severe cases result in end-stage renal disease. The most common causes of parenchymal kidney injury are described in **Table 1**.

Table 1
Parenchymal (intrinsic) kidney injury

Ischemic injury/ATN	Any of the prerenal causes if prolonged Patient is at risk for further kidney injury throughout the injury and recovery phases, so avoid additional insults as much as possible Perinatal asphyxia/hypoxic-ischemic injury Endothelial and tubular cell damage may trigger a systemic inflammatory response that causes distant organ dysfunction[14,48,49]
Nephrotoxic medications	
Direct tubular injury	Aminoglycosides, amphotericin, intravenous contrast Aminoglycosides: primarily proximal tubular cell damage;[50] use with caution in any patient with preexisting AKI, concomitant nephrotoxic medication use, or poor renal perfusion. Usually nonoliguric AKI Amphotericin B: causes renal tubular acidosis and increased urinary potassium excretion. Reported levels of toxicity vary widely[51,52]
Decreased renal perfusion	ACE inhibitors, NSAIDs (indomethacin), diuretics Indomethacin: commonly associated with increased SCr concentrations, decreased urine output, hyponatremia. Usually reversible[47,53]
Tubular obstruction	Acyclovir
Sepsis and other infections	Decreased renal blood flow and subsequent ATN from shock/hypotension Sepsis-associated AKI Microvascular dysfunction associated with normal or increased renal blood flow that manifests with decreased GFR and tubular dysfunction; histologically distinct from ATN[54] Pyelonephritis Congenital infections
Vascular lesions	Renal vein and artery thrombosis Perinatal event; risk factors include perinatal asphyxia, dehydration, infection, prematurity, maternal diabetes, and underlying hypercoagulable state[55]

Abbreviations: ACE, angiotensin-converting enzyme; NSAIDs, nonsteroidal antiinflammatory drugs.

The issue of nephrotoxic medications deserves special mention here. Several recent studies have highlighted the risk of AKI associated with nephrotoxic medications in critically ill, non–critically ill, and oupatient pediatric patients.[56–60] Rhone and colleagues[61] retrospectively reviewed nephrotoxic medication exposure among 107 VLBW infants. Exposure was nearly universal, with 87% of infants receiving at least one nephrotoxic medication during their NICU stay and most receiving gentamicin (86% of infants). Infants with lower gestational age and birth weight received more nephrotoxic medications. Infants exposed to nephrotoxic medications had higher rates of AKI. This degree of potentially harmful medication exposure is of particular concern in preterm infants, because the harmful effects of nephrotoxic medications may disrupt the ongoing nephrogenesis that occurs after birth. Injury during this time may lead to reduced nephron mass and long-term CKD.[62]

Urinary Tract Obstruction (Postrenal)

Urinary tract obstruction requires prompt recognition and restoration of urinary flow in order to reverse AKI. Interventions may include a urinary catheter or a percutaneous nephrostomy tube, depending on the nature of the obstruction. Obstruction that occurs early in fetal development (eg, posterior urethral valves) may not completely reverse because of prenatal renal injury. Possible causes of obstruction include congenital malformations (posterior urethral valves, neurogenic bladder, urethral stricture); occluded or malpositioned urinary catheter; medication-related urinary retention (eg, morphine); and, very rarely, fungal balls or kidney stones.

DIAGNOSTIC EVALUATION
History and Risk Factors

The maternal, birth, and clinical histories should be reviewed for any of the events described earlier. Review the prenatal history for abnormalities of the urinary tract on prenatal ultrasonography, oligohydramnios, and maternal medication use (angiotensin-converting enzyme inhibitors, nonsteroidal antiinflammatory drugs, illicit drugs). Renal hypoperfusion may occur during resuscitation; it is important to review the need for chest compression or vasoactive medications. Nephrotoxic medication exposure, including blood levels of aminoglycosides, should be ascertained.

Physical Examination

A primary focus of the physical examination is assessment of volume status so that the appropriate fluid management strategies may be used. Signs of dehydration include tachycardia, hypotension, sunken fontanel, sunken eyes, or dry mucous membrane. Signs of fluid overload may include tachypnea, worsening oxygenation status and escalation of ventilatory support, and clinical edema (chest wall; dependent areas such as the posterior scalp, scrotum, and labia). The cumulative fluid balance should be estimated and compared with the daily weight trend. Ensure that all inputs are recorded (flushes, intermittently dosed medications) and that all losses (including chest tubes and drains) are noted. Infants may have large insensible losses (eg, with phototherapy) that cannot be accounted for in daily totals. In addition, it is important to monitor the total quantity of urine output relative to total inputs as well as the urine output trend. There may be relative oliguria with urine output of 2 mL/kg/h if the patient is receiving large quantities of fluids for resuscitation, nutrition, medications, and blood products.

Laboratory and Radiology Findings

Laboratory values to be monitored in the infant with AKI include serum sodium, potassium, chloride, bicarbonate, calcium, phosphorus, magnesium, BUN, creatinine, glucose, albumin, blood gases, hemoglobin and platelets, urinalysis, and urine culture. These values should be obtained as soon as an AKI event is recognized. Frequency of monitoring going forward depends on the degree of derangements at baseline as well as the severity of the AKI episode and quantity of urine output.

Random urine sodium and urine creatinine for calculation of the fractional excretion of sodium (FENa) may help in the evaluation if there is uncertainty about whether a prerenal state exists. If renal perfusion is low and tubular function is intact, sodium will be avidly retained, making the FENa low. In the context of an increasing SCr, a FENa in a term newborn is less than 2% in prerenal states and greater than 3% with ATN or intrinsic kidney dysfunction. Normal FENa in preterm infants born at less than 32 weeks of gestation is usually higher than 3%,[63] although varying degrees of tubular immaturity may make FENa difficult to interpret. FENa is not valid when an infant is receiving diuretics.

Renal and bladder ultrasonography should be performed to evaluate for underlying congenital kidney abnormalities and urinary tract obstruction. Doppler ultrasonography of the renal vessels should be performed to evaluate for renal vascular lesions if suspected. A chest radiograph should be reviewed to help assess for pulmonary edema or congestive heart failure in patients with clear signs of fluid overload.

MEDICAL MANAGEMENT OF AKI IN THE NEONATE

There are currently no specific therapies for the treatment or prevention of AKI. Thus, management of AKI in neonates remains supportive. Keys to managing the infant with AKI include identifying and correcting any modifiable risk factors and minimizing additional kidney insults. Determination of the AKI cause is based on clinical interpretation of history, physical examination, and laboratory and radiology findings.

Urinary tract obstruction should be corrected as quickly as possible, either via the urethra with a urinary catheter or via the renal pelvis with percutaneous nephrostomy tubes. Polyuria with electrolyte losses may occur following the relief of the obstruction. Close monitoring of serum electrolytes (especially sodium, potassium, and bicarbonate) is necessary, every 2 to 4 hours in some cases, with replacement of electrolytes as needed.

If there is suspicion for renal hypoperfusion, the patient should be challenged with a 10-mL/kg bolus of an isotonic fluid. Large chest tube and gastrointestinal tract losses may need to be replaced using an appropriate fluid determined by the electrolyte composition of the losses. Infants with congestive heart failure or a prior urinary outlet obstruction may not tolerate multiple fluid boluses. Frequent reassessment of the patient following each intervention enables appropriate restoration of intravascular volume but avoids excessive fluid administration that may lead to volume overload.

Fluid management in the critically ill neonate with AKI can be difficult, especially when the infant is oliguric. These infants may require large volumes of intravenous nutrition, blood products, and medications. An oliguric or anuric child may develop volume overload. Severe fluid restriction, such as limiting intake to insensible, urine output, and extrarenal losses, may severely limit nutritional intake or may not be adequate to avoid volume overload. At this point, renal replacement therapy should be considered.

Electrolyte and Mineral Homeostasis

Electrolyte abnormalities vary depending on the cause of AKI. For example, severe oliguric/anuric AKI may lead to marked hyponatremia, hyperkalemia, and hyperphosphatemia, whereas nonoliguric AKI and proximal tubular dysfunction, as occurs with aminoglycoside toxicity, may result in hypokalemia and hypomagnesemia. Patients require careful assessment and reassessment of the electrolyte composition of enteral and parenteral fluids.

Hyponatremia may occur during the course of AKI and is typically the result of total body volume overload rather than total body sodium depletion. Attention to fluid status is critical when determining the cause and proper treatment of hyponatremia. Hypervolemic hyponatremia (serum sodium concentrations usually between 120 and 130 mEq/L) often requires restriction of free water intake. Symptomatic (lethargy or seizures) or severe hyponatremia (serum Na <120 mEq/L) may require use of normal saline or 3% sodium chloride.

Severe hyperkalemia is a life-threatening medical emergency. Frequent review of the electrolyte composition of all fluids is critical for prevention. Potassium should be removed from all intravenous fluids if the infant becomes anuric or if the serum potassium is increasing rapidly. Enteral formulas with lower potassium contents include breast milk, Similac PM 60/40, and Nestle Good Start. Breast milk, if available, is also an excellent option as it's content of potassium and phosphorous are similar to these "renal" formulas. Formulas may be pretreated with sodium polystyrene to decrease the potassium content before the formula is given to the patient.[64] Pretreatment with sodium polystyrene also decreases the calcium content and increases the sodium content of the formula. Loop diuretics may be used to enhance urinary potassium excretion if the patient is not anuric. Treatment options to address hyperkalemia emergently include maneuvers to shift potassium from the extracellular to the intracellular compartments (eg, albuterol inhalation, sodium bicarbonate, and insulin plus glucose). If medical management fails, then renal replacement therapy may be required.

Hyperphosphatemia is common in AKI caused by impaired renal excretion of phosphorus. Enteral feeding options that are low in phosphorus are the same as those that are low in potassium. Calcium carbonate may be used as an enteral phosphate-binding agent. Formula or breast milk may also be pretreated with phosphate-binding agents such as sevelamer hydrochloride.[65] Ongoing collaboration with an NICU or renal dietician is an important part of care for these patients.

Acid-Base Homeostasis

Non–anion gap metabolic acidosis is common in infants with AKI, because normal acid/base homeostasis depends on the kidneys' ability to excrete acid and reabsorb filtered bicarbonate. Preterm infants also have immature renal tubules that do not reabsorb bicarbonate appropriately.[36] Base supplementation with either bicarbonate or acetate is indicated in those with AKI and metabolic acidosis. In infants with severe respiratory failure, large doses of bicarbonate should be avoided because they can cause carbon dioxide retention.

Therapeutics

At present, there are insufficient data to determine whether specific therapies improve outcomes in neonates with AKI. Several therapies, including dopamine, diuretics, theophyline, and fenoldopam, have been studied but none can have enough evidence to justify widespread use (**Table 2**).

Other Medications

Consultation with pharmacists and nephrologists familiar with drug dosing in renal failure is recommended to avoid side effects of drug accumulation as well as additional nephrotoxicity. Medication lists should be reviewed frequently to ensure correct dosing based on the level of renal failure.

Renal Supportive Therapy

Absolute indications for the initiation of renal supportive therapy are the same as for other patients (eg, severe hyperkalemia). However, waiting for late indicators of severe renal dysfunction to occur is likely not appropriate for the infant with AKI, and consideration for renal replacement therapy should occur earlier in the course of illness than for patients with end-stage renal disease who are initiating chronic dialysis.[80] Data on fluid overload in pediatric and adult patients show that those with higher fluid overload at the time of dialysis initiation have worse survival, even when controlling for severity

Table 2 Therapeutics	
Dopamine	Widely used for support of systemic blood pressure in preterm and term infants,[66–68] although no survival benefit or decreased length of hospital stay has been shown in adult patients[69–72]
Diuretics	Used to augment urine output in oliguric patients; useful in small patients for whom placing dialysis access presents technical challenges. No evidence to suggest that diuretics prevent or reverse AKI once it has occurred.[69,73] Long-term furosemide therapy has several potential side effects: ototoxicity, interstitial nephritis, osteopenia, nephrocalcinosis, hypotension, and persistence of patent ductus arteriosus[74]
Fenoldopam	Selective dopamine-1 receptor agonist; causes vasodilation of renal and splanchnic vasculature, increased renal blood flow, and increased GFR. Not clinically approved for the treatment of AKI. Use in augmenting urine output in neonates with AKI has been explored in several single-center analyses.[75,76] Used in 2 prospective studies of infants undergoing cardiopulmonary bypass; some modest benefit seen with high-dose fenoldopam (1 µg/kg/min)[77,78]
Theophylline	Recent meta-analysis including 4 randomized trials on full-term asphyxiated infants suggests that prophylactic theophylline significantly reduces the incidence of severe renal dysfunction.[79] However, there is little evidence on the long-term renal and neurodevelopmental outcomes or adverse effects at various measured levels, so prudence with clinical use of prophylactic theophylline is required. In addition, the trials were before the therapeutic hypothermia era

of illness.[81–84] There are now some limited data in neonates[85] that show the same association. These data suggest that prevention of fluid overload and early initiation of renal support therapy could improve outcomes in patients with AKI. In practical terms, marked edema creates technical challenges for dialysis access placement and makes fluid management and general support much more difficult.

NOVEL BIOMARKERS

As discussed previously, SCr-based AKI definitions have multiple shortcomings, especially in the neonatal population. Most importantly, SCr estimates glomerular function, not damage, and takes days to increase after an injury has occurred. Studies in VLBW infants,[86,87] infants who undergo cardiopulmonary bypass surgery,[3,88–93] and other sick newborns admitted to the NICU[94] suggest that a variety of biomarkers can detect infants who will later have an increase in SCr. However, before these biomarkers are available at the bedside, large studies are needed to determine whether they can predict important clinical outcomes such as mortality and CKD. In premature infants, it is important to recognize that normal levels of urine biomarkers differ by gestational age, probably because of different degrees of tubular immaturity. At present, bedside tests for serum and urine NGAL and kidney injury biomarker-1 are available in Europe and are undergoing testing and review by the US Food and Drug Administration.

LONG-TERM OUTCOMES

Carmody and Charlton[62] reviewed the relationship between prematurity and low birth weight and CKD in adulthood. Preterm delivery disrupts nephrogenesis, which is normally not complete until around 34 to 36 weeks' gestation. A small number of autopsy studies suggest that nephrogenesis after premature birth continues for only a short time.[95–97] The remaining nephrons hypertrophy to compensate for decreased nephron mass, but this response (hyperfiltration) eventually becomes deleterious and leads to glomerulosclerosis with sodium retention, systemic hypertension, proteinuria, and progressive CKD (Brenner hypothesis[98]). Thus, these infants are already primed for kidney injury and CKD based on their premature birth. The impact of superimposed AKI in the NICU on long-term kidney outcomes is unknown.

It used to be assumed that patients who survived an episode of AKI would recover kidney function without long-term sequelae; however, recent data from animals,[99] critically ill children,[100,101] and adults[102–114] with AKI suggest that survivors are at risk for development of CKD. A meta-analysis showed that adults with AKI have higher risk of developing incident CKD (pooled adjusted hazard ratio [HR], 8.8; 95% confidence interval [CI], 3.1–25.5), end-stage kidney disease (pooled adjusted HR, 3.1; 95% CI, 1.9–5.0), and mortality (pooled adjusted HR, 2.0; 95% CI, 1.3–3.1) compared with patients without AKI.[115]

Several case reports document that CKD occurs in infants who sustain AKI; however, these studies are small single-center retrospective reports.[46,116] Human autopsy and animal studies suggest that AKI affects postnatal nephron development. In an autopsy study, Rodriguez and colleagues[96] showed that premature infants with AKI have fewer nephrons than term neonates. Sutherland and colleagues[117] showed that premature baboons exposed to ibuprofen had decreased nephrogenic zone width. Studies designed to determine which factors are associated with long-term CKD are needed to define the most appropriate surveillance protocols to identify patients at most risk.

FUTURE DIRECTIONS

There has been an increase in neonatal AKI research that has led to greater recognition about the potential impact of AKI on patient outcomes. In order to reduce morbidity and mortality and improve outcomes for these patients, neonatologists and nephrologists must work together to develop better AKI definitions using newer, more precise biomarkers in conjunction with SCr and urine output criteria. Any new biomarkers require testing against hard clinical end points (eg, need for renal replacement therapy, mortality, hospital length of stay). Therapies designed to reduce the incidence and severity of AKI should be assessed using these biomarkers and hard clinical outcomes. In addition, there needs to be ongoing emphasis on the development of renal support technology designed specifically for the smallest patients. At present, a continuous renal replacement therapy (CRRT) machine designed specifically for neonates,[118] and smaller filters for current CRRT machines, are being tested. Extensive progress is anticipated in neonatal AKI in the coming years that will ultimately improve outcomes.

REFERENCES

1. Koralkar R, Ambalavanan N, Levitan EB, et al. Acute kidney injury reduces survival in very low birth weight infants. Pediatr Res 2011;69:354–8.
2. Gadepalli SK, Selewski DT, Drongowski RA, et al. Acute kidney injury in congenital diaphragmatic hernia requiring extracorporeal life support: an insidious problem. J Pediatr Surg 2011;46:630–5.
3. Krawczeski CD, Woo JG, Wang Y, et al. Neutrophil gelatinase-associated lipocalin concentrations predict development of acute kidney injury in neonates and children after cardiopulmonary bypass. J Pediatr 2011;158:1009–15.e1001.

4. Askenazi DJ, Griffin R, McGwin G, et al. Acute kidney injury is independently associated with mortality in very low birthweight infants: a matched case-control analysis. Pediatr Nephrol 2009;24:991–7.
5. Blinder JJ, Goldstein SL, Lee VV, et al. Congenital heart surgery in infants: effects of acute kidney injury on outcomes. J Thorac Cardiovasc Surg 2012; 143:368–74.
6. Selewski DT, Jordan BK, Askenazi DJ, et al. Acute kidney injury in asphyxiated newborns treated with therapeutic hypothermia. J Pediatr 2013;162:725–9.e721.
7. Askenazi DJ, Ambalavanan N, Goldstein SL. Acute kidney injury in critically ill newborns: what do we know? What do we need to learn? Pediatr Nephrol 2009;24:265–74.
8. Jetton JG, Askenazi DJ. Update on acute kidney injury in the neonate. Curr Opin Pediatr 2012;24:191–6.
9. Karlowicz MG, Adelman RD. Nonoliguric and oliguric acute renal failure in asphyxiated term neonates. Pediatr Nephrol 1995;9:718–22.
10. Kaur S, Jain S, Saha A, et al. Evaluation of glomerular and tubular renal function in neonates with birth asphyxia. Ann Trop Paediatr 2011;31:129–34.
11. Gupta BD, Sharma P, Bagla J, et al. Renal failure in asphyxiated neonates. Indian Pediatr 2005;42:928–34.
12. Aggarwal A, Kumar P, Chowdhary G, et al. Evaluation of renal functions in asphyxiated newborns. J Trop Pediatr 2005;51:295–9.
13. Picca S, Principato F, Mazzera E, et al. Risks of acute renal failure after cardiopulmonary bypass surgery in children: a retrospective 10-year case-control study. Nephrol Dial Transplant 1995;10:630–6.
14. Sorof JM, Stromberg D, Brewer ED, et al. Early initiation of peritoneal dialysis after surgical repair of congenital heart disease. Pediatr Nephrol 1999;13:641–5.
15. Alabbas A, Campbell A, Skippen P, et al. Epidemiology of cardiac surgery-associated acute kidney injury in neonates: a retrospective study. Pediatr Nephrol 2013;28:1127–34.
16. Morgan CJ, Zappitelli M, Robertson CM, et al, Western Canadian Complex Pediatric Therapies Follow-Up Group. Risk factors for and outcomes of acute kidney injury in neonates undergoing complex cardiac surgery. J Pediatr 2013;162:120–7.e1.
17. Shaheen IS, Harvey B, Watson AR, et al. Continuous venovenous hemofiltration with or without extracorporeal membrane oxygenation in children. Pediatr Crit Care Med 2007;8:362–5.
18. Cavagnaro F, Kattan J, Godoy L, et al. Continuous renal replacement therapy in neonates and young infants during extracorporeal membrane oxygenation. Int J Artif Organs 2007;30:220–6.
19. Meyer RJ, Brophy PD, Bunchman TE, et al. Survival and renal function in pediatric patients following extracorporeal life support with hemofiltration. Pediatr Crit Care Med 2001;2:238–42.
20. Weber TR, Connors RH, Tracy TF Jr, et al. Prognostic determinants in extracorporeal membrane oxygenation for respiratory failure in newborns. Ann Thorac Surg 1990;50:720–3.
21. Sell LL, Cullen ML, Whittlesey GC, et al. Experience with renal failure during extracorporeal membrane oxygenation: treatment with continuous hemofiltration. J Pediatr Surg 1987;22:600–2.
22. Askenazi DJ, Ambalavanan N, Hamilton K, et al. Acute kidney injury and renal replacement therapy independently predict mortality in neonatal and pediatric

noncardiac patients on extracorporeal membrane oxygenation. Pediatr Crit Care Med 2011;12:e1–6.

23. Zwiers AJ, de Wildt SN, Hop WC, et al. Acute kidney injury is a frequent complication in critically ill neonates receiving extracorporeal membrane oxygenation: a 14-year cohort study. Crit Care 2013;17:R151.

24. Askenazi DJ, Koralkar R, Hundley HE, et al. Fluid overload and mortality are associated with acute kidney injury in sick near-term/term neonate. Pediatr Nephrol 2012;28(4):661–6.

25. Mathur NB, Agarwal HS, Maria A. Acute renal failure in neonatal sepsis. Indian J Pediatr 2006;73:499–502.

26. Mehta RL, Kellum JA, Shah SV, et al, Acute Kidney Injury Network. Acute Kidney Injury Network: report of an initiative to improve outcomes in acute kidney injury. Crit Care 2007;11:R31.

27. Endre ZH, Kellum JA, Di Somma S, et al. Differential diagnosis of AKI in clinical practice by functional and damage biomarkers: workgroup statements from the tenth Acute Dialysis Quality Initiative Consensus Conference. Contrib Nephrol 2013;182:30–44.

28. Zappitelli M, Parvex P, Joseph L, et al. Derivation and validation of cystatin C-based prediction equations for GFR in children. Am J Kidney Dis 2006;48: 221–30.

29. Mishra J, Ma Q, Prada A, et al. Identification of neutrophil gelatinase-associated lipocalin as a novel early urinary biomarker for ischemic renal injury. J Am Soc Nephrol 2003;14:2534–43.

30. Devarajan P. Review: neutrophil gelatinase-associated lipocalin: a troponin-like biomarker for human acute kidney injury. Nephrology (Carlton) 2010;15:419–28.

31. Devarajan P. Neutrophil gelatinase-associated lipocalin: a promising biomarker for human acute kidney injury. Biomark Med 2010;4:265–80.

32. Devarajan P. Biomarkers for the early detection of acute kidney injury. Curr Opin Pediatr 2011;23:194–200.

33. Guignard JP, Drukker A. Why do newborn infants have a high plasma creatinine? Pediatrics 1999;103:e49.

34. Miall LS, Henderson MJ, Turner AJ, et al. Plasma creatinine rises dramatically in the first 48 hours of life in preterm infants. Pediatrics 1999;104:e76.

35. Auron A, Mhanna MJ. Serum creatinine in very low birth weight infants during their first days of life. J Perinatol 2006;26:755–60.

36. Chevalier RL. Developmental renal physiology of the low birth weight pre-term newborn. J Urol 1996;156:714–9.

37. Bruel A, Roze JC, Flamant C, et al. Critical serum creatinine values in very pre-term newborns. PLoS One 2013;8:e84892.

38. Bellomo R, Ronco C, Kellum JA, et al, Acute Dialysis Quality Initiative work-group. Acute renal failure - definition, outcome measures, animal models, fluid therapy and information technology needs: the Second International Consensus Conference of the Acute Dialysis Quality Initiative (ADQI) Group. Crit Care 2004; 8:R204–12.

39. Akcan-Arikan A, Zappitelli M, Loftis LL, et al. Modified RIFLE criteria in critically ill children with acute kidney injury. Kidney Int 2007;71:1028–35.

40. Kellum JA, Lameire N, for the KAKIGWG. Diagnosis, evaluation, and management of acute kidney injury: a KDIGO summary (Part 1). Crit Care 2013; 17:204.

41. Chertow GM, Burdick E, Honour M, et al. Acute kidney injury, mortality, length of stay, and costs in hospitalized patients. J Am Soc Nephrol 2005;16:3365–70.

42. Palevsky PM, Liu KD, Brophy PD, et al. KDOQI US commentary on the 2012 KDIGO clinical practice guideline for acute kidney injury. Am J Kidney Dis 2013;61:649–72.
43. Gallini F, Maggio L, Romagnoli C, et al. Progression of renal function in preterm neonates with gestational age < or = 32 weeks. Pediatr Nephrol 2000;15: 119–24.
44. Andreoli SP. Acute renal failure. Curr Opin Pediatr 2002;14:183–8.
45. Moghal NE, Brocklebank JT, Meadow SR. A review of acute renal failure in children: incidence, etiology and outcome. Clin Nephrol 1998;49:91–5.
46. Andreoli SP. Acute renal failure in the newborn. Semin Perinatol 2004;28:112–23.
47. Leonhardt A, Strehl R, Barth H, et al. High efficacy and minor renal effects of indomethacin treatment during individualized fluid intake in premature infants with patent ductus arteriosus. Acta Paediatr 2004;93:233–40.
48. Li X, Hassoun HT, Santora R, et al. Organ crosstalk: the role of the kidney. Curr Opin Crit Care 2009;15:481–7.
49. Awad AS, Okusa MD. Distant organ injury following acute kidney injury. Am J Physiol Renal Physiol 2007;293:F28–9.
50. Giuliano RA, Paulus GJ, Verpooten GA, et al. Recovery of cortical phospholipidosis and necrosis after acute gentamicin loading in rats. Kidney Int 1984;26: 838–47.
51. Baley JE, Kliegman RM, Fanaroff AA. Disseminated fungal infections in very low-birth-weight infants: therapeutic toxicity. Pediatrics 1984;73:153–7.
52. Le J, Adler-Shohet FC, Nguyen C, et al. Nephrotoxicity associated with amphotericin B deoxycholate in neonates. Pediatr Infect Dis J 2009;28:1061–3.
53. Cifuentes RF, Olley PM, Balfe JW, et al. Indomethacin and renal function in premature infants with persistent patent ductus arteriosus. J Pediatr 1979;95: 583–7.
54. Gomez H, Ince C, De Backer D, et al. A unified theory of sepsis-induced acute kidney injury: inflammation, microcirculatory dysfunction, bioenergetics, and the tubular cell adaptation to injury. Shock 2014;41:3–11.
55. Brandao LR, Simpson EA, Lau KK. Neonatal renal vein thrombosis. Semin Fetal Neonatal Med 2011;16:323–8.
56. Pannu N, Nadim MK. An overview of drug-induced acute kidney injury. Crit Care Med 2008;36:S216–23.
57. Moffett BS, Goldstein SL. Acute kidney injury and increasing nephrotoxic-medication exposure in noncritically-ill children. Clin J Am Soc Nephrol 2011;6: 856–63.
58. Zappitelli M, Moffett BS, Hyder A, et al. Acute kidney injury in non-critically ill children treated with aminoglycoside antibiotics in a tertiary healthcare centre: a retrospective cohort study. Nephrol Dial Transplant 2011;26:144–50.
59. Misurac JM, Knoderer CA, Leiser JD, et al. Nonsteroidal anti-inflammatory drugs are an important cause of acute kidney injury in children. J Pediatr 2013;162: 1153–9, 1159.e1.
60. Lindle KA, Dinh K, Moffett BS, et al. Angiotensin-converting enzyme inhibitor nephrotoxicity in neonates with cardiac disease. Pediatr Cardiol 2014;35(3): 499–506.
61. Rhone ET, Carmody JB, Swanson JR, et al. Nephrotoxic medication exposure in very low birth weight infants. J Matern Fetal Neonatal Med 2013. [Epub ahead of print].
62. Carmody JB, Charlton JR. Short-term gestation, long-term risk: prematurity and chronic kidney disease. Pediatrics 2013;131:1168–79.

63. Ellis EN, Arnold WC. Use of urinary indexes in renal failure in the newborn. Am J Dis Child 1982;136:615–7.

64. Cameron JC, Kennedy D, Feber J, et al. Pretreatment of infant formula with sodium polystyrene sulfonate: focus on optimal amount and contact time. Paediatr Drugs 2013;15:43–8.

65. Ferrara E, Lemire J, Reznik VM, et al. Dietary phosphorus reduction by pretreatment of human breast milk with sevelamer. Pediatr Nephrol 2004;19:775–9.

66. Seri I. Cardiovascular, renal, and endocrine actions of dopamine in neonates and children. J Pediatr 1995;126:333–44.

67. Seri I, Abbasi S, Wood DC, et al. Regional hemodynamic effects of dopamine in the sick preterm neonate. J Pediatr 1998;133:728–34.

68. Seri I, Abbasi S, Wood DC, et al. Regional hemodynamic effects of dopamine in the indomethacin-treated preterm infant. J Perinatol 2002;22:300–5.

69. Bellomo R, Chapman M, Finfer S, et al. Low-dose dopamine in patients with early renal dysfunction: a placebo-controlled randomised trial. Australian and New Zealand Intensive Care Society (ANZICS) Clinical Trials Group. Lancet 2000;356:2139–43.

70. Friedrich JO, Adhikari N, Herridge MS, et al. Meta-analysis: low-dose dopamine increases urine output but does not prevent renal dysfunction or death. Ann Intern Med 2005;142:510–24.

71. Hoste EA, Clermont G, Kersten A, et al. RIFLE criteria for acute kidney injury are associated with hospital mortality in critically ill patients: a cohort analysis. Crit Care 2006;10:R73.

72. Marik PE. Low-dose dopamine: a systematic review. Intensive Care Med 2002; 28:877–83.

73. Bagshaw SM, Delaney A, Haase M, et al. Loop diuretics in the management of acute renal failure: a systematic review and meta-analysis. Crit Care Resusc 2007;9:60–8.

74. Karlowicz MG, Adelman RD. Acute renal failure in the neonate. Clin Perinatol 1992;19:139–58.

75. Yoder SE, Yoder BA. An evaluation of off-label fenoldopam use in the neonatal intensive care unit. Am J Perinatol 2009;26(10):745–50.

76. Moffett BS, Mott AR, Nelson DP, et al. Renal effects of fenoldopam in critically ill pediatric patients: a retrospective review. Pediatr Crit Care Med 2008;9:403–6.

77. Ricci Z, Luciano R, Favia I, et al. High-dose fenoldopam reduces postoperative neutrophil gelatinase-associated lipocaline and cystatin C levels in pediatric cardiac surgery. Crit Care 2011;15:R160.

78. Ricci Z, Stazi GV, Di Chiara L, et al. Fenoldopam in newborn patients undergoing cardiopulmonary bypass: controlled clinical trial. Interact Cardiovasc Thorac Surg 2008;7:1049–53.

79. Al-Wassia H, Alshaikh B, Sauve R. Prophylactic theophylline for the prevention of severe renal dysfunction in term and post-term neonates with perinatal asphyxia: a systematic review and meta-analysis of randomized controlled trials. J Perinatol 2013;33:271–7.

80. Walters S, Porter C, Brophy PD. Dialysis and pediatric acute kidney injury: choice of renal support modality. Pediatr Nephrol 2009;24:37–48.

81. Goldstein SL, Somers MJ, Baum MA, et al. Pediatric patients with multi-organ dysfunction syndrome receiving continuous renal replacement therapy. Kidney Int 2005;67:653–8.

82. Sutherland SM, Zappitelli M, Alexander SR, et al. Fluid overload and mortality in children receiving continuous renal replacement therapy: the prospective

pediatric continuous renal replacement therapy registry. Am J Kidney Dis 2010; 55:316–25.

83. Foland JA, Fortenberry JD, Warshaw BL, et al. Fluid overload before continuous hemofiltration and survival in critically ill children: a retrospective analysis. Crit Care Med 2004;32:1771–6.

84. Gillespie RS, Seidel K, Symons JM. Effect of fluid overload and dose of replacement fluid on survival in hemofiltration. Pediatr Nephrol 2004;19:1394–9.

85. Hazle MA, Gajarski RJ, Yu S, et al. Fluid overload in infants following congenital heart surgery. Pediatr Crit Care Med 2013;14:44–9.

86. Askenazi DJ, Montesanti A, Hunley H, et al. Urine biomarkers predict acute kidney injury and mortality in very low birth weight infants. J Pediatr 2011;159(6): 907–12.e1.

87. Lavery AP, Meinzen-Derr JK, Anderson E, et al. Urinary NGAL in premature infants. Pediatr Res 2008;64:423–8.

88. Portilla D, Dent C, Sugaya T, et al. Liver fatty acid-binding protein as a biomarker of acute kidney injury after cardiac surgery. Kidney Int 2008;73:465–72.

89. Zappitelli M, Krawczeski CD, Devarajan P, et al. Early postoperative serum cystatin C predicts severe acute kidney injury following pediatric cardiac surgery. Kidney Int 2011;80:655–62.

90. Hall IE, Koyner JL, Doshi MD, et al. Urine cystatin C as a biomarker of proximal tubular function immediately after kidney transplantation. Am J Nephrol 2011; 33:407–13.

91. Parikh CR, Devarajan P, Zappitelli M, et al. Postoperative biomarkers predict acute kidney injury and poor outcomes after pediatric cardiac surgery. J Am Soc Nephrol 2011;22:1737–47.

92. Nguyen MT, Dent CL, Ross GF, et al. Urinary aprotinin as a predictor of acute kidney injury after cardiac surgery in children receiving aprotinin therapy. Pediatr Nephrol 2008;23:1317–26.

93. Ramesh G, Krawczeski CD, Woo JG, et al. Urinary netrin-1 is an early predictive biomarker of acute kidney injury after cardiac surgery. Clin J Am Soc Nephrol 2010;5:395–401.

94. Askenazi DJ, Koralkar R, Hundley HE, et al. Urine biomarkers predict acute kidney injury in newborns. J Pediatr 2012;161(2):270–5.e1.

95. Faa G, Gerosa C, Fanni D, et al. Marked interindividual variability in renal maturation of preterm infants: lessons from autopsy. J Matern Fetal Neonatal Med 2010;23(Suppl 3):129–33.

96. Rodriguez MM, Gomez AH, Abitbol CL, et al. Histomorphometric analysis of postnatal glomerulogenesis in extremely preterm infants. Pediatr Dev Pathol 2004;7:17–25.

97. Sutherland MR, Gubhaju L, Moore L, et al. Accelerated maturation and abnormal morphology in the preterm neonatal kidney. J Am Soc Nephrol 2011;22:1365–74.

98. Brenner BM, Garcia DL, Anderson S. Glomeruli and blood pressure. Less of one, more the other? Am J Hypertens 1988;1:335–47.

99. Basile DP. The endothelial cell in ischemic acute kidney injury: implications for acute and chronic function. Kidney Int 2007;72:151–6.

100. Askenazi DJ, Feig DI, Graham NM, et al. 3-5 year longitudinal follow-up of pediatric patients after acute renal failure. Kidney Int 2006;69:184–9.

101. Mammen C, Al Abbas A, Skippen P, et al. Long-term risk of CKD in children surviving episodes of acute kidney injury in the intensive care unit: a prospective cohort study. Am J Kidney Dis 2012;59:523–30.

102. Weiss AS, Sandmaier BM, Storer B, et al. Chronic kidney disease following non-myeloablative hematopoietic cell transplantation. Am J Transplant 2006;6: 89–94.
103. Wald R, Quinn RR, Luo J, et al, Group UoTAKIR. Chronic dialysis and death among survivors of acute kidney injury requiring dialysis. JAMA 2009;302: 1179–85.
104. Newsome BB, Warnock DG, McClellan WM, et al. Long-term risk of mortality and end-stage renal disease among the elderly after small increases in serum creatinine level during hospitalization for acute myocardial infarction. Arch Intern Med 2008;168:609–16.
105. Lo LJ, Go AS, Chertow GM, et al. Dialysis-requiring acute renal failure increases the risk of progressive chronic kidney disease. Kidney Int 2009;76:893–9.
106. Lafrance JP, Djurdjev O, Levin A. Incidence and outcomes of acute kidney injury in a referred chronic kidney disease cohort. Nephrol Dial Transplant 2010;25: 2203–9.
107. James MT, Hemmelgarn BR, Wiebe N, et al. Glomerular filtration rate, proteinuria, and the incidence and consequences of acute kidney injury: a cohort study. Lancet 2010;376:2096–103.
108. James MT, Ghali WA, Tonelli M, et al. Acute kidney injury following coronary angiography is associated with a long-term decline in kidney function. Kidney Int 2010;78:803–9.
109. Ishani A, Xue JL, Himmelfarb J, et al. Acute kidney injury increases risk of ESRD among elderly. J Am Soc Nephrol 2009;20:223–8.
110. Ishani A, Nelson D, Clothier B, et al. The magnitude of acute serum creatinine increase after cardiac surgery and the risk of chronic kidney disease, progression of kidney disease, and death. Arch Intern Med 2011;171:226–33.
111. Hsu CY, Chertow GM, McCulloch CE, et al. Nonrecovery of kidney function and death after acute on chronic renal failure. Clin J Am Soc Nephrol 2009;4:891–8.
112. Choi AI, Li Y, Parikh C, et al. Long-term clinical consequences of acute kidney injury in the HIV-infected. Kidney Int 2010;78:478–85.
113. Ando M, Ohashi K, Akiyama H, et al. Chronic kidney disease in long-term survivors of myeloablative allogeneic haematopoietic cell transplantation: prevalence and risk factors. Nephrol Dial Transplant 2010;25:278–82.
114. Amdur RL, Chawla LS, Amodeo S, et al. Outcomes following diagnosis of acute renal failure in U.S. veterans: focus on acute tubular necrosis. Kidney Int 2009; 76:1089–97.
115. Coca SG, Singanamala S, Parikh CR. Chronic kidney disease after acute kidney injury: a systematic review and meta-analysis. Kidney Int 2011;81(5):442–8.
116. Abitbol CL, Bauer CR, Montane B, et al. Long-term follow-up of extremely low birth weight infants with neonatal renal failure. Pediatr Nephrol 2003;18:887–93.
117. Sutherland MR, Yoder BA, McCurnin D, et al. Effects of ibuprofen treatment on the developing preterm baboon kidney. Am J Physiol Renal Physiol 2012;302: F1286–92.
118. Ronco C, Davenport A, Gura V. The future of the artificial kidney: moving towards wearable and miniaturized devices. Nefrologia 2011;31:9–16.

Chronic Kidney Disease in the Neonate

Joshua J. Zaritsky, MD, PhD[a],*, Bradley A. Warady, MD[b]

KEYWORDS

- Chronic kidney disease • Neonate • Dialysis • Nutrition

KEY POINTS

- The definition of chronic kidney disease (CKD) in neonates differs from that of children older than 2 years. In addition, kidney function during the neonatal period is characterized as normal, moderately reduced, or severely reduced, based on the age-adjusted glomerular filtration rate (GFR).
- Nutritional management is a key component of the care provided to the neonate with CKD. Optimal nutrition is mandatory if the best possible outcomes in terms of height, weight, and brain development are to be achieved by the neonate or young infant experiencing impaired kidney function.
- Historically, the morbidity and mortality rates of neonates with CKD have been poor, with the presence of nonrenal disease being the most important predictor of mortality. Over the last decade, however, there has been steady improvement in patient survival, even in those patients initiated on chronic dialysis as neonates.

DEFINING CKD IN THE NEONATE

Although the diagnosis of chronic kidney disease (CKD) is applicable to patients of all ages, its definition in neonates has some clear distinctions from that made in older children and adults. Specifically, the criterion established by KDOQI (Kidney Disease Outcomes Quality Initiative)[1] and expanded by KDIGO (Kidney Disease: Improving Global Outcomes)[2] that the duration of kidney disease be longer than 3 months does not apply to neonates. Instead, it is recognized that many of the developmental renal abnormalities that can account for decreased kidney function (see the next section) have lifelong consequences. Thus, it is possible to classify many children as having CKD within the first few days of life.

The diagnosis of CKD in the neonatal period is typically made a priori after a renal ultrasonogram, first performed in the prenatal period and repeated soon after birth,

Disclosures: None.
[a] Department of Pediatrics, Nemours/A.I. duPont Hospital for Children, 1600 Rockland Road, Wilmington, DE 19803, USA; [b] Department of Pediatrics, Children's Mercy Hospital, 2401 Gillham Road, Kansas City, MO 64108, USA
* Corresponding author.
E-mail address: Joshua.zaritsky@nemours.org

Clin Perinatol 41 (2014) 503–515
http://dx.doi.org/10.1016/j.clp.2014.05.002
0095-5108/14/$ – see front matter © 2014 Elsevier Inc. All rights reserved.

reveals disorganized renal architecture or a significant urologic abnormality accompanied by abnormal kidney function; this is in stark contrast to adult CKD, which is usually the result of an episode of acute kidney injury (AKI) or a long-standing metabolic (ie, diabetes) or cardiovascular (ie, hypertension) condition. Clearly some neonates who suffer AKI shortly after birth as a result of perinatal asphyxia, hypoxia, sepsis, or hypovolemia will also go on to have long-standing kidney damage and CKD, although the time period that passes before the diagnosis can be made remains variable.[3]

It is important to recognize that the additional diagnostic criterion for CKD as per KDOQI of a glomerular filtration rate (GFR) of less than 60 mL/min/1.73 m^2 does not apply until age greater than 2 years when the body surface area–adjusted GFR is comparable with values achieved by older children and adults. The normal GFR in the newborn period is significantly less than 60 mL/min/1.73 m^2, and increases rapidly owing to enhancement of renal perfusion via a combination of increased mean arterial pressure accompanied by a decrease in renal vascular resistance.[4] Increases in glomerular size and capillary permeability coupled with a redistribution of intrarenal blow flow to more superficial cortical nephrons also contribute to the characteristic increase in GFR that occurs throughout the neonatal period and early infancy.[5]

Thus, the definition of normal kidney function in the neonatal period (and conversely CKD) must take into account age-appropriate values of GFR. There are several published references for normative GFR values in both preterm infants[6,7] and neonates[4,8,9] (**Table 1**). GFR approximation is often made based on serum creatinine levels via a GFR-estimating equation for clinical care. At present the updated Schwarz equation, derived using iohexol clearance and enzymatically measured creatinine, appears to be the most robust,[10] although none of the data that formed the basis for this equation were derived from neonates. In addition, estimated GFRs cannot be used in the setting of AKI when the serum creatinine is rapidly changing.

Given these limitations, attempting to classify a neonate based on the traditional 5 KDOQI stages of CKD is potentially misleading and, therefore, not recommended.

Table 1	
Glomerular filtration rate (GFR) in healthy infants as assessed by inulin clearance	
Age	**Mean GFR ± SD (mL/min/1.73 m^2)**
Preterm babies	
1–3 d	14.0 ± 5
1–7 d	18.7 ± 5.5
4–8 d	44.3 ± 9.3
3–13 d	47.8 ± 10.7
8–14 d	35.4 ± 13.4
1.5–4 mo	67.4 ± 16.6
Term babies	
1–3 d	20.8 ± 5.0
3–4 d	39.0 ± 15.1
4–14 d	36.8 ± 7.2
6–14 d	54.6 ± 7.6
15–19 d	46.9 ± 12.5
1–3 mo	85.3 ± 35.1

Abbreviation: SD, standard deviation.
Adapted from Schwartz GJ, Furth SL. Glomerular filtration rate measurement and estimation in chronic kidney disease. Pediatr Nephrol 2007;22(11):1840.

Instead, the KDIGO guidelines[2] recommend a CKD classification scheme for patients younger than 2 years, which takes into consideration normative data and the inherent variation associated with the GFR measurement method (ie, urine collection, clearance of exogenous marker). In turn, the kidney function of neonates can be classified as normal, moderately reduced, or severely reduced based on the age-adjusted GFR (**Table 2**).

INCIDENCE AND COMMON CAUSES

Despite an increased awareness of the capacity to care for neonates with CKD, and a significant increase in the frequency of detection of the at-risk and affected population with prenatal ultrasonography,[11,12] data regarding the incidence of CKD in neonates are limited. Much of the published data have examined the incidence and management of infants with end-stage renal disease (ESRD), in contrast to less severe CKD, and has considered a much broader age range of birth to 24 months. Wedekin and colleagues[13] estimated a CKD incidence of 1:10,000 in a single-center retrospective analysis of infants younger than 1 year with a serum creatinine level greater than 1.13 mg/dL (100 μmol/L). The gender distribution (male-to-female ratio of 2.8:1) was expected as a result of the male-dominated contribution of obstructive uropathy (eg, posterior urethral valves) as a frequent cause of CKD. More than 50% of the infants with CKD were premature, a figure significantly higher than in the study's total infant population. More recently, Greenbaum and colleagues[14] reported that 17% of children enrolled in the Chronic Kidney Disease in Children (CKiD) study had a low birth weight compared with an overall rate of approximately 8% in the general United States population. Carey and colleagues,[15] using data from the dialysis registry of the North American Pediatric Renal Trials and Collaborative Studies (NAPTRCS), estimated the incidence of ESRD in neonates to be only 0.045 cases per million population per year, or 0.32 cases per 100,000 live births. This rate is roughly comparable with that seen in the United Kingdom, where the annual infant incidence is estimated at 3 cases per million population.[16] The incidence rate for neonates is substantially lower than the overall incidence of ESRD during the first 4 years of life based on data from the United States Renal Data System (USRDS), which reported an incidence of approximately 10 cases per million population in the 0- to 4-year age group over the last decade.[17] This difference is likely a result of the fact that one of the most common causes of CKD in the neonatal period (see later discussion), congenital renal dysplasia, does not typically compromise kidney function so severely that dialysis is required in the newborn period.

With the growing awareness of the frequent occurrence of AKI in this population, it must be noted that although the exact incidence of CKD after AKI remains unknown, it is likely substantial and parallels that seen in adults.[18] In a retrospective study of

Table 2	
KDIGO classification schemata for CKD for ages less than 2 years	
Neonatal CKD Classification	**GFR**
Normal GFR	GFR ≤1 SD below the mean
Moderately reduced GFR	GFR >1 SD to ≤2 SD below the mean
Severely reduced GFR	GFR >2 SD below the mean

Abbreviations: KDIGO, Kidney Disease: Improving Global Outcomes; SD, standard deviation.

Adapted from Kidney Disease: Improving Global Outcomes (KDIGO) 2012 clinical practice guideline for the evaluation and management of chronic kidney disease. Kidney International Supplements 2013;3(1). Jan 1; with permission.

older children who suffered from AKI (median age of 6.5 years at AKI event), Askenazi and colleagues[19] found that more than 50% developed some form of CKD 3 to 5 years later.

A variety of kidney disorders can result in neonatal CKD (**Box 1**). However, most studies examining the frequency of these disorders have focused on those that result in the need for chronic renal replacement therapy. In the cohort of neonatal patients needing dialysis (N = 193) examined by Carey and colleagues,[15] the most frequent renal disorders were congenital renal hypoplasia/dysplasia and obstructive uropathy (eg, posterior urethral valves) (**Table 3**).[20] Similarly, Warady and Martz[21] reviewed the causes of ESRD in 85 neonates who were entered into the NAPRTCS database from 2000 to 2010, and found the same 2 diagnoses predominant. These and other structural abnormalities of the urinary tract account for nearly 60.0% of cases of chronic dialysis in neonates, with the next most common diagnosis being polycystic kidney disease (PKD). In an Italian registry including 20 infants who began peritoneal dialysis (PD) during the first month of life, congenital anomalies of the kidney and urinary tract (CAKUT) accounted for half of the cases, followed by autosomal recessive PKD.[22] Finally, recent data from 4 separate registries on a combined total of 264 neonates from 32 countries who received dialysis during the first month of life showed that CAKUT was the most common cause of ESRD (54.6%), followed by cystic kidneys (13.2%) and cortical necrosis (11.4%).[23]

ETHICAL CONSIDERATIONS

One of the most difficult issues that families and health care providers are confronted with is the decision regarding when and if chronic dialysis therapy should be initiated for the neonate with ESRD. Despite advances in dialysis technology and clinical expertise that now makes it possible to provide dialysis to this patient population safely and effectively, the concept of proceeding with a lifetime of ESRD care is unavoidably complex. Comorbidities such as neurocognitive delay, growth delay, and the almost universal need for supplemental tube feeding and multiple hospitalizations contribute to the ethical dilemma experienced by many. Often complicating the situation is the presence of significant nonrenal abnormalities, such as pulmonary hypoplasia, which are present in up to one-third of infants with ESRD and are

---

Box 1
Disorders resulting in neonatal CKD

Aplastic/hypoplastic/dysplastic kidneys[a]

Autosomal dominant polycystic kidney disease

Autosomal recessive polycystic kidney disease[a]

Obstructive uropathy (posterior urethral valves)[a]

Pyelonephritis

Reflux nephropathy

Renal infarct[a]

Syndrome of agenesis of abdominal musculature[a]

[a] May result in need for dialysis in neonatal period.
  Adapted from Flynn JT, Mitsnefes M, Pierce C, et al. Blood pressure in children with chronic kidney disease: a report from the Chronic Kidney Disease in Children study. Hypertension 2008;52(4):631–7.

Table 3	
Diagnosis of neonates with end-stage renal disease	
Diagnosis	**n (%)**
Renal dysplasia	72 (37.3)
Obstructive uropathy	39 (20.2)
ARPKD	23 (11.9)
Congenital nephrotic syndrome	3 (1.5)
Other	56 (29)

Abbreviation: ARPKD, autosomal recessive polycystic kidney disease.
Adapted from Carey WA, Talley LI, Sehring SA, et al. Outcomes of dialysis initiated during the neonatal period for treatment of end-stage renal disease: a North American Pediatric Renal Trials and Collaborative Studies special analysis. Pediatrics 2007;119(2):e470.

associated with an increased risk for mortality.[24] In fact, the mortality rate of the youngest infants (0–2 years) who have received chronic dialysis has historically been poor, with 2-year mortality rates as high as 30%, although recent data have revealed somewhat better outcomes (see later discussion).[15,25]

In adult patients the 4 principles of medical ethics, namely autonomy, beneficence, nonmaleficence, and justice, are characteristically applied to decisions on whether to withhold or withdraw dialysis.[26] In the case of neonates and young infants, the wishes of the parents, who are entitled to make decisions regarding the medical care their children receive, must also be taken into account. This type of ethical dilemma is not all that uncommon in the neonatal intensive care unit and occurs in other situations as well, such as in the case of the neonate with hypoplastic left heart syndrome.[27,28] Ideally the decision of whether to provide dialysis represents a consensus opinion of the parents, nephrologist, neonatologist, and other members of a multidisciplinary team. The decision should be made only after a thorough review of the patient's clinical status and the family's desires is conducted, along with a review of the limited data that exist within the medical literature on the outcome of young infants with ESRD. Despite the best efforts to this end, there remains the substantial potential for disagreement regarding the best course of action to take because of the multiple patient and social factors that often exist, along with the different prior experiences of health care team members with similar patient scenarios. All of this can result in an emotionally charged environment. Nonetheless, it is most desirable for all nephrology team members who are involved in the patient's care to have the opportunity to weigh in on the decision process. Although the nephrology team and family members most often come to a conclusion that is agreeable to all, on occasion a hospital ethics committee may be consulted for their opinion.

More than a decade ago, Geary[29] surveyed the opinions of pediatric caregivers from around the globe regarding the decision process surrounding the initiation of chronic dialysis in infants younger than 1 year. In that survey, a substantial percentage (50%) of physicians responded that it was usually acceptable for parents to refuse dialysis for children younger than 1 month, in contrast to the situation when children were 1 to 12 months of age at presentation, at which time dialysis refusal was less acceptable. Factors thought to be most influential by the physicians with respect to their opinions regarding withholding dialysis were the presence of "coexistent serious medical abnormalities" and the "anticipated morbidity for the child." As a follow-up to this survey, Teh and colleagues[30] and many of the same investigators recently reported on the results of a similar multination survey of both nephrologists and nurses on this topic. The survey was conducted to determine whether the perspectives of health care providers had changed over the subsequent decade in association with the advances in care that had taken place, and additional personal and published experiences. Of note, only 30% of the 270 nephrologists who responded indicated that they offer chronic dialysis to all children younger than 1 month, whereas 50% stated that they recommend the therapy to all children aged 1 to 12 months. The figure of 30% was decreased from the 41% figure reported in the prior survey. Ninety-eight percent of physicians responding to the recent survey stated they would offer dialysis to some infants younger than 1 month, compared with 93% 10 years ago. In the recent assessment, a minority of physicians (27%) believed that the parents should not be given the option to refuse dialysis for infants younger than 1 month, a figure that increased to 50% for children aged 1 to 12 months. Not surprisingly, and as was reported in the initial survey, the most influential factor contributing to a decision not to offer dialysis was the presence of a coexisting nonrenal abnormality. One additional and potentially troubling finding in terms of generating the all-important consensus within the health care team was the presence of significant differences in the responses of physicians and nurses with respect to dialysis initiation in the neonate. Specifically, nurses were more likely to consider the presence of oliguria or anuria as a contraindication to initiating dialysis, and placed more emphasis on the parent's right to decide.

The topic of ethics is undoubtedly in need of additional study, supported by the accumulation of data from clinicians and affected family members. The influence of advances in dialysis care, more recent data on short-term and long-term patient outcomes, and cultural differences must be considered in any future analysis.[23]

NUTRITIONAL MANAGEMENT

In the setting of neonatal CKD, the provision of adequate nutrition takes on particular importance because the neonatal period is typically characterized by accelerated brain growth and a linear growth rate of nearly 25 cm per year. Remarkably, approximately half of postnatal brain growth takes place in the first year of life, and one-third of the normal final adult height is achieved during the initial 2 years of life.[31,32]

Infants with severe CKD can lose more than 2 standard deviations of height and forever affect their final height if their clinical status is compromised by suboptimal care and/or complications of their disorder.[33,34] One single-center retrospective study by Karlberg and colleagues[34] of 71 children with early-onset ESRD found that one-third of the reduction in height occurred during the first postnatal months. There are also data linking poor growth with mortality in children with ESRD. Both Wong and colleagues[35] and Furth and colleagues[36] demonstrated an independent association between a decrease in height standard deviation score (SDS) and an increased risk of death, with impaired growth likely serving as a surrogate of overall well-being.

Most noteworthy is that this early period of linear growth primarily depends on the provision of optimal nutrition, with the growth hormone/insulin-like growth factor (IGF) axis having less importance in comparison with its role later in life. Updated KDOQI pediatric nutrition guidelines have recently been published that provide recommendations for the parameters of growth and nutritional status to be monitored in infants and young children with CKD, and how frequently the monitoring should take place (**Table 4**). The guidelines addressing dietary intake include recommendations for 100% of the estimated energy requirements for chronologic age, with adjustments based on changes in either weight or linear growth,[1,37] and 100% to 140% of the dietary reference intake (DRI) for protein in those patients with CKD and not yet on dialysis.[1]

Table 4
Recommended parameters and frequency of nutritional assessment for neonates with CKD

Measure	Minimal Interval (mo)		
	Normal GFR	Moderately Reduced GFR	Severely Reduced GFR
Dietary intake	0.5–3	0.5–3	0.5–2
Height or length velocity-for-age percentile or SDS	0.5–1.5	0.5–1.5	0.5–1
Height or length-for-age percentile or SDS	0.5–2	0.5–2	0.5–1
Estimated dry weight and weight-for-age	0.5–1.5	0.5–1.5	0.25–1
BMI-for-height-age percentile or SDS	0.5–1.5	0.5–1.5	0.5–1
Head circumference-for-age percentile or SDS	0.5–1.5	0.5–1.5	0.5–1

Abbreviations: BMI, body mass index; SDS, standard deviation score.
Adapted from KDOQI clinical practice guideline for nutrition in children with CKD: 2008 update. Executive summary. Am J Kidney Dis 2009;53(3 Suppl 2):S16; with permission.

There are several additional nutritional considerations that need to be addressed when PD is conducted. Specifically, neonates and infants can experience excessive losses of protein across the peritoneal membrane, with studies demonstrating average losses of 250 mg of protein per kilogram of body weight per day.[38] To avoid the negative consequences of protein depletion, current guidelines recommend a dietary protein intake of 1.8 g/kg/d for the first 6 months of life, a value that takes into account the DRI and peritoneal losses.[1]

Neonates and infants who receive PD also experience excessive sodium losses across the peritoneal membrane because of the need for high ultrafiltration rates in relation to body weight. Both breast milk and standard formulas contain 7 to 8 mmol of sodium per liter, which is inadequate for the replacement of ongoing losses. Without adequate supplementation (~3–5 mEq/kg/d), the consequences of the resultant hyponatremia and low intravascular volume can be catastrophic, and include both blindness caused by anterior ischemic optic neuropathy and cerebral edema.[39,40]

In most cases, the nutritional targets for neonates with moderately to severely reduced GFR are not achievable without the implementation of either nasogastric (NG) or gastrostomy tube feeding. Children with advanced CKD suffer from poor appetite and early satiety that, in part, may be due to elevated circulating cytokines.[41,42] Compounding the problem is the frequent presence of poor gastrointestinal motility and gastroesophageal reflux, which can lead to the loss of up to one-third of feedings via emesis.[42–45] In turn, the provision of nocturnal feedings by slow, continuous drip, along with intermittent bolus feedings during the day, is often required to meet the nutritional goals (**Table 5**). Historically, NG tubes were preferentially used because of the simplicity of placement (although not necessarily simple from the perspective of the parent and patient) with no disruption of any ongoing PD. However, frequently associated complications of this approach to therapy (in addition to the unsightly appearance) include recurrent emesis, nasal trauma associated with tube replacement, and inhibition of the normal development of oral motor skills.[46] The latter problem needs to be addressed with oral and occupational therapy. On the other hand, gastrostomy tubes and buttons, which were championed early on by Watson and Coleman, are not

Table 5 Suggested rates for initiating and advancing tube feedings for neonates with CKD			
Method	Initial Hourly Infusion	Daily Increases	Goal
Continuous feedings	1–2 mL/kg/h	1 mL/kg/h	6 mL/kg/h
Bolus feedings	10–15 mL/kg/feed	20–40 mL every 4 h	20–30 mL/kg/feed

Adapted from KDOQI clinical practice guideline for nutrition in children with CKD: 2008 update. Executive summary. Am J Kidney Dis 2009;53(3 Suppl 2):S91; with permission.

associated with the development of altered oral motor skills, are not regularly associated with emesis, are not visible, and offer the additional advantage of being available for prolonged use during the postrenal transplant period when they can help ensure proper hydration and medication administration.[47] It is for these reasons that gastrostomy tubes and buttons have supplanted NG tubes as the preferred route of enteral tube support in many centers.

Data from single-center studies have repeatedly shown that the provision of tube feedings facilitates both height and weight gain. Kari and colleagues,[33] in a review of 81 tube-fed infants with a GFR less than 20 mL/min/1.73 m² during the first 6 months of life or placed on dialysis during the first 2 years of life, found that 81% of subjects achieved a normal height SDS after 1 year of follow-up. Subsequent evaluation of this same cohort 10 years later revealed that the intensive feeding regimen combined with early transplantation resulted in a normal mean adult height in those patients without comorbidities.[48] Ramage and colleagues[49] demonstrated that the use of enteral feedings in 8 infants receiving PD arrested the decline in height SDS traditionally reported, while Ledermann and colleagues[50] demonstrated that enteral feeding resulted in significant improvements in weight, height, and head circumference SDS at both 1 and 2 years of age in 12 infants receiving PD. The most recent data are derived from the International Pediatric Peritoneal Dialysis Network (IPPN), which has provided further evidence of the benefit of supplemental tube feedings in terms of height and weight gain in children younger than 2 years and on PD, with marked global variation in the use of tube feedings during infancy.[51]

OUTCOMES

Published data on the outcomes of neonates with CKD are sparse. In a retrospective analysis of 1461 preterm infants that included 2-year follow-up data, Bruel and colleagues[52] found that creatinine values greater than 1.6, 1.1, and 1.0 mg/dL at 24 to 27, 28 to 29, and 30 to 32 weeks of gestation, respectively, after adjustment for gestational age, birth weight, sex, and other renal failure risk factors, were significantly associated with neonatal mortality (odds ratio of 8.55 [95% confidence interval 4.23–17.28], $P<.01$). Interestingly the same values were also highly predictive (odds ratio 2.06 [95% confidence interval 1.26–3.36]) of poor neurodevelopmental outcomes (defined as a diagnosis of cerebral palsy or neurologic signs of abnormal movement during independent walking) at 2 years.

However, as with the information pertaining to incidence and etiology, much of the limited data on the outcome of neonates with CKD come from those treated with chronic dialysis. Carey and colleagues[15] used the NAPRTCS database to evaluate the outcomes of 193 infants who initiated dialysis before 1 month of age. The most frequent reason for dialysis termination in this cohort was renal transplantation

(46%). Termination for reasons of death or recovery of kidney function accounted for 10.8% and 14.6% of patients, respectively. In a recent analysis of contemporary NAPRTCS data from 2000 to 2010 conducted by Warady and Martz and as was seen by Carey and colleagues, the largest percentage of patients who terminated dialysis (45%) did so to receive a kidney transplant. Termination for reasons of death or recovery of kidney function accounted for 4.7% and 8.2% of patients, respectively.[21] Most importantly, survival when starting dialysis in the neonatal period has significantly improved in comparison with historical data, with a 3-year patient survival of 93.9% (K. Martz, personal communication, 2013). Data from the Italian Registry, by contrast, showed a mortality rate of 20% by age 1 year among those infants beginning PD within the first month of life.[22] Finally, recent international data from 240 neonates with ESRD[23] show 2- and 5-year survival rates of 81.2% and 76.4%, respectively **(Fig. 1)**. The major complications noted during 2 years of follow-up were growth retardation (63%), anemia (55%), and hypertension (57%). At 48 months, 22% of patients had discontinued dialysis for transplantation. Noteworthy is the finding that 2 recent studies have shown no differences in mortality rates of PD patients who initiated dialysis at younger than 1 month versus 2 to 24 months of age **(Fig. 2)**.[15,53] These data are complemented by the fact that the transplant outcome of young patients is the best among the pediatric population, with a 10-year survival of 86.5% and 80.6% for those transplanted at ages less than 1 year or 1 to 5 years, respectively.[54] Data from a Canadian registry mirror this experience, with a mortality rate of only 0.3 per 100 patient-years for those transplanted before age 2 years.[55]

What persists, however, is the finding that the most important predictor of mortality in this patient age group remains the presence of nonrenal disease.[33,56–58] Years ago, Wood and colleagues[56] clearly showed that comorbidities such as anuria, pulmonary hypoplasia, and severe developmental delay were associated with the greatest risk of mortality in infants undergoing dialysis. Data from a recent publication of the IPPN revealed that the presence of at least 1 comorbidity was associated with a 4-year survival of 73% versus 90% survival in those without a comorbidity ($P<.001$).[24] Data on the influence of comorbidities on survival are likely affected by regional difference, as countries with a lower gross national income seem to be more restrictive in terms

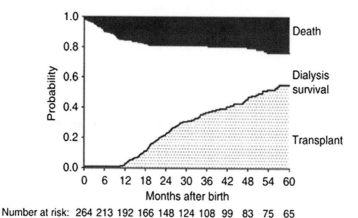

Fig. 1. Two-year survival after start of renal replacement therapy and subsequent renal transplant probability. (*From* van Stralen KJ, Borzych-Duzalka D, Hataya H, et al. Survival and clinical outcomes of children starting renal replacement therapy in the neonatal period. Kidney Int 2014;86(1):169; with permission.)

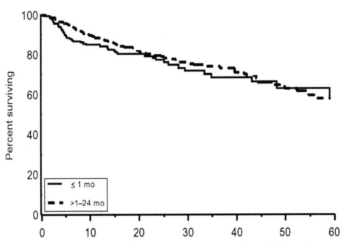

Fig. 2. Kaplan-Meier survival curve for neonates versus older children. Both groups had similar survival within 5 years of dialysis initiation. (*From* Carey WA, Talley LI, Sehring SA, et al. Outcomes of dialysis initiated during the neonatal period for treatment of end-stage renal disease: a North American Pediatric Renal Trials and Collaborative Studies special analysis. Pediatrics 2007;119(2):e468–73; with permission. Copyright © 2007 AAP.)

of making PD available to very young patients (<3 years of age) and those with significant extrarenal complications.[59]

REFERENCES

1. KDOQI Work Group. KDOQI clinical practice guideline for nutrition in children with CKD: 2008 update. Executive summary. Am J Kidney Dis 2009;53(3 Suppl 2):S11–104.
2. Kidney Disease: Improving Global Outcomes (KDIGO) 2012 clinical practice guideline for the evaluation and management of chronic kidney disease. Kidney International Supplements 2013;3(1). Jan 1.
3. Jetton JG, Askenazi DJ. Update on acute kidney injury in the neonate. Curr Opin Pediatr 2012;24(2):191–6.
4. Guignard JP, Torrado A, Da Cunha O, et al. Glomerular filtration rate in the first three weeks of life. J Pediatr 1975;87(2):268–72.
5. Haycock GB. Development of glomerular filtration and tubular sodium reabsorption in the human fetus and newborn. Br J Urol 1998;81(Suppl 2):33–8.
6. Gallini F, Maggio L, Romagnoli C, et al. Progression of renal function in preterm neonates with gestational age < or = 32 weeks. Pediatr Nephrol 2000;15(1–2): 119–24.
7. Bueva A, Guignard JP. Renal function in preterm neonates. Pediatr Res 1994; 36(5):572–7.
8. Schwartz GJ, Brion LP, Spitzer A. The use of plasma creatinine concentration for estimating glomerular filtration rate in infants, children, and adolescents. Pediatr Clin North Am 1987;34(3):571–90.
9. Schwartz GJ, Furth SL. Glomerular filtration rate measurement and estimation in chronic kidney disease. Pediatr Nephrol 2007;22(11):1839–48.
10. Schwartz GJ, Munoz A, Schneider MF, et al. New equations to estimate GFR in children with CKD. J Am Soc Nephrol 2009;20(3):629–37.

11. Carr MC. Prenatal management of urogenital disorders. Urol Clin North Am 2004;31(3):389–97, vii.
12. Hubert KC, Palmer JS. Current diagnosis and management of fetal genitourinary abnormalities. Urol Clin North Am 2007;34(1):89–101.
13. Wedekin M, Ehrich JH, Offner G, et al. Aetiology and outcome of acute and chronic renal failure in infants. Nephrol Dial Transplant 2008;23(5):1575–80.
14. Greenbaum LA, Munoz A, Schneider MF, et al. The association between abnormal birth history and growth in children with CKD. Clin J Am Soc Nephrol 2011;6(1): 14–21.
15. Carey WA, Talley LI, Sehring SA, et al. Outcomes of dialysis initiated during the neonatal period for treatment of end-stage renal disease: a North American Pediatric Renal Trials and Collaborative Studies special analysis. Pediatrics 2007; 119(2):e468–73.
16. Coulthard MG, Crosier J. Outcome of reaching end stage renal failure in children under 2 years of age. Arch Dis Child 2002;87(6):511–7.
17. Atlas of ESRD: United States Renal Data System (USRDS), 2010. Available at: http://www.usrds.org/2010/pdf/v2_08.pdf. Accessed August 7, 2010.
18. Chertow GM, Soroko SH, Paganini EP, et al. Mortality after acute renal failure: models for prognostic stratification and risk adjustment. Kidney Int 2006; 70(6):1120–6.
19. Askenazi DJ, Feig DI, Graham NM, et al. 3-5 year longitudinal follow-up of pediatric patients after acute renal failure. Kidney Int 2006;69(1):184–9.
20. Annual Report of the North American Pediatric Renal Trials and Collaborative Studies (NAPRTCS). 2008. Available at: https://web.emmes.com/study/ped/annlrept/Annual%20Report%20-2008.pdf. Accessed September 7, 2010.
21. Warady BA, Martz K. Providing or withholding dialysis for neonates: a report of the NAPRTCS. Denver (CO): Pediatric Academic Societies; 2011.
22. Vidal E, Edefonti A, Murer L, et al. Peritoneal dialysis in infants: the experience of the Italian Registry of Paediatric Chronic Dialysis. Nephrol Dial Transplant 2012; 27(1):388–95.
23. van Stralen KJ, Borzych-Duzalka D, Hataya H, et al. Survival and clinical outcomes of children starting renal replacement therapy in the neonatal period. Kidney Int 2014;86(1):168–74.
24. Neu AM, Sander A, Borzych-Dużałkac D, et al. Co-morbidities in chronic pediatric peritoneal dialysis patients: a report of the International Pediatric Peritoneal Dialysis Network (IPPN). Perit Dial Int 2012;32(4):410–8.
25. Brunner FP, Fassbinder W, Broyer M, et al. Survival on renal replacement therapy: data from the EDTA Registry. Nephrol Dial Transplant 1988;3(2):109–22.
26. Beauchamp TL, Childress JF. Principles of biomedical ethics. 5th edition. Oxford (NY): Oxford University Press; 2001. p. 454, xi.
27. Mavroudis C, Mavroudis CD, Farrell RM, et al. Informed consent, bioethical equipoise, and hypoplastic left heart syndrome. Cardiol Young 2011;21(Suppl 2):133–40.
28. Zeigler VL. Ethical principles and parental choice: treatment options for neonates with hypoplastic left heart syndrome. Pediatr Nurs 2003;29(1):65–9.
29. Geary DF. Attitudes of pediatric nephrologists to management of end-stage renal disease in infants. J Pediatr 1998;133(1):154–6.
30. Teh JC, Frieling ML, Sienna JL, et al. Attitudes of caregivers to management of end-stage renal disease in infants. Perit Dial Int 2011;31(4):459–65.
31. Reed RB, Stuart HC. Patterns of growth in height and weight from birth to eighteen years of age. Pediatrics 1959;24:904–21.

32. Lowrey G. Growth and development of children. 7th edition. Chicago: Year Book Medical Publishers; 1978.
33. Kari JA, Gonzalez C, Ledermann SE, et al. Outcome and growth of infants with severe chronic renal failure. Kidney Int 2000;57(4):1681–7.
34. Karlberg J, Schaefer F, Hennicke M, et al. Early age-dependent growth impairment in chronic renal failure. European Study Group for Nutritional Treatment of Chronic Renal Failure in Childhood. Pediatr Nephrol 1996;10(3):283–7.
35. Wong CS, Hingorani S, Gillen DL, et al. Hypoalbuminemia and risk of death in pediatric patients with end-stage renal disease. Kidney Int 2002;61(2): 630–7.
36. Furth SL, Stablein D, Fine RN, et al. Adverse clinical outcomes associated with short stature at dialysis initiation: a report of the North American Pediatric Renal Transplant Cooperative Study. Pediatrics 2002;109(5):909–13.
37. Food and Nutrition Board. Dietary reference intakes for energy, carbohydrate, fiber, fat, fatty acids, cholesterol, protein, and amino acids (macronutrients). Food and Nutrition Board. Washington, DC: National Academies; 2002.
38. Quan A, Baum M. Protein losses in children on continuous cycler peritoneal dialysis. Pediatr Nephrol 1996;10(6):728–31.
39. Lapeyraque AL, Haddad E, Andre JL, et al. Sudden blindness caused by anterior ischemic optic neuropathy in 5 children on continuous peritoneal dialysis. Am J Kidney Dis 2003;42(5):E3–9.
40. Bunchman TE. Chronic dialysis in the infant less than 1 year of age. Pediatr Nephrol 1995;9(Suppl):S18–22.
41. Bellisle F, Dartois AM, Kleinknecht C, et al. Alteration of the taste for sugar in renal insufficiency: study in the child. Nephrologie 1995;16(2):203–8.
42. Mak RH, Cheung W, Cone RD, et al. Leptin and inflammation-associated cachexia in chronic kidney disease. Kidney Int 2006;69(5):794–7.
43. Rees L. Long-term peritoneal dialysis in infants. Perit Dial Int 2007;27(Suppl 2): S180–4.
44. Daschner M, Tonshoff B, Blum WF, et al. Inappropriate elevation of serum leptin levels in children with chronic renal failure. European Study Group for Nutritional Treatment of Chronic Renal Failure in Childhood. J Am Soc Nephrol 1998;9(6): 1074–9.
45. Ruley EJ, Bock GH, Kerzner B, et al. Feeding disorders and gastroesophageal reflux in infants with chronic renal failure. Pediatr Nephrol 1989;3(4):424–9.
46. Dello Strologo L, Principato F, Sinibaldi D, et al. Feeding dysfunction in infants with severe chronic renal failure after long-term nasogastric tube feeding. Pediatr Nephrol 1997;11(1):84–6.
47. Wong H, Mylrea K, Cameron A, et al. Caregiver attitudes towards gastrostomy removal after renal transplantation. Pediatr Transplant 2005;9(5):574–8.
48. Mekahli D, Shaw V, Ledermann SE, et al. Long-term outcome of infants with severe chronic kidney disease. Clin J Am Soc Nephrol 2010;5(1):10–7.
49. Ramage IJ, Geary DF, Harvey E, et al. Efficacy of gastrostomy feeding in infants and older children receiving chronic peritoneal dialysis. Perit Dial Int 1999;19(3): 231–6.
50. Ledermann SE, Spitz L, Moloney J, et al. Gastrostomy feeding in infants and children on peritoneal dialysis. Pediatr Nephrol 2002;17(4):246–50.
51. Rees L, Azocar M, Borzych D, et al. Growth in very young children undergoing chronic peritoneal dialysis. J Am Soc Nephrol 2011;22(12):2303–12.
52. Bruel A, Roze JC, Flamant C, et al. Critical serum creatinine values in very preterm newborns. PLoS One 2013;8(12):e84892.

53. Wedekin M, Ehrich JH, Offner G, et al. Renal replacement therapy in infants with chronic renal failure in the first year of life. Clin J Am Soc Nephrol 2010;5(1):18–23.
54. Annual Report of the US Organ Procurement and Transplantation Network and the Scientific Registry of Transplant Recipients. Transplant data 1994-2009. Rockville (MD); Richmond (VA); Ann Arbor (MI): Department of Health and Human Services, Health Resources and Services Administration, Healthcare Systems Bureau, Division of Transplantation; United Network for Organ Sharing; University Renal Research and Education Association; 2010.
55. Alexander RT, Foster BJ, Tonelli MA, et al. Survival and transplantation outcomes of children less than 2 years of age with end-stage renal disease. Pediatr Nephrol 2012;27(10):1975–83.
56. Wood EG, Hand M, Briscoe DM, et al. Risk factors for mortality in infants and young children on dialysis. Am J Kidney Dis 2001;37(3):573–9.
57. Ledermann SE, Scanes ME, Fernando ON, et al. Long-term outcome of peritoneal dialysis in infants. J Pediatr 2000;136(1):24–9.
58. Shroff R, Rees L, Trompeter R, et al. Long-term outcome of chronic dialysis in children. Pediatr Nephrol 2006;21(2):257–64.
59. Schaefer F, Borzych D, Azocar M, et al. Impact of global economic disparities on practices and outcomes of chronic peritoneal dialysis in children: insights from the International Pediatric Peritoneal Dialysis Network Registry. Perit Dial Int 2012;32(4):399–409.

Renal Replacement Therapy in Neonates

Ahmad Kaddourah, MD, MS, Stuart L. Goldstein, MD*

KEYWORDS

- Acute kidney injury • Continuous renal replacement therapy • Peritoneal dialysis
- Hyperammonemia • Neonates

KEY POINTS

- Dialysis is an effective therapy for treating neonates with acute kidney injury and hyperammonemia.
- Peritoneal dialysis is the most common modality for treating acute kidney injury in neonates, although continuous renal replacement therapy is an increasingly utilized alternative.
- Early initiation of dialysis may improve outcomes in neonates with kidney failure and volume overload.
- Hyperammonemia requires rapid intervention with dialysis to decrease neurologic toxicity.

Video of PD catheter accompanies this article at http://www.perinatology.theclinics.com/

INTRODUCTION

Recent advances in the technology and safety of renal replacement therapy (RRT) have changed the practice of pediatric nephrologists significantly in the last 2 decades. In the 1990s, only 53% of pediatric nephrologists offered RRT for infants younger than 1 year of age, and only 41% offered RRT to infants younger than 1 month of age.[1] In 2011, initiation of dialysis in the first year of life represented up to 9.4% of all children who required maintenance dialysis according to the North American Pediatric Renal Trials and Collaborative Studies (NAPRTCS) report. This initiation rate was the highest of any year in the first 18 years of life.[2] Providing RRT is the expected standard of care for newborns when it is indicated. This article reviews the available acute RRT options for neonates to treat acute kidney injury (AKI) and inborn errors of metabolism

Dr Kaddourah was sponsored in the Cincinnati Children's Hospital Pediatric Acute Care Nephrology and Dialysis Fellowship by an unrestricted educational grant from Gambro Renal Products.
Center for Acute Care Nephrology, Cincinnati Children's Hospital Medical Center (CCHMC), MLC 7022, 3333 Burnet Avenue, Cincinnati, OH 45229-3039, USA
* Corresponding authors.
E-mail address: stuart.goldstein@cchmc.org

with hyperammonemia. RRT for chronic end-stage renal disease is beyond the scope of this review.

RRT FOR AKI

AKI is one of the most important independent risk factors for mortality in hospitalized children[3,4] and adults.[5-7] The AKI incidence rate is high in neonatal intensive care units (NICUs) among specific populations such as very low-birth weight infants (18%),[8] neonates undergoing cardiopulmonary bypass (23%–52%),[9,10] and neonates receiving extracorporeal membrane oxygenation (ECMO) (71%).[11] Unfortunately, although AKI has been recognized as an important mortality risk factor, the current universal clinical practice is limited to treating the complications of AKI rather than preventing it. Trials to study the effect of different medications such as fenoldopam[12,13] and rasburicase[14] to prevent AKI have had equivocal results. With the current lack of effective pharmacologic approaches to treat or prevent AKI, RRT is the main intervention to manage its consequences. The common modalities of RRT in the NICU to support neonates with AKI include acute peritoneal dialysis (PD), continuous renal replacement therapy (CRRT), and intermittent hemodialysis (HD). There are no randomized clinical trials to favor one modality; hence, the choice of modality is based on patient condition, physician expertise, and institutional resources.[15]

Acute PD for AKI in Neonates

Unlike older children, in whom CRRT has become the preferred modality for the management of AKI,[16-18] acute PD is the most common modality of RRT provided to neonates. The principal advantages of PD are the relatively easy technique in terms of surgical insertion of a PD catheter and lack of need for vascular access and an extracorporeal blood circuit, which represent the most challenging technical problems for HD and CRRT, especially for low birth-weight neonates.

The requirements for effective PD are a functioning PD catheter, an intact peritoneal membrane, which represents the filter for dialysis, dialysis fluids, and connecting tubing and drainage bags.

PD access

In acute situations, where the clinical scenario requires only a temporary need of dialysis for clearance or volume overload, most neonates receive a temporary peritoneal catheter placed in the true pelvis. There are many commercially available temporary catheters including Tenckhoff (Quinton peritoneal catheters; Kendall Co, Mansfield, MA, USA), Mac-Loc multipurpose drainage (Cook Inc, Bloomington, IN, USA) and Teflon rigid (Cook Inc, Bloomington, IN, USA) catheters, with equivocal evidence of superiority of one over the others.[19] Although these temporary catheters have a higher risk of leak and dialysis failure compared with permanent tunneled PD catheters, they are usually effective and thus recommended as the initial approach.

PD fluids

The dialysis fluid is generally composed of an osmotic agent, a buffer, and electrolytes. These components can be modified to affect blood purification (ie, clearance) and fluid removal (ie, ultrafiltration). **Table 1** shows the components' concentration ranges of the standard commercially available PD fluids.

Osmotic agents Dextrose monohydrate (the bioavailable D-form of glucose) is the conventional osmotic agent used in dialysis fluids. The supraphysiologic concentrations (1500–4250 mg/dL) of dextrose create an osmotic gradient via the peritoneal

Table 1
Components' concentration ranges in the standard commercially available PD fluids

Osmotic Agent	
Dextrose	1.5–4.5 g/dL
Icodextrin	7.5 g/dL
Amino acids	1.1 g/dL
Buffer	
Lactate	30–40 mmol/L
Bicarbonate	34 mmol/L
Lactate/bicarbonate	15/25 mmol/L
Electrolytes	
Sodium	132–134 mmol/L
Calcium	1.25–1.75 mmol/L
Magnesium	0.25–0.75 mmol/L
Chloride	95–103.5 mmol/L

Data from Verrina EE, Perfumo F. Comprehensive pediatric nephrology. Philadelphia: Elsevier; 2008.

membrane to achieve ultrafiltration (the movement of water molecules) from the peritoneal capillaries to the peritoneal cavity via osmotic pressure. Solutions that utilize amino acids or icodextrin as osmotic agents were developed to decrease the toxic effects of the dextrose on the peritoneal membrane in the setting of chronic dialysis; however, they are generally not used in acute situations.

Buffers Lactate, the metabolic precursor of bicarbonate, was the only buffer available for PD solutions until recently (and remains so in the United States). Lactate is rapidly absorbed and metabolized to bicarbonate by the liver. The net buffer gain is counterbalanced by the simultaneous loss of blood bicarbonate into the relatively acidotic (pH 5.5–6.5) dialysis fluid.[20] In recent years, advances in foil technology and use of double-chamber PD solutions have made it possible to produce stable PD fluid bags containing either pure bicarbonate or a mixture of bicarbonate and lactate buffer.[21] Bicarbonate-containing PD fluids have demonstrated better correction of metabolic acidosis[22] and lower peritoneal inflammatory markers[23] than lactate-only PD fluids in the pediatric chronic dialysis setting.

Electrolytes The sodium concentration in PD dialysis fluids ranges from 132 to 134 mmol/L, which is slightly lower than the normal plasma sodium concentration. The slight difference of sodium concentration between the dialysis and the capillary vessels enhances the diffusion of sodium from the plasma to the dialysate fluids. This movement of sodium parallels ultrafiltration of water, and thus the increased diffusion of sodium prevents the development of hypernatremia. The standard PD solutions have 2 different calcium concentrations: high-calcium (1.75 mmol/L) and low-calcium (1.25 mmol/L) dialysis fluids. The calcium concentration of the high-calcium dialysis fluids is higher than the normal serum ionized calcium level and thus will cause a positive calcium balance. Unless hypercalcemia is present, high-calcium dialysis fluids are usually preferred, because they provide the positive calcium balance needed for neonatal growth. However, high dialysate calcium may cause hypercalcemia if other sources of calcium are not adjusted appropriately (eg, continuous intravenous infusions of calcium and total parental nutrition). Accordingly, a collaborative approach between the neonatal intensivist, nephrologist, and nutritionist should be established to choose the appropriate dialysate calcium concentration.

ACUTE PD PRESCRIPTION

Once the temporary nontunneled peritoneal catheter is placed, PD initiation is guided by the severity of the kidney dysfunction and patient clinical status. If needed, the PD can be started immediately. Typically, PD is initiated using low-fill volumes such as 10 to 20 mL/kg[24,25] or 600 to 800 mL/m^2 of body surface area (BSA).[26] This low-volume approach can provide the appropriate blood purification and ultrafiltration to manage the newborn without increasing the risk of complications of starting PD early, such as dialysate leak around the exit site. There are no specific guidelines designed to direct acute PD, and current practice is based on the chronic PD literature.[27]

SPECIAL CASE: ACUTE PD FOR NEONATAL AKI AFTER CARDIOPULMONARY BYPASS

There has been significant research focusing on AKI after cardiac surgery. AKI following cardiopulmonary bypass (CPB) has been a productive area for defining the role of urinary biomarkers to detect early AKI and to investigate potential therapeutic and prophylactic approaches in this population.[28] The single insulting factor of CPB causing the kidney injury, the known timing of the AKI, and high post-CPB AKI rates render this clinical AKI setting as ideal for clinical and translational research.

Newborns and infants undergoing CPB are at significant risk of developing AKI and subsequently needing RRT. The reported incidence of AKI after CPB has ranged from 23% to 52%.[9,10] This wide range incidence is partially due to varying definitions of AKI. The reported need of RRT ranges between 2.1% and 17%,[29–33] with a mortality rate up to 40%[30] in infants requiring RRT. PD is the most commonly used RRT modality to treat the consequences of AKI in this population. Despite awareness of the significant incidence of AKI following CPB, there is no universally applied predictive approach to prevent the consequences of AKI and oliguria. Until recently, the approach was limited to careful observation and RRT initiation when neonates developed significant volume overload compromising the recovery process of the congenital heart surgery repair. This practice started to change due to the growing evidence of the beneficiary approach of starting RRT early in the course of AKI. This evidence evolved from observational prospective studies in adults.[34–36] Despite using different definitions of early RRT and different RRT modalities, these studies concluded that starting RRT early after cardiac surgeries using CPB is associated with decreased in-hospital mortality, decreased hospital stay, shorter duration of RRT and lower dialysis dependence. Two neonatal studies generated the same favorable results of the early strategy for RRT in neonates. Bojan and colleagues[33] compared the outcomes of starting peritoneal dialysis in the first day versus second day or later after the cardiac surgery in a total of 146 newborns weighing 3.5 ($\pm$1.2) kg. Patients in the early PD group had a lower 30-day mortality (23% vs 43% [P = .02]) and a lower 90-day mortality rate (28% vs 51.3% [P = .02]) when compared with the delayed PD group.

Sasser and colleagues[37] prospectively compared 2 cohorts of neonates following CPB. The first cohort was managed with passive peritoneal drainage and diuretics (controls); the second cohort was started on prophylactic PD in the immediate postoperative period (the PD cohort). The median net fluid balance was more negative in the PD cohort at 24 hours and 48 hours than in the controls. In addition, the PD cohort had a lower mean inotrope score at 24 hours, earlier sternal closure, shorter duration of mechanical ventilation, and lower serum concentrations of inflammatory cytokines (interleukin-6 [IL-6] and IL-8) at 24 hours than the control cohort.

At the authors' institution, patients scheduled to have heart surgery requiring CPB are screened, and they are classified into high-, moderate-, and low-risk AKI groups to determine the need to prophylactically place a temporary PD catheter in the operating room (**Table 2**). The PD catheter is surgically placed through the thoracic cavity (Video 1). The authors reported improved outcomes with this approach, showing earlier attainment of negative fluid balance, greater prevention of volume overload, and earlier discontinuation of mechanical ventilation.[38]

CRRT for AKI in Neonates

Although PD is usually efficient at blood purification and fluid removal, it cannot be utilized in a significant proportion of neonates. PD is technically impossible or undesirable in cases of abdominal wall defects or recent abdominal surgical operations and skin infections. Moreover, some neonates, especially if severely overloaded with high fluid intake, do not have adequate ultrafiltration with PD. CRRT has become more widely used in neonates because of technological advances.[18]

In a report from the Prospective Pediatric Continuous Renal Replacement Therapy registry, the mortality rate was 57% among infants weighing no more than 10 kg and 36% in infants weighing more than 10 kg of weight.[39] The mortality rate did not defer among patients less than 5 kg and 5 to 10 kg. Survivors in this report were more likely to start CRRT sooner after ICU admission and were less fluid overloaded at CRRT initiation than nonsurvivors. Moreover, infants who were able to achieve dry weight during their CRRT course were more likely to survive than children remaining fluid overloaded. These data suggest that clinical management strategies to prevent fluid overload and early initiation of CRRT for ultrafiltration may improve the outcome in these infants.

CRRT technique

One of the key benefits of the CRRT is the gradual and adjustable rate of solute and fluid removal, which makes it ideal for patients with hemodynamic instability. CRRT treatment requires an access line; hemofilter and tubing; anticoagulation; and replacement and dialysate fluids.

Table 2
Cincinnati Children's Hospital Medical Center protocol to identify the risk of AKI following CPB surgeries

Risk Category	Patients' Criteria	Action
High risk of AKI	a. Neonates ≤3 mo undergoing any heart surgery using CPB b. Patients ≤6 mo of age undergoing heart transplantation c. Patients ≤4 mo of age undergoing tetralogy of Fallot or double-outlet right ventricular repair	Plan to prophylactically place a temporary peritoneal dialysis catheter in the operating room
Moderate risk of AKI	a. Patients >6 mo of age undergoing heart transplantation b. Patients >4 mo of age undergoing tetralogy of Fallot or double-outlet right ventricular repair c. CPB time >120 min	Consider placing peritoneal dialysis catheter prophylactically based on the patient's condition in the operating room and the surgeon's assessment
Low risk of AKI	Patients do not meet the high- or the low-risk of AKI as above	Peritoneal dialysis catheter placement is not indicated

Access line The presence of a functional and optimally sized vascular access line is a critical component of successful CRRT treatment. To maximize blood flow, the largest gauge catheter that can be placed safely is ideal.[40] A 7 French dialysis catheter can usually be placed successfully in 3 to 6 kg infants, and an 8 French catheter can be used for 6 to 12 kg infants in either the femoral or internal jugular veins. Subclavian catheters should be avoided because of the risk of venous stenosis that may limit chronic HD options if needed. Both double- and triple-lumen catheters are acceptable; however, triple-lumen catheters are preferred, because they provide a third venous access that can be used for blood access and medications infusion.

Hemofilter and tubing The goal is to use the smallest possible circuit volume to minimize the extracorporeal blood volume. Most neonates require a blood prime, which is necessary if the extracorporeal circuit exceeds 10% to 15% of the total blood volume (total blood volume is approximately 80 mL/kg).[41]

Anticoagulation CRRT circuits used in neonates are likely to clot because of the relatively slow blood flow rates and small vascular access. The 2 most common anticoagulation protocols are systemic heparin and circuit regional anticoagulation using citrate. When heparin is used, serial activated clotting times are typically followed to adjust the heparin infusion.[40]

Replacement and dialysate fluids CRRT utilizes either a replacement fluid or a dialysis fluid to provide solute clearance. Both forms of clearance can be used simultaneously if high clearance rates are needed.

CRRT prescription
CRRT has 4 different modalities:

- Slow continuous ultra filtration (SCUF). This is used for fluid removal, but produces minimal solute removal.
- Continuous veno-venous hemofiltration (CVVH). A replacement fluid is used to provide solute removal.
- Continuous veno-venous hemodialysis (CVVHD). Dialysate fluid is used to provide solute removal.
- Continuous veno-venous hemodiafiltration (CVVHDF). Both a replacement fluid and a dialysis fluid are used to provide solute removal.

There is no evidence that one of these techniques is superior. **Box 1** summarizes recommendations for pediatric CRRT prescription.[40,42]

CRRT circuit ECMO
Children on ECMO are at high risk for AKI, and may need RRT for volume overload or electrolyte removal. In 1 study, only 23% of children on ECMO did not require RRT.[43] Although any form of RRT can be used in children on ECMO, CRRT is usually used in this population because of the hemodynamic instability of these patients and the advantage of an already existing anticoagulated circuit. CRRT using the ECMO circuit can be applied using 1 of 2 different methods[44,45]: using a hemofilter in-line with the ECMO circuit or connecting a CRRT machine to the ECMO circuit in parallel (integrated ultrafiltration). In the in-line method, intravenous pumps are used to run the dialysis fluid and control the ultrafiltration. While the first method has the advantage of simplicity and low cost, the integrated RRT provides more accurate fluid management during the ECMO course. The use of integrated ultrafiltration has been associated with shorter duration of ECMO (384 vs 583 h, $P<.001$) RRT (185 vs 477 h, $P<.001$) than hemofilter in-line ECMO patients.[45] With

---

Box 1
CRRT prescription

Blood Flow Rate

- Neonate/infants: 8–12 mL/kg/min
- Toddlers: 6–8 mL/kg/min
- Older children: 3–6 mL/kg/min

Combined Dialysis and Convection Dose

- 2000–3000 mL/h/1.73 m^2

Anticoagulation

Citrate: (ACD-A; Baxter Healthcare, McGaw Park, Illinois)

- Start rate (mL/h) = Blood flow rate (mL/min) × 1.5
- Adjust the rate to keep the circuit ionized calcium between 0.2 and 0.5 mmol/L

Heparin:

- Bolus: 10–20 U/kg upon starting CRRT
- Continuous infusion: 10 U/kg/h, the dose to be adjusted to keep the anticoagulation time between 140 and 180 seconds for patients without evidence of systemic bleeding and between 120 and 160 seconds for patients with evidence of systemic bleeding

Calcium Infusion (If citrate is used as anticoagulation)

- Calcium chloride (8 g/L of 0.9% sodium chloride) (mL/h): blood flow rate (mL/min) × 0.6
- Calcium gluconate (50 g/L of 0.9% sodium chloride) (mL/h): blood flow rate (mL/min) × 0.3

---

either method, the return from the hemofilter or CRRT device should be placed before the ECMO oxygenator, so that any clot or air will be trapped in the oxygenator[41] before traveling to the patient.

CRRT challenges in neonates and the future

Despite significant advances in critical care technology, the available CRRT systems are designed for adult patients, and almost all CRRT machines are used off label in the United States when treating small children. Current CRRT machines are not designed to treat a small infant who requires accurate blood flow rates in the range of 10 to 30 mL/min and ultrafiltration error of less than 5 mL/hour. The ultrafiltration volume error range of some CRRT machines is 20 to 190 mL.[46] Although this error might be inconsequential to a 70 kg adult, it is enormous for a 3 kg neonate. The Cardio-Renal, Pediatric Dialysis Emergency Machine (CARPEDIEM) was developed for the treatment of neonates between 2.0 and 9.9 kg with circuit volumes not exceeding 41.5 mL.[47] In in vitro testing, the error of ultrafiltration was about 1 mL/h. In addition, a low-volume CRRT circuit (HF20, Gambro Renal Products) has been designed to provide the low extracorporeal volume (50 mL) needed for neonates to decrease the hemodynamic challenges observed with using other circuits. This circuit has been in the non-US market since 2011[48] and has been used for neonates weighing as little as 2.3 kg.

Intermittent Hemodialysis for AKI in Neonates

Although intermittent hemodialysis (IHD) in children was described as early as 1955,[49] the utilization of IHD in neonates and small infants has been limited. IHD produces solute clearance via diffusion across a semipermeable membrane. The high blood flow and dialysate rates make IHD the most rapid modality to clear solutes and remove fluid. As opposed to CRRT or PD, IHD can provide substantial clearance in several hours. Despite superior clearance, other RRT modalities are preferred in many centers given the technical challenges of IHD in small newborns. These challenges include inability to precisely control ultrafiltration, intradialytic hypotension rates that can be as high as 64%,[50] the requirement of highly skilled personnel, the large extracorporeal blood volume, and the risk of the disequilibrium syndrome in uremic children secondary to the rapid clearance of solutes.

The reported experience with IHD in newborns with AKI is sparse. Sadowski and colleagues reported on neonatal IHD in 33 infants with AKI, hyperammonemia, and chronic kidney disease. The survival in the AKI group was only 33%, but more than 70% in the remainder of the patients. Hypotension requiring intervention occurred in 61% of the neonates with AKI.

IHD requires vascular access, anticoagulation, a dialyzer with tubing system, and dialysate fluids.

RRT FOR NEONATES WITH HYPERAMMONEMIA

Neonatal hyperammonemia is the most common non-AKI indication of RRT in NICUs. Ammonia (NH_3) is the end product of multiple inborn errors of metabolism such as urea cycle defects, organic acidurias, and fatty acid oxidation defects. Ammonia is a potent neurotoxin and may cause fulminant cerebral edema and death when its serum concentrations exceed 800 μmol/L for more than 24 hours.[51] The cornerstone of managing neonates with hyperammonemia is administration of a combination preparation of sodium phenylacetate and sodium benzoate and initiation of arginine, carnitine, hydroxycobalamin, and biotin to decrease NH_3 production. However, pharmacologic therapy does not produce the rapid decrease in the ammonia level needed to prevent permanent neurologic damage in some patients. RRT should be initiated as soon as possible when the ammonia level is greater than 400 μmol/L,[52] with the goal to decrease the level to less than 200 μmol/L. IHD provides the most efficient RRT modality to rapidly clear ammonia; however, IHD is limited by the need for systemic anticoagulation and the rapid rebound in ammonia levels after stopping IHD; this need leads to repeated courses of IHD. A combined approach of initial IHD for 2 hours followed by CRRT is an approach that provides rapid ammonia reduction by IHD followed by ongoing ammonia clearance via CRRT.[51] An alternative strategy is exclusive use of CVVH.[53] With this approach, 85% of the neonates achieved an ammonia level of less than 200 μmol/L in 24 hours or less using a replacement fluid rate of 2000 mL/h/1.73 m². An alternative approach is the use of high dose-dose CRRT.[52] In this case series, 2 patients with an ammonia level greater than 1000 μmol/L received CVVHDF and CVVHD doses of 8000 mL/h/1.73 m² (4 times higher than the regular CRRT prescription of AKI). The ammonia level decreased to less than 200 μmol/L in less than 6 hours, with corresponding ammonia clearance of 1000 mL/h compared with 1800 mL/hour if IHD were used with the same blood flow rate. When citrate is used as regional anticoagulation for CRRT, it should be started at 50% of the usual rate due to decreased hepatic metabolism.[40]

Some centers use ECMO with hemodialysis. This technique provides very high flow rates (170–200 mL/min) and rapidly reduces ammonia levels, but with greater morbidity associated with surgical vascular access. Despite the more rapid removal of plasma ammonia with extracorporeal dialysis, PD may be effective in newborns with less severe hyperammonemia[54] and should be started if IHD or CRRT is not available at a particular center.

SUPPLEMENTARY DATA

Supplementary data related to this article can be found online at http://dx.doi.org/10.1016/j.clp.2014.05.003.

REFERENCES

1. Geary DF. Attitudes of pediatric nephrologists to management of end-stage renal disease in infants. J Pediatr 1998;133(1):154–6.
2. Studies NAPRTaC. NAPRTCS 2011 Annual Dialysis Report 2011. Available at: https://web.emmes.com/study/ped/annlrept/annualrept2011.pdf.
3. Akcan-Arikan A, Zappitelli M, Loftis LL, et al. Modified RIFLE criteria in critically ill children with acute kidney injury. Kidney Int 2007;71(10):1028–35.
4. Zappitelli M, Parikh CR, Akcan-Arikan A, et al. Ascertainment and epidemiology of acute kidney injury varies with definition interpretation. Clin J Am Soc Nephrol 2008;3(4):948–54.
5. Li PK, Burdmann EA, Mehta RL, et al. Acute kidney injury: global health alert. Transplantation 2013;95(5):653–7.
6. Cuhaci B. More data on epidemiology and outcome of acute kidney injury with AKIN criteria: benefits of standardized definitions, AKIN and RIFLE classifications. Crit Care Med 2009;37(9):2659–61.
7. Uchino S. Outcome prediction for patients with acute kidney injury. Nephron Clin Pract 2008;109(4):C217–23.
8. Koralkar R, Ambalavanan N, Levitan EB, et al. Acute kidney injury reduces survival in very low birth weight infants. Pediatr Res 2011;69(4):354–8.
9. Krawczeski CD, Woo JG, Wang Y, et al. Neutrophil gelatinase-associated lipocalin concentrations predict development of acute kidney injury in neonates and children after cardiopulmonary bypass. J Pediatr 2011;158(6):1009–15.e1.
10. Blinder JJ, Goldstein SL, Lee VV, et al. Congenital heart surgery in infants: effects of acute kidney injury on outcomes. J Thorac Cardiovasc Surg 2012;143(2):368–74.
11. Gadepalli SK, Selewski DT, Drongowski RA, et al. Acute kidney injury in congenital diaphragmatic hernia requiring extracorporeal life support: an insidious problem. J Pediatr Surg 2011;46(4):630–5.
12. Ricci Z, Stazi GV, Di Chiara L, et al. Fenoldopam in newborn patients undergoing cardiopulmonary bypass: controlled clinical trial. Interact Cardiovasc Thorac Surg 2008;7(6):1049–53.
13. Moffett BS, Mott AR, Nelson DP, et al. Renal effects of fenoldopam in critically ill pediatric patients: a retrospective review. Pediatr Crit Care Med 2008;9(4):403–6.
14. Hobbs DJ, Steinke JM, Chung JY, et al. Rasburicase improves hyperuricemia in infants with acute kidney injury. Pediatr Nephrol 2010;25(2):305–9.
15. Walters S, Porter C, Brophy PD. Dialysis and pediatric acute kidney injury: choice of renal support modality. Pediatr Nephrol 2009;24(1):37–48.
16. Sutherland SM, Alexander SR. Continuous renal replacement therapy in children. Pediatr Nephrol 2012;27(11):2007–16.
17. Belsha CW, Kohaut EC, Warady BA. Dialytic management of childhood acute renal failure: a survey of North American pediatric nephrologists. Pediatr Nephrol 1995;9(3):361–3.
18. Warady BA, Bunchman T. Dialysis therapy for children with acute renal failure: survey results. Pediatr Nephrol 2000;15(1–2):11–3.

19. Auron A, Warady BA, Simon S, et al. Use of the multipurpose drainage catheter for the provision of acute peritoneal dialysis in infants and children. Am J Kidney Dis 2007;49(5):650–5.
20. Schmitt CP, Haraldsson B, Doetschmann R, et al. Effects of pH-neutral, bicarbonate-buffered dialysis fluid on peritoneal transport kinetics in children. Kidney Int 2002;61(4):1527–36.
21. Schmitt CP. Pediatric dialysis. New York: Springer; 2012.
22. Haas S, Schmitt CP, Arbeiter K, et al. Improved acidosis correction and recovery of mesothelial cell mass with neutral-pH bicarbonate dialysis solution among children undergoing automated peritoneal dialysis. J Am Soc Nephrol 2003; 14(10):2632–8.
23. Fusshoeller A, Plail M, Grabensee B, et al. Biocompatibility pattern of a bicarbonate/lactate-buffered peritoneal dialysis fluid in APD: a prospective, randomized study. Nephrol Dial Transplant 2004;19(8):2101–6.
24. Goldstein SL. Overview of pediatric renal replacement therapy in acute renal failure. Artif Organs 2003;27(9):781–5.
25. Shaheen IS, Watson AR, Harvey B. Acute renal failure in children: etiology, treatment and outcome. Saudi J Kidney Dis Transpl 2006;17(2):153–8.
26. Fischbach M, Haraldsson B. Dynamic changes of the total pore area available for peritoneal exchange in children. Journal of the American Society of Nephrology: JASN 2001;12(7):1524–9.
27. White CT, Gowrishankar M, Feber J, et al. Clinical practice guidelines for pediatric peritoneal dialysis. Pediatr Nephrol 2006;21(8):1059–66.
28. Goldstein SL. A novel use for novel acute kidney injury biomarkers: fenoldopam's effect on neutrophil gelatinase-associated lipocalin and cystatin C. Crit Care 2011;15(4):177.
29. Pedersen KR, Povlsen JV, Christensen S, et al. Risk factors for acute renal failure requiring dialysis after surgery for congenital heart disease in children. Acta Anaesthesiol Scand 2007;51(10):1344–9.
30. Boigner H, Brannath W, Hermon M, et al. Predictors of mortality at initiation of peritoneal dialysis in children after cardiac surgery. Ann Thorac Surg 2004; 77(1):61–5.
31. Chan KL, Ip P, Chiu CS, et al. Peritoneal dialysis after surgery for congenital heart disease in infants and young children. Ann Thorac Surg 2003;76(5):1443–9.
32. Kuitunen A, Vento A, Suojaranta-Ylinen R, et al. Acute renal failure after cardiac surgery: evaluation of the RIFLE classification. Ann Thorac Surg 2006;81(2): 542–6.
33. Bojan M, Gioanni S, Vouhe PR, et al. Early initiation of peritoneal dialysis in neonates and infants with acute kidney injury following cardiac surgery is associated with a significant decrease in mortality. Kidney Int 2012;82(4):474–81.
34. Elahi MM, Lim MY, Joseph RN, et al. Early hemofiltration improves survival in postcardiotomy patients with acute renal failure. Eur J Cardiothorac Surg 2004;26(5): 1027–31.
35. Bagshaw SM, Uchino S, Bellomo R, et al. Timing of renal replacement therapy and clinical outcomes in critically ill patients with severe acute kidney injury. J Crit Care 2009;24(1):129–40.
36. Bent P, Tan HK, Bellomo R, et al. Early and intensive continuous hemofiltration for severe renal failure after cardiac surgery. Ann Thorac Surg 2001;71(3):832–7.
37. Sasser WC, Dabal RJ, Askenazi DJ, et al. Prophylactic peritoneal dialysis following cardiopulmonary bypass in children is associated with decreased inflammation and improved clinical outcomes. Congenit Heart Dis 2014;9(2):106–15.

38. Kwiatkowski DM, Menon S, Krawczeski CD, et al. Improved outcomes with peritoneal dialysis catheter placement after cardiopulmonary bypass in infants. J Thorac Cardiovasc Surg 2013. [Epub ahead of print].
39. Askenazi DJ, Goldstein SL, Koralkar R, et al. Continuous renal replacement therapy for children </=10 kg: a report from the prospective pediatric continuous renal replacement therapy registry. J Pediatr 2013;162(3):587–92.e3.
40. Bunchman TE, Brophy PD, Goldstein SL. Technical considerations for renal replacement therapy in children. Semin Nephrol 2008;28(5):488–92.
41. Bridges BC, Askenazi DJ, Smith J, et al. Pediatric renal replacement therapy in the intensive care unit. Blood Purif 2012;34(2):138–48.
42. Brophy PD, Somers MJ, Baum MA, et al. Multi-centre evaluation of anticoagulation in patients receiving continuous renal replacement therapy (CRRT). Nephrol Dial Transplant 2005;20(7):1416–21.
43. Fleming GM, Askenazi DJ, Bridges BC, et al. A multicenter international survey of renal supportive therapy during ECMO: the Kidney Intervention During Extracorporeal Membrane Oxygenation (KIDMO) group. ASAIO J 2012;58(4):407–14.
44. Askenazi DJ, Selewski DT, Paden ML, et al. Renal replacement therapy in critically ill patients receiving extracorporeal membrane oxygenation. Clin J Am Soc Nephrol 2012;7(8):1328–36.
45. Symons JM, McMahon MW, Karamlou T, et al. Continuous renal replacement therapy with an automated monitor is superior to a free-flow system during extracorporeal life support. Pediatr Crit Care Med 2013;14(9):e404–8.
46. Ronco C, Garzotto F, Ricci Z. CA.R.PE.DI.E.M. (Cardio-Renal Pediatric Dialysis Emergency Machine): evolution of continuous renal replacement therapies in infants. A personal journey. Pediatr Nephrol 2012;27(8):1203–11.
47. Ronco C, Ricci Z, Bellomo R, et al. Management of fluid balance in CRRT: a technical approach. International J Artif Organs 2005;28(8):765–76.
48. Rodl S, Marschitz I, Mache CJ, et al. One-year safe use of the Prismaflex HF20((R)) disposable set in infants in 220 renal replacement treatment sessions. Intensive Care Med 2011;37(5):884–5.
49. Mateer FM, Greenman L, Danowski TS. Hemodialysis of the uremic child. AMA Am J Dis Child 1955;89(6):645–55.
50. Sadowski RH, Harmon WE, Jabs K. Acute hemodialysis of infants weighing less than five kilograms. Kidney Int 1994;45(3):903–6.
51. Bunchman TE, Barletta GM, Winters JW, et al. Phenylacetate and benzoate clearance in a hyperammonemic infant on sequential hemodialysis and hemofiltration. Pediatr Nephrol 2007;22(7):1062–5.
52. Spinale JM, Laskin BL, Sondheimer N, et al. High-dose continuous renal replacement therapy for neonatal hyperammonemia. Pediatr Nephrol 2013;28(6):983–6.
53. Westrope C, Morris K, Burford D, et al. Continuous hemofiltration in the control of neonatal hyperammonemia: a 10-year experience. Pediatr Nephrol 2010;25(9):1725–30.
54. Pela I, Seracini D, Donati MA, et al. Peritoneal dialysis in neonates with inborn errors of metabolism: is it really out of date? Pediatr Nephrol 2008;23(1):163–8.

Neonatal Hypertension

Donald L. Batisky, MD

KEYWORDS

- Neonatal • Hypertension • Blood pressure • Oscillometric

KEY POINTS

- The incidence of neonatal hypertension remains low, at less than 2%, and the etiology of hypertension is varied.
- The most common cause of neonatal hypertension is renovascular disease, with umbilical artery catheter placement as a consistent risk factor. Most of the causes are determined by history and basic clinical investigations.
- Strict definitions of hypertension in neonates are unavailable, and the decision to treat is based on opinion rather than evidence guided by well-designed large, multicenter studies with definitive outcomes.
- More studies are needed to define normal blood pressure in this age group and to refine current reference values.
- Treatment is guided by clinical judgment and expert opinion, given the limited number of clinical trials.

INTRODUCTION

Neonatal hypertension (HTN) has been recognized for many decades.[1–3] HTN in the neonate is a difficult issue to define well, owing to a lack of good normative data. Nevertheless, there are clearly neonates with HTN, which may be severe with the potential for significant morbidity. This article focuses on diagnostic approaches to neonatal HTN and reviews treatment options.

SCOPE OF THE PROBLEM

The incidence of HTN in the neonatal period is low, and seems to range between 0.2% and 3%.[1,2,4–6] A recent study of infants admitted to a neonatal intensive care unit (NICU) used billing data to evaluate the incidence of HTN, risk factors associated with HTN, and patterns of use of antihypertensive medications in the NICU. Excluding infants with congenital cardiac disorders, approximately 1% of infants were coded for

Disclosure: Dr D.L. Batisky receives research support from the National Institutes of Health (Lande, R01 HL098332) and participates in clinical trials sponsored by Novartis and Takeda.
Pediatric Hypertension Program, Children's Healthcare of Atlanta, Emory - Children's Center, 2015 Uppergate Drive North East, Atlanta, GA 30322, USA
E-mail address: dbatisk@emory.edu

0095-5108/14/$ – see front matter © 2014 Elsevier Inc. All rights reserved.

HTN. Risks for HTN on multivariate analysis included those with a high All-Patient Refined Diagnosis-Related Groups (APR-DRG) severity of illness assessment, exposure to extracorporeal membranous oxygenation, underlying renal disease, and history of renal failure. Nearly 60% of these infants were on antihypertensive medications, and nearly half received more than 1 medication.[7]

MEASURING BLOOD PRESSURE IN A NEONATE

Blood pressure (BP) is a constantly changing vital sign. There may be several factors that influence BP that must be considered, such as gestational age at birth, the infant's postnatal and postconceptual age, and the size of the infant relative to the gestational age. Maternal factors and perinatal events also contribute to the newborn's BP. The circumstances of the given infant must be considered when assessing the BP value obtained.[8]

Intra-arterial monitoring is considered to be the gold standard method for measuring BP in infants, and the common sites used for placement of a catheter include the umbilical artery, the radial artery, and the posterior tibial artery.[9] An extremely ill infant may warrant invasive monitoring, but most infants in a NICU will have BP measured indirectly with oscillometric devices. Ultrasonic Doppler monitoring is another method used in the NICU, but palpation and auscultation are not considered practical in this setting. The oscillometric technique of BP measurement is most commonly used.[10,11] With this method, a BP cuff is placed on a limb and inflated above the expected systolic pressure. The cuff deflates at timed intervals and the cuff detects vibrations or oscillations in the artery to determine the mean arterial pressure (MAP). The BP device then uses an algorithm to calculate systolic and diastolic BP. Comparisons between oscillometric BP and radial artery pressures have shown good correlation, which has been shown even in premature infants.[12] A suggested protocol for measuring BP in infants in a NICU was proposed by Nwankwo and colleagues,[13] and the elements of their protocol are listed in **Box 1**.

BP data from more than 300 infants on the first day of life have defined the mean and upper and lower 95% confidence intervals for BP.[14] This study showed that increases in BP occurred with both increasing gestational age and birth weight. More recently, Pejovic and colleagues[15] analyzed BP in stable premature and term infants admitted to the NICU, and showed that BP on the first day of life correlated with gestational age and birth weight. Premature newborns show a more rapid increase in BP over the first

---

Box 1
Method for standard neonatal blood pressure measurement

- Method: use oscillometric device
- Time of reading:
  - 1.5 hours after feeding for medical intervention/procedure
  - After cuff is placed, wait 15 minutes
- Position: prone or supine
- Extremity: right upper arm
- Infant state: asleep or quietly awake
- Number of readings: 3, at 2-minute intervals

Adapted from Nwankwo M, Lorenz J, Gardiner J. A standard protocol for blood pressure measurement in the newborn. Pediatrics 1997;99(6):E10.

few of weeks of life.[14,15] An Australian study by Kent and colleagues showed continued increases in BP for infants of less than 31 weeks' gestation, but only over the first week in those of more than 31 weeks gestational age.

In infants who are born at term, birth weight and appropriateness for gestational age seem to influence BP, although there are many conflicting reports in the literature.

A recent report that compared oscillometric and intra-arterial BP measurements in ill preterm infants and full-term neonates aimed to determine the accuracy of oscillometric measurements and evaluate BP distributions in ill neonates. The investigators evaluated almost 1500 simultaneously obtained BP measurements using either umbilical artery catheter (UAC) or radial arterial lines, and also looked at more than 125,000 intra-arterial BP readings to evaluate the BP distribution. There was a statistically significant difference between oscillometric and radial artery mean arterial BP, systolic BP, and diastolic BP. There was also a difference between oscillometric and UAC systolic BP and diastolic BP. The MAP increased with weight, postmenstrual age, and advanced gestational age at birth.[16]

DIAGNOSIS OF HYPERTENSION

The Fourth Report defines HTN in older children, and provides well-defined standards stratified by gender, age, and stature.[17] However, this is not the case in the newborn infant, whether premature or full term. One set of standards for premature infants was derived from a synthesis of published data (**Table 1**). Premature infants with BP values that persist above the 99th percentile warrant further investigation and possible treatment with pharmacologic therapy.

In term infants, there are similar issues of lack of normative data. The Second Task Force on Blood Pressure, published in 1987, included normative BP data for infants from birth to 12 months, but the data were derived from a small group of infants.[23] These data are clearly limited and may not be generalizable. There is also a set of reference curves that may be useful for assessing BP in term newborns and during infancy.[22]

ETIOLOGY OF HYPERTENSION

There are many causes of HTN in the newborn infant (**Table 2**).[5,9] More common causes of HTN in the neonate include the antenatal administration of corticosteroids, maternal history of HTN, placement of a UAC, acute kidney injury postnatally, and chronic lung disease of the newborn.[8,24–35] In the ill newborn, UAC-associated thromboembolism that affects the aorta and/or the renal arterial supply is the most common cause.[9] There has been long-standing debate about whether a "low" or "high" umbilical artery line is more likely to cause HTN. A recent Cochrane review concluded that there were fewer ischemic events such as necrotizing enterocolitis with high lines, but the incidence of HTN was the same.[36] This finding suggests that line placement, perhaps via endothelial injury, may be the cause of thromboembolism leading to HTN. Longer duration of UAC placement is an additional risk factor for thromboembolism. After UAC-related issues, congenital renal anomalies are the second most common cause of HTN in newborns. This large category of conditions includes a variety of congenital anomalies such as obstructive uropathy and cystic kidney disease.

CLINICAL INVESTIGATION

As with any patient, a complete evaluation includes a comprehensive history and a thorough physical examination followed by diagnostic testing, which is crucial in defining causes that may require specific therapy.

Table 1
Estimated values for blood pressures after 2 weeks of age in infants from 26 to 44 weeks postconceptual age

Postconceptual Age (wk)	50th Percentile	95th Percentile	99th Percentile
26			
Systolic	55	72	77
Diastolic	30	50	56
Mean	38	57	63
28			
Systolic	60	75	80
Diastolic	38	50	54
Mean	45	58	63
30			
Systolic	65	80	85
Diastolic	40	55	60
Mean	48	63	68
32			
Systolic	68	83	88
Diastolic	40	55	60
Mean	49	64	69
34			
Systolic	70	85	90
Diastolic	40	55	60
Mean	50	65	70
36			
Systolic	72	87	92
Diastolic	50	65	70
Mean	57	72	77
38			
Systolic	77	92	97
Diastolic	50	65	70
Mean	59	74	79
40			
Systolic	80	95	100
Diastolic	50	65	70
Mean	60	75	80
42			
Systolic	85	98	102
Diastolic	50	65	70
Mean	62	76	81
44			
Systolic	88	105	110
Diastolic	50	68	73
Mean	63	80	85

The 95th and 99th percentile values are intended to serve as a reference to identify infants with persistent hypertension who may require treatment.
    Data from Refs.[14,15,18–22]

Table 2
Causes of neonatal hypertension

Renovascular	Medications/intoxications
Thromboembolism	Infant
Renal artery stenosis	Dexamethasone
Midaortic coarctation	Adrenergic agents
Renal venous thrombosis	Vitamin D intoxication
Compression of renal artery	Theophylline
Idiopathic arterial calcification	Caffeine
Congenital rubella syndrome	Pancuronium
Renal parenchymal disease	Phenylephrine
Congenital	Maternal
Polycystic kidney disease	Cocaine
Multicystic dysplastic kidney disease	Heroin
Tuberous sclerosis	Neoplasia
Ureteropelvic junction obstruction	Wilms tumor
Unilateral renal hypoplasia	Mesoblastic nephroma
Congenital nephrotic syndrome	Neuroblastoma
Renal tubular dysgenesis	Pheochromocytoma
Acquired	Neurologic
Acute tubular necrosis	Pain
Cortical necrosis	Intracranial hypertension
Interstitial nephritis	Seizures
Hemolytic-uremic syndrome	Familial dysautonomia
Obstruction (stones, tumors)	Subdural hematoma
Pulmonary	Miscellaneous
Bronchopulmonary dysplasia	Total parenteral nutrition
Pneumothorax	Closure of abdominal wall defect
Cardiac	Adrenal hemorrhage
Thoracic aortic coarctation	Hypercalcemia
Endocrine	Traction
Congenital adrenal hyperplasia	Extracorporeal membrane oxygenation
Hyperaldosteronism	Birth asphyxia
Hyperthyroidism	Nephrocalcinosis
Pseudohypoaldosteronism type II	

Adapted from Skalina ME, Kliegman RM, Fanaroff AA. Epidemiology and management of severe symptomatic neonatal hypertension. Am J Perinatol 1986;3:235–9, with permission; and Dionne JM, Abitbol CL, Flynn JT. Hypertension in infancy: diagnosis, management and outcome. Pediatr Nephrol 2012;27(1):17–32. http://dx.doi.org/10.1007/s00467-010-1755-z, with permission.

Although **Table 2** lists many causes of HTN in the neonate, the diagnostic evaluation is usually fairly focused initially, given that a limited number of causes lead to most cases of neonatal HTN.

The perinatal history may provide important diagnostic clues, with important elements including prenatal exposures (medications, maternal diabetes), results of prenatal imaging, and immediate postnatal complications such as hypotension or meconium aspiration. UAC placement is a crucial part of the history. Medications should be reviewed for direct effects on BP (eg, corticosteroids) or renal toxicity (eg, aminoglycosides). The BP readings since birth should be reviewed to determine the timing and severity of HTN.

The physical examination should include at least 1 determination of BPs in the 4 extremities to evaluate for possible coarctation of the aorta. The technique of BP measurement and placement of the BP cuff should be reviewed. The general appearance of the infant should be assessed for dysmorphic features suggesting a specific diagnosis. The cardiac examination should include assessment for a murmur consistent with coarctation but also an evaluation for signs of cardiac target organ damage (ie, congestive heart failure). The abdominal examination (mass) and genitourinary examination (anomaly or virilization) may provide an important diagnostic clue.[8]

Beyond the history and physical examination, there will likely be a need for laboratory investigation. Basic tests to evaluate the kidneys should include blood urea nitrogen, creatinine, and a urinalysis. Abnormal electrolytes may suggest an endocrine cause of HTN such as congenital adrenal hypoplasia (hypokalemia) or pseudohypoaldosteronism type II (hyperkalemia). A complete blood count may provide useful information. For example, thrombocytopenia suggests the possibility of renal vein thrombosis. Further evaluation for thrombophilia may be necessary if renal thrombosis is identified.[37] If there is suggestive history or physical examination findings, hormonal levels such as thyroid studies, cortisol levels, and aldosterone may be helpful. Plasma renin levels are not very helpful in screening, as they are usually high in infancy, especially in premature infants. A plasma renin measurement may be helpful if there are findings consistent with a renal tubular disorder such as hypokalemia.[37,38]

Radiologic imaging is typically warranted in the hypertensive infant. A chest radiograph is helpful to look at heart size. An echocardiogram will assess structural lesions that can lead to HTN (ie, coarctation of the aorta), cardiac function, and left ventricular size. Given that renal disease or renal vascular disease are the leading causes of HTN in infants, ultrasonography of the urinary tract is helpful, and one may consider using Doppler to assess the renal vessels noninvasively. The ultrasonography scan may be helpful in identifying renal venous thrombosis, urinary tract obstruction, and even aortic thrombi.[5,9] It is difficult to obtain accurate results in nuclear imaging studies of infants, and often these studies are deferred. Other advanced imaging techniques may be considered, including computed tomographic angiography and magnetic resonance imaging, but one must balance the risks and benefits of performing such tests on neonates. Traditional angiography under fluoroscopy is the gold standard for assessing the renal vasculature, but is technically challenging in neonates and thus is generally deferred.[39,40]

TREATMENT

Given the lack of data, most published treatment recommendations are based on a few published case series and expert opinion.[9,41] Correctable causes of HTN should be addressed when possible, including iatrogenic causes of HTN such as inotropic medications, hypercalcemia, pain, and excessive volume.[9] Endocrine causes of hypertension frequently have specific therapy.

There are no definitive recommendations on when to initiate pharmacologic intervention. Clearly all infants with evidence of target organ dysfunction such as congestive heart failure or seizures require medical therapy. Expert opinion suggests that drug therapy should be initiated when the infant's BP is consistently at the 99th percentile or greater, mainly because sustained BP elevation may have renal, cardiac, and central nervous system effects. Using intravenous or oral medications will be determined by clinical circumstances.[9,42]

Several classes of antihypertensive medications may be used in the setting of neonatal HTN. **Table 3** lists medications and recommended guidelines for initiating and titrating therapy. The choice of agent may depend on the clinical condition of the infant and local experience with certain agents.

A hypertensive emergency is the combination of hypertension and acute target organ damage. Prompt reduction is necessary, and this often leads to the use of shorter-acting and intravenous medications.[43–45] Sodium nitroprusside has been used for decades, but requires special handling and careful titration to achieve the desired target level of BP. Cyanide and thiocyanate accumulation can occur, especially in infants with renal impairment. Enalaprilat is the only intravenous angiotensin-converting enzyme (ACE) inhibitor. One case series demonstrates a high number of side effects; given the importance of the renin-angiotensin-aldosterone system (RAAS) in newborns, its use should be avoided. Labetalol, a combined α- and β-blocker, has been used effectively for many years.[46] It seems to have equal efficacy and safety when compared with intravenous nitroprusside and nicardipine. Esmolol, a short-acting intravenous β-blocker, has been used in young infants undergoing cardiac surgery with good safety and efficacy.[47]

Hydralazine is another option, which may be given orally or intravenously.[1,48] Nifedipine may be used with caution and is difficult to dose in small infants. Nifedipine, a short-acting calcium-channel blocker, is effective, but concerns have been raised about transient neurologic effects, likely attributable to hypotension.[49] Isradipine is a newer short-acting calcium-channel blocker that seems to be easier to dose and is effective.[50–52]

The RAAS is very important in the developing neonate, and drugs that affect this system may be effective in controlling BP. However, they must be used with caution. Captopril, the initial ACE inhibitor, is short acting and much more potent in neonates so may require a smaller dose, and yet is also best absorbed on an empty stomach, which rarely happens in a small neonate. Overly aggressive use of any antihypertensive medication, especially ACE inhibitors, may be associated with acute kidney injury and neurologic compromise. Caution should be used with all ACE inhibitors, including the longer-acting ones such as lisinopril, benazepril, enalapril, and quinapril.[53–55]

A longer-acting calcium-channel blocker such as amlodipine, which is a third-generation dihydropyridine, seems to be safe and effective in older children. It may be compounded into a liquid formulation, which allows for ease of administration. Isradipine, another calcium-channel blocker, has been used with good effect in hospitalized infants, and may also be compounded into a liquid preparation.[9] Diuretics are sometimes needed for fluid retention in infants and may help with BP control, but are typically not first-line agents in BP management, unless lung disease with fluid retention seems to be a primary cause of the elevated BP.

Since the 1970s, hydralazine has been the most commonly used medication for neonatal HTN.[1] In a study from Australia, neonatal HTN was treated during the initial hospitalization in 82% of patients and the most commonly used medications were, from most to least commonly used, hydralazine, captopril, labetalol, and atenolol. In a more recent review of a neonatal database, the most commonly used classes of medications were vasodilators (64.2%), ACE inhibitors (50.8%), calcium-channel blockers (24%), combined α- and β-blockers (18.4%), and clonidine (5%). Other interesting findings include that medications were prescribed at a median age of 15 days of age, the median duration of therapy was 10 days, and almost half (45%) of infants were treated with 2 or more medications.[7]

Table 3
Treatment options

Drug Class	Medication (Route)	Dosing	Interval	Comments
Direct-acting vasodilators	Sodium nitroprusside (IV)	Initial: 0.25 µg/kg/min Max: 8 µg/kg/min	Infusion	May cause hypotension, tachycardia. Monitor for cyanide toxicity. Caution in renal failure
	Hydralazine (IV) (PO)	0.2–1.0 mg/kg/dose 0.25–1.0 mg/kg/dose Max: 5 mg/kg/d	Every 4–6 h TID to QID	May cause tachycardia, fluid retention, diarrhea, emesis, agranulocytosis
	Minoxidil (PO)	0.05–2.0 mg/kg/d	BID	May cause tachycardia, fluid retention, hypertrichosis
ACE inhibitors	Captopril (PO)	Neonates: Initial: 0.01 mg/kg/dose Max: 1.5 mg/kg/d Infants: Initial: 0.1–0.3 mg/kg/dose Max: 6 mg/kg/d	TID to QID BID to TID	May cause hypotension, oliguria, acute renal failure, hyperkalemia, neurologic complications
	Enalapril (PO)	Infants: 0.1–0.6 mg/kg/d	Daily to BID	All may cause hypotension, oliguria, acute renal failure, hyperkalemia, agranulocytosis, angioedema. Caution in preterm neonates
	Lisinopril (PO)	0.1–0.5 mg/kg/d	Daily	
	Quinapril (PO)	0.1–0.2 mg/kg/d	Daily	
Calcium-channel blockers	Nicardipine (IV)	0.5–4 µg/kg/min	Infusion (central line)	May cause hypotension, tachycardia, and flushing. Caution in perinatal asphyxia
	Amlodipine (PO)	Initial: 0.1 mg/kg/dose Max: 0.6 mg/kg/d	Daily to BID	May cause edema, tachycardia, gingival hypertrophy
	Isradipine (PO)	Initial: 0.05–0.15 mg/kg/dose Max: 0.8 mg/kg/d	TID to QID	May cause hypotension, tachycardia, edema. Caution with QTc prolongation
	Nifedipine (PO)	Initial: 0.25 mg/kg/dose Max: 2.5 mg	Every 4–6 h	May cause hypotension, tachycardia, transient neurologic changes

Category	Drug	Dose	Frequency	Adverse effects
Combined α- and β-antagonists	Labetalol (IV)	0.2–1.0 mg/kg/dose 0.25–3.0 mg/kg/h	Load Infusion	May cause hypotension, hyperkalemia. Caution in chronic lung disease, heart block, unstable heart failure
	Labetalol (PO)	1.0–10 mg/kg/d	BID	May cause hypotension, bradycardia, edema, hyperglycemia
	Carvedilol (PO)	0.05–0.4 mg/kg/dose	BID to TID	
β-Antagonists	Esmolol (TV)	125–1000 μg/kg/min	Infusion	All may cause hypotension, bradycardia. Caution in chronic lung disease, unstable heart failure
	Propranolol (IV)	0.01–0.15 mg/kg/dose		
	Propranolol (PO)	0.5–6 mg/kg/d		
α-Antagonist	Prazosin (PO)	Initial: 5 μg/kg/dose 25–400 μg/kg/d	TID to QID	May cause hypotension, somnolence
Central α-agonist	Clonidine (PO)	2–10 μg/kg/d	QID	May cause hypotension, bradycardia, rebound hypertension, somnolence, xerostomia
Diuretics	Amiloride (PO)	0.4–0.625 mg/kg/d	Daily to BID	May cause hyperkalemia. Caution in renal failure
	Furosemide (PO)	1–6 mg/kg/dose	Daily to QID	May cause hyponatremia, hypokalemia, ototoxicity, nephrocalcinosis
	Hydrochlorothiazide (PO)	1–3 mg/kg/d	BID	May cause hyponatremia, hypokalemia, alkalosis
	Spironolactone (PO)			May cause hyperkalemia. Caution in renal failure

Abbreviations: ACE, angiotensin-converting enzyme; BID, twice daily; IV, intravenous; Max, maximum; PO, oral; QID, 4 times daily; TID, 3 times daily.

Adapted from Skalina ME, Kliegman RM, Fanaroff AA. Epidemiology and management of severe symptomatic neonatal hypertension. Am J Perinatol 1986;3:235–9; and Dionne JM, Abitbol CL, Flynn JT. Hypertension in infancy: diagnosis, management and outcome. Pediatr Nephrol 2012;27(1):17–32.

SURGICAL INTERVENTIONS

Issues that may warrant surgical intervention for HTN are uncommon but warrant some discussion.[56,57] Infants with urinary tract obstruction, coarctation of the aorta, and renal artery stenosis are most likely to require surgical intervention.[58] In the setting of renovascular disease, the infant will likely need to be managed medically before surgery is done to correct a lesion, but in rare instances severe, refractory HTN may require unilateral nephrectomy.[59,60] Wilms tumor or neuroblastoma in infancy may require surgical intervention. Renal thrombosis, either arterial or venous, may result in the need for surgical intervention, but most cases are managed medically with thrombolytic agents. Very rarely the removal of a multicystic dysplastic kidney may be needed to control BP, and bilateral nephrectomy is occasionally needed to control malignant HTN associated with autosomal recessive polycystic kidney disease.

OUTCOMES

Limited data have been published on outcomes of neonatal HTN, which are likely to depend on the underlying etiology. Older studies suggest that HTN associated with UAC placement will resolve with time.[1,61] A recent study from Australia showed that more than 40% of hypertensive neonates were discharged home from the NICU on antihypertensive medications, but only 15% were on therapy 3 to 6 months after discharge. There are no data on longer-term follow-up, but most patients do not require prolonged treatment. However, patients with renal or renovascular disease are most likely to require long-term management.[62]

Infants with chronic lung disease discharged from the NICU are more likely to have resolution of HTN, with one study demonstrating resolution of the HTN at a mean of 7.8 months with a range from less than a month to more than 2 years.[63] By contrast, infants with autosomal recessive polycystic kidney disease who survived the neonatal period have increasing use of antihypertensive medications: almost 40% required antihypertensive therapy by 1 year, 50% by 3 years, and 60% by 15 years of age. Renal venous thrombosis is also a risk factor for the need to receive long-term therapy for HTN. Several studies have demonstrated poor renal outcomes regardless of therapy, with 66% to 90% having irreversible renal damage at follow-up and 19% to 34% having elevated BP.[64]

There is also concern about development of HTN in high-risk infants following discharge from the NICU. The Victorian Infant Collaborative Study Group is attempting to address this issue, and recently reported on a comparison between young adult survivors born at less than 28 weeks' gestation and term controls. At the age of 18 years, those born extremely premature (EP; <28 weeks' gestation) were compared with those born at term, and underwent 24-hour ambulatory BP monitoring. EP subjects had a mean systolic BP difference over the entire 24-hour period of 3.2 mm Hg. The investigators concluded that young adult EP survivors have higher BP than their term gestation counterparts, and therefore longer follow-up must be considered in assessing the risk for HTN in these individuals.[65]

SUMMARY

There are many challenges in neonatal hypertension, including lack of clear definitions and limited data on effective medications. Fortunately, neonatal hypertension is relatively uncommon, and many cases will resolve. Renovascular disease associated with UAC placement is the most common cause. A variety of medications are available for treating neonatal hypertension, with intravenous medications frequently used in hypertensive emergencies.

REFERENCES

1. Adelman RD. Neonatal hypertension. Pediatr Clin North Am 1978;25:99–110.
2. Watkinson M. Hypertension in the newborn baby. Arch Dis Child Fetal Neonatal Ed 2002;86:F78–88.
3. Flynn JT. Neonatal hypertension: diagnosis and management. Pediatr Nephrol 2000;14:332–41.
4. Buchi KF, Siegler RL. Hypertension in the first month of life. J Hypertens 1986;4: 525–8.
5. Skalina ME, Kliegman RM, Fanaroff AA. Epidemiology and management of severe symptomatic neonatal hypertension. Am J Perinatal 1986;3:235–9.
6. Singh HP, Hurley RM, Myers TF. Neonatal hypertension: incidence and risk factors. Am J Hypertens 1992;5:51–5.
7. Blowey DL, Duda PJ, Stokes P, et al. Incidence and treatment of hypertension in the neonatal intensive care unit. J Am Soc Hypertens 2011;5(6):478–83. http://dx.doi.org/10.1016/j.jash.2011.08.001.
8. Flynn JT. Hypertension in the neonatal period. Curr Opin Pediatr 2012;24(2): 197–204. http://dx.doi.org/10.1097/MOP.0b013e32834f8329.
9. Dionne JM, Abitbol CL, Flynn JT. Hypertension in infancy: diagnosis, management and outcome. Pediatr Nephrol 2012;27(1):17–32. http://dx.doi.org/10.1007/s00467-010-1755-z.
10. Kimble K, Darnall R, Yelderman M, et al. An automated oscillometric technique for estimating mean arterial pressure in critically ill newborns. Anesthesiology 1981;54:423–5.
11. Park M, Menard S. Accuracy of blood pressure measurement by the Dinamap monitor in infants and children. Pediatrics 1987;79:907–14.
12. Butt W, Whyte H. Blood pressure monitoring in neonates: comparison of umbilical and peripheral artery catheter measurements. J Pediatr 1984;105: 630–2.
13. Nwankwo M, Lorenz J, Gardiner J. A standard protocol for blood pressure measurement in the newborn. Pediatrics 1997;99(6):E10.
14. Zubrow AB, Hulman S, Kushner H, et al. Determinants of blood pressure in infants admitted to neonatal intensive care units: a prospective multicenter study. J Perinatol 1995;15:470–9.
15. Pejovic B, Peco-Antic A, Marinkovic-Eric J. Blood pressure in noncritically ill preterm and full-term neonates. Pediatr Nephrol 2007;22:249–57.
16. Lalan S, Blowey D. Comparison between oscillometric and intra-arterial blood pressure measurements in ill preterm and full-term neonates. J Am Soc Hypertens 2014;8(1):36–44. http://dx.doi.org/10.1016/j.jash.2013.10.003.
17. National High Blood Pressure Education Program Working Group on High Blood Pressure in Children and Adolescents. The fourth report on the diagnosis, evaluation, and treatment of high blood pressure in children and adolescents. Pediatrics 2004;114(2 Suppl 4th Report):555–76.
18. de Swiet M, Fayers P, Shineboume EA. Systolic blood pressure in a population of infants in the first year of life: the Brompton study. Pediatrics 1980;65: 1028–35.
19. Kent A, Kecskes Z, Shadbolt B, et al. Normative blood pressure data in the early neonatal period. Pediatr Nephrol 2007;22:1335–41.

20. Kent A, Meske S, Falk M, et al. Normative blood pressure data in non-ventilated premature neonates from 28-36 weeks gestation. Pediatr Nephrol 2009;24: 141–6.

21. Lurbe E, Garcia-Vicent C, Torro I, et al. First-year blood pressure increase steepest in low birthweight newborns. J Hypertens 2007;25:81–6.

22. Kent A, Kecskes Z, Shadbolt B, et al. Blood pressure in the first year of life in healthy infants born at term. Pediatr Nephrol 2007;22:1743–9.

23. Report of the Second Task Force on Blood Pressure Control in Children–1987. Task Force on Blood Pressure Control in Children. National Heart, Lung and Blood Institute, Bethesda, Maryland. Pediatrics 1987;79(1):1–25.

24. Been JV, Kornelisse RF, Rours IG, et al. Early postnatal blood pressure in preterm infants: effects of chorioamnionitis and timing of antenatal steroids. Pediatr Res 2009;66:571–6.

25. Kent AL, Shadbolt B, Hu E, et al. Do maternal- or pregnancy-associated disease states affect blood pressure in the early neonatal period? Aust N Z J Obstet Gynaecol 2009;49:364–70.

26. Neal WA, Reynolds JW, Jarvis CW, et al. Umbilical artery catheterization: demonstration of arterial thrombosis by aortography. Pediatrics 1972;50:6–13.

27. Seibert JJ, Taylor BJ, Williamson SL, et al. Sonographic detection of neonatal umbilical artery thrombosis: clinical correlation. Am J Roentgenol 1987;148: 965–8.

28. Ford KT, Teplick SK, Clark RE. Renal artery embolism causing neonatal hypertension. Radiology 1974;113:169–70.

29. Bauer SB, Feldman SM, Gellis SS, et al. Neonatal hypertension: a complication of umbilical-artery catheterization. N Engl J Med 1975;293:1032–3.

30. Plumer LB, Kaplan GW, Mendoza SA. Hypertension in infants - a complication of umbilical arterial catheterization. J Pediatr 1976;89:802–5.

31. Merten DF, Vogel JM, Adelman RD, et al. Renovascular hypertension as a complication of umbilical arterial catheterization. Radiology 1978;126:751–7.

32. Brooks WG, Weibley RE. Emergency department presentation of severe hypertension secondary to complications of umbilical artery catheterization. Pediatr Emerg Care 1987;3:104–6.

33. Goetzman BW, Stadalnik RC, Bogren HG, et al. Thrombotic complications of umbilical artery catheters: a clinical and radiographic study. Pediatrics 1975; 56:374–9.

34. Wesstrom G, Finnstrom O, Stenport G. Umbilical artery catheterization in newborns I. Thrombosis in relation to catheter type and position. Acta Paediatr Scand 1979;68:575–81.

35. Boo NY, Wong NC, Zulkifli SS, et al. Risk factors associated with umbilical vascular catheter-associated thrombosis in newborn infants. J Paediatr Child Health 1999;35:460–5.

36. Barrington KJ. Umbilical artery catheters in the newborn: effects of catheter materials. Cochrane Database Syst Rev 2010;1:CD000505.

37. Proesmans W, van de Wijdeven P, Van Geet C. Thrombophilia in neonatal renal venous thrombosis. Pediatr Nephrol 2005;20:241–2.

38. Vahaskari VM. Heritable forms of hypertension. Pediatr Nephrol 2009;24: 1929–37.

39. Mustafa AE, Bloom DA, Valentini RP, et al. MR angiography in the evaluation of a renovascular cause of neonatal hypertension. Pediatr Radiol 2008;38:158–61.

40. Tullus K, Brennan E, Hamilton G, et al. Renovascular hypertension in children. Lancet 2008;371:1453–63.

41. Flynn JT. Neonatal hypertension. In: Flynn JT, Ingelfinger J, Portman R, editors. Pediatric hypertension. 2nd edition. New York: Humana Press Inc; 2011. p. 375–96.
42. James L, Ito S. Neonatal pharmacology: rational therapeutics for the most vulnerable. Clin Pharmacol Ther 2009;86:573–7.
43. Flynn JT, Tullus K. Severe hypertension in children and adolescents: pathophysiology and treatment. Pediatr Nephrol 2009;24:1101–12.
44. Roth CG, Spottswood SE, Chan JC, et al. Evaluation of the hypertensive infant: a rational approach to diagnosis. Radiol Clin North Am 2003;41:931–44.
45. Adelman RD, Cappo R, Dillon MJ. The emergency management of severe hypertension. Pediatr Nephrol 2000;14:422–7.
46. Thomas CA, Moffett BS, Wagner JL, et al. Safety and efficacy of intravenous labetalol for hypertensive crisis in infants and small children. Pediatr Crit Care Med 2010. http://dx.doi.org/10.1097/PCC.ObO13e3181e328d8.
47. Wiest DB, Gamer SS, Uber WE, et al. Esmolol for the management of pediatric hypertension after cardiac operations. J Thorac Cardiovasc Surg 1998;115:890–7.
48. Ueda H, Yagi S, Kaneko Y. Hydralazine and plasma renin activity. Arch Intern Med 1968;122(5):387–91. http://dx.doi.org/10.1001/archinte.1968.00040010387001.
49. Flynn JT. Safety of short-acting nifedipine in children with severe hypertension. Expert Opin Drug Saf 2003;2:133–9.
50. Flynn JT, Warnick SJ. Isradipine treatment of hypertension in children: a single-center experience. Pediatr Nephrol 2002;17:748–53.
51. Miyashita Y, Peterson D, Rees JM, et al. Isradipine treatment of acute hypertension in hospitalized children and adolescents. J Clin Hypertens 2010;12:850–5.
52. MacDonald JL, Johnson CE, Jacobson P. Stability of isradipine in an extemporaneously compounded oral liquid. Am J Hosp Pharm 1994;51:2409–11.
53. O'Dea RF, Mirkin BL, Alward CT, et al. Treatment of neonatal hypertension with captopril. J Pediatr 1998;113:403–6.
54. Tack ED, Perlman JM. Renal failure in sick hypertensive premature infants receiving captopril therapy. J Pediatr 1998;112:805–10.
55. Guron G, Friberg P. An intact renin-angiotensin system is a prerequisite for normal renal development. J Hypertens 2000;18:123–37.
56. Hendren WH, Kim SH, Herrin JT, et al. Surgically correctable hypertension of renal origin in childhood. Am J Surg 1982;143:432–42.
57. Rajpoot DK, Duel B, Thayer K, et al. Medically resistant neonatal hypertension: revisiting the surgical causes. J Perinatol 1999;19:582–3.
58. Seirafi PA, Warner KG, Geggel RL, et al. Repair of coarctation of the aorta during infancy minimizes the risk of late hypertension. Ann Thorac Surg 1998;66:1378–82.
59. Kiessling SG, Wadhwa N, Kriss VM, et al. An unusual case of severe therapy-resistant hypertension in a newborn. Pediatrics 2007;119:e301–4.
60. Stanley JC, Zelenock GB, Messina LM, et al. Pediatric renovascular hypertension: a thirty-year experience of operative treatment. J Vasc Surg 1995;21:212–27.
61. Caplan MS, Cohn RA, Langman CB, et al. Favorable outcome of neonatal aortic thrombosis and renovascular hypertension. J Pediatr 1989;115:291–5.
62. Seliem WA, Falk MC, Shadbolt B, et al. Antenatal and postnatal risk factors for neonatal hypertension and infant follow-up. Pediatr Nephrol 2007;22:2081–7.
63. Anderson AH, Warady BA, Daily DK, et al. Systemic hypertension in infants with severe bronchopulmonary dysplasia: associated clinical factors. Am J Perinatol 1993;10(3):190–3.

64. Roy S, Dillon MJ, Trompeter RS, et al. Autosomal recessive polycystic kidney disease: long-term outcome of neonatal survivors. Pediatr Nephrol 1997;11: 302–6.
65. Roberts G, Lee KJ, Cheong JL, et al, Victorian Infant Collaborative Study Group. Higher ambulatory blood pressure at 18 years in adolescents born less than 28 weeks' gestation in the 1990s compared with term controls. J Hypertens 2014; 32(3):620–6. http://dx.doi.org/10.1097/HJH.0000000000000055.

Neonatal Polycystic Kidney Disease

Priya Verghese, MD, MPH[a],*, Yosuke Miyashita, MD, MPH[b]

KEYWORDS

- Polycystic kidney • ARPKD • ADPKD • Multicystic dysplastic kidney • Renal cyst

KEY POINTS

- Neonatal polycystic kidney disease (PKD) is most commonly due to autosomal recessive PKD (ARPKD), multicystic dysplastic kidney disease (MCDK), cystic dysplasia, or, rarely, autosomal dominant PKD (ADPKD).
- ARPKD and ADPKD are inherited disorders involving bilateral renal cysts *without* dysplasia, unlike MCDK, which is classically unilateral, nonhereditary, and associated with dysplasia of intervening tissue.
- Ultrasonography is the diagnostic test of choice for neonatal PKD. MCDK must be differentiated from severe ureteropelvic junction obstruction by a renogram, as emergent surgical therapy may be indicated in the latter to preserve any residual renal function.
- There is no medication to prevent cyst formation for any neonatal PKD, but the complications of ARPKD and ADPKD must be carefully managed (hypertension, chronic kidney disease, or congenital hepatic fibrosis).
- MCDK must be followed clinically to ensure involution with normal compensatory hypertrophy and functioning of contralateral kidney.

INTRODUCTION

Due to an evolving trend for increased imaging in gestational care, prenatal ultrasound has increased the detection rate of fetal genitourinary abnormalities.[1] Although renal cysts occur in a variety of diseases in children, neonatal polycystic kidney disease (PKD) is a unique entity with a wide differential diagnosis often requiring prompt diagnostic and therapeutic interventions. Therefore, it is important that practicing perinatologists have a comprehensive understanding of neonatal cystic kidney disease.

Disclosures: None.
Conflicts of Interest: None.
[a] Division of Pediatric Nephrology, Department of Pediatrics, Amplatz Children's Hospital, University of Minnesota, 2450 Riverside Avenue, MB 682, Minneapolis, MN 55454, USA; [b] Division of Pediatric Nephrology, Department of Pediatrics, Children's Hospital of Pittsburgh of UPMC, University of Pittsburgh School of Medicine, 4401 Penn Avenue, Pittsburgh, PA 15224, USA
* Corresponding author.
E-mail address: pverghes@umn.edu

Neonatal cysts can occur as an isolated finding or they may occur as a part of a syndrome. The cysts could be hereditary or nonhereditary fetal malformations. We aim to provide an up-to-date comprehensive review on this area with emphasis on the clinical manifestations, diagnostic techniques, and potential therapeutic approaches to neonatal PKD. Notably, cystic kidneys are a feature of numerous genetic syndromes not covered in this review, such as Bardet-Biedl, Beckwith-Wiedemann, Ivemark, Jeune, juvenile nephronophthisis, Von-Hippel-Lindau, Hajdu-Cheney, Meckel-Gruber, orofacial-digital syndrome type 1, or Zellweger cerebrohepatorenal syndrome.[2] However since the most common genetic syndromes associated with cystic kidney are ARPKD and ADPKD, these rare genetic syndromes have not been included in this review.

Hereditary PKD

Background
Although PKD is a pathologic description of a kidney with multiple cysts, the term is most often used to describe an inherited disorder involving bilateral renal cysts *without* dysplasia. PKD is broadly divided into 2 forms depending on its mode of inheritance and genetic mutation.

- Autosomal recessive PKD (ARPKD)
- Autosomal dominant PKD (ADPKD)

PKD begins with conception, and ARPKD and ADPKD can have renal cysts present at any time in a person's life, ranging as early as antenatally to adolescence or older. Most often, ARPKD presents in the neonatal period or childhood with rare reports of initial presentation in late adolescence and early adulthood.[3,4] ADPKD most often presents in adults aged 20 to 40 years, but increasingly there are reports of ADPKD presenting in childhood and even in utero.[5] Both forms of PKD affect all racial and ethnic groups and they affect male and female individuals equally.

ARPKD
ARPKD is a rare cilia-related disorder primarily affecting the kidneys and liver with less frequent extrarenal manifestations occurring at any age. It is classically characterized by cystic dilation of renal collecting ducts associated with hepatic abnormalities of varying degrees, including biliary dysgenesis and periportal fibrosis. In 1994, the ARPKD gene was localized to the short arm of chromosome 6 (*PKHD1*). Fibrocystin/polyductin, a protein that is encoded by this gene, is expressed on the cilia of renal and bile duct epithelial cells and is thought to be crucial in maintaining normal tubular architecture of renal tubules and bile ducts. Different combinations of mutations in *PKHD1* and its resulting changes in fibrocystin may partially explain the wide phenotypic variance in this disease. However, there is also wide intrafamilial clinical variability among affected siblings that cannot be explained by genotypic differences.[6]

ARPKD is characterized by nonobstructive, bilateral, symmetric dilation and elongation of 10% to 90% of the renal collecting ducts, accounting for a wide variability of renal dysfunction. With an increase in the number of ducts involved, the kidneys enlarge but the reniform shape is maintained, as the abnormality is in the collecting ducts and the cysts are usually minute (<3 mm). Gross examination of an autopsied kidney shows multiple minute cystic spaces throughout the capsular surfaces. Cut sections of the kidney show that these cystic structures are subcapsular extensions of radially oriented cylindrical or fusiform ectatic spaces with poor corticomedullary differentiation due to the extension of the elongated and dilated collecting ducts from the medulla to the cortex. In all patients with ARPKD, there is congenital hepatic fibrosis (CHF), which results from ductal plate malformations with cystic dilation of intrahepatic and extrahepatic bile ducts. The liver biopsy also shows enlarged, fibrotic portal tracts and normal hepatocytes. The ductules can show true cystic changes and when this is macroscopic, it can be indistinguishable from Caroli disease. The portal hypertension (HTN) that occurs secondary to the CHF can be clinically debilitating, as detailed in the Clinical Manifestations section.

Frequency
The exact incidence is unknown due to varying reports in autopsied patients versus survivors, as well as possibility of affected children dying perinatally without a definitive diagnosis. Prevalence is likely 1 in 20,000 live births, although the frequency of the gene in the general population is estimated to be 1 in 70.[7] Carriers or heterozygotes are asymptomatic.

Clinical manifestations
ARPKD is most often diagnosed by third trimester antenatal ultrasounds that may demonstrate oligohydramnios, large renal masses, or absence of fetal bladder filling. If undiagnosed antenatally, neonates may present with large palpable flank masses that may cause difficulty in delivery. Neonates often have pulmonary hypoplasia with respiratory distress due to oligohydramnios, worsened by large renal masses. Secondary to oligohydramnios, infants have Potter facies with low-set flattened ears, short snubbed nose, deep eye creases, and micrognathia. Clubfoot also is commonly seen secondary to oligohydramnios due to the pressure effect in utero. Hepatic involvement is present in all children with ARPKD but may not manifest in neonates (50%–60%).

If undiagnosed in the antenatal period, parents or pediatricians usually discover abdominal masses with impaired renal function in 70% to 80% of infants, which often improves as the pulmonary function recovers. If the diagnosis is delayed and occurs in older children/adults, the primary presentation is usually portal HTN/hepatic fibrosis, including hepatosplenomegaly with normal liver function until late stages of the disease.[4] Many patients progress to end-stage renal disease (ESRD) within the first decade of life. Ascending cholangitis is a serious and frequent complication, and manifestations of portal HTN can be life threatening, including splenomegaly, hypersplenism, varices, protein-losing enteropathy, and gastrointestinal hemorrhage. Portal HTN occurs early, with 60% of children younger than 5 years having splenomegaly. Esophageal varices occur in 5% to 37% of patients. In all age groups, there may be systemic HTN, which can be severe, and if poorly managed cause cardiac hypertrophy and congestive heart failure. Hyponatremia related to fluid overload and other electrolyte abnormalities, such as metabolic acidosis, are possible due to oliguric renal failure and renal tubular concentrating defects.

Diagnostic testing
Blood and urine studies are useful in the management of but are not diagnostic in ARPKD.

Ultrasonography Ultrasonography is the primary radiographic modality for the evaluation of ARPKD, especially during the perinatal and neonatal periods. It is often diagnostic (**Fig. 1**) and manifestations vary depending on age of testing (**Table 1**). Portal HTN is characterized on ultrasound by decreased blood flow in the visualized portal vein with minimal undulation, splenomegaly, and the presence of varices.

Radiography Although radiographs are not a diagnostic test of choice, an abdominal radiograph may show enlarged neonatal kidneys, abdominal distension, or centrally

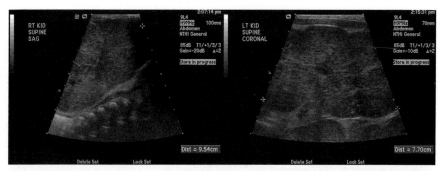

Fig. 1. Longitudinal sonogram of ARPKD in a neonate. Both kidneys are enlarged and echogenic with loss of corticomedullary differentiation. There is maintenance of the reniform shape of the kidney. Distinct cysts are not visualized in this image and classically do not occur in ARPKD. If discrete cysts are present, they usually occur later and are no more than 1 to 2 cm in diameter, unlike ADPKD.

deviated gas-filled bowel loops. Chest radiograph shows pulmonary hypoplasia that manifests as a small thorax. Pneumothorax can occur in infants after birth.

Magnetic resonance imaging (MRI) and computed tomography (CT) scans These tests are not considered first-line diagnostic tests in ARPKD due to cost, radiation exposure, and risks, with contrast administration in renal insufficiency. If performed in the neonatal period, a noncontrast computed tomography (CT) scan would demonstrate smooth, enlarged kidneys, and with intravenous contrast, kidneys have a striated appearance due to accumulation of contrast in dilated tubules. Depending on degree of renal insufficiency, there is a proportionate delay in arrival of contrast to kidneys. Macrocysts may appear as well-circumscribed lucent defects. The bladder may be opacified. Over time, kidneys and cysts often progress in size. If there is a cyst hemorrhage, it can be observed as high-density cysts. An magnetic resonance

Table 1	
Ultrasonographic findings in pediatric cases of autosomal recessive polycystic kidney disease	
Antenatally	Bilaterally enlarged echogenic kidneys Small/nonvisualized bladder with absence of urine Oligohydramnios Usually *not* observed before 30 wk of gestation
Neonatally	Bilaterally smooth, enlarged, diffusely echogenic kidneys with poor corticomedullary differentiation Microcysts that are difficult to visualize and account for the diffuse echogenicity Hypoechoic macrocysts may be visualized in worsening disease Hepatic parenchymal echogenicity may be diffusely increased with fibrous tissue causing poor depiction of peripheral portal veins
Older children	Enlarged kidneys with echogenic medulla due to focal tubular cysts Renal macrocysts Liver often enlarged with heterogeneously or homogeneously increased echogenicity Macrocysts in liver and pancreas often visualized Splenomegaly Reversal of hepatic venous blood flow on Doppler suggestive of portal hypertension. Biliary duct dilation is indistinguishable from Caroli disease when present

imaging (MRI) would show enlarged kidneys, with T2-weighted imaging showing increased signal intensity and a characteristic hyperintense, linear, radial pattern in cortex and medulla.

Genetic testing Genetic diagnosis of ARPKD is challenging because of the length and allelic heterogeneity of the *PKHD1* gene. Therefore, currently DNA analysis of *PKHD1* is most often reserved for confirming the diagnosis of ARPKD in complicated cases and for prenatal diagnosis. Previously, genetic testing was done by linkage analysis. This method was useful to identify disease and carrier status in the fetus or newborn, but it requires at least one established index case of ARPKD in the family. More recently, haplotype analysis and direct gene testing are possible, making the diagnosis easier, but *PKHD1* sequencing data must be used cautiously if being used for clinical decisions.[6] The role of the recently developed next-generation sequencing in the diagnosis of ARPKD remains to be established.

Treatment

Survival of neonates with ARPKD depends mainly on the degree of pulmonary hypoplasia. If the large size of the kidneys is worsening the respiratory compromise in the neonatal period or if neonates have failure to thrive due to bilateral nephromegaly preventing appropriate nourishment, oftentimes a unilateral or bilateral nephrectomy is undertaken. Fluid overload can be managed with diuretics/renal replacement therapy/nephrectomy to optimize ventilation. Electrolyte abnormalities and systemic HTN should be treated appropriately. Multidrug therapy is frequently required for HTN. Angiotensin-converting enzyme (ACE) inhibitors are the first choice, although they have not been formally studied[8] and their safety in neonates is debatable (see ADPKD Treatment section). Calcium channel blockers, beta-blockers, and judicious use of diuretics are also potential antihypertensive therapies. Because of increased risk of urinary tract infections, surveillance and prompt antibiotic therapy is important. Surveillance and management of the sequelae of CKD will need to be managed by pediatric nephrologists: anemia with iron and erythropoietin, correction of acidosis and electrolyte abnormalities, prevention of metabolic bone disease with calcium supplements, phosphate binders, and parathyroid suppressing medication. Dialysis and kidney transplantation are performed when patients are in ESRD.

With improving pulmonary and renal care, hepatic complications are presenting an increasing degree of mortality and morbidity in ARPKD.[2,9] After kidney transplantation, 78% of patients had clinically significant portal HTN and 38% had gastrointestinal bleeding rarely leading to mortality.[10] A large number of hepatic complications require surgical management, which is fairly complicated; therefore, regular esophageal gastroduodenal monitoring to prevent recurrent esophageal bleeding is essential. Endoscopic band ligation is an effective prophylaxis and therapy for esophageal varices with reduced mortality and decreased complications.[11] Sclerotherapy is an alternative but has increased complications. Nonselective beta-blockers with or without band ligation may reduce the mortality of portal HTN but there are insufficient data on whether this is justified in children. Hypersplenism with cytopenias and splenic rupture, a dreaded and potentially fatal complication of ARPKD, as well as protein-losing enteropathy cannot be alleviated by band therapy, so sometimes portosystemic shunting becomes necessary. Hemorrhoids can be treated with band ligation. Therefore, in patients with ARPKD who have ESRD or advanced CKD, kidney transplantation can be performed alone or, if patients have associated portal HTN not amenable to therapy or recurrent cholangitis or sepsis, they may be candidates for a combined liver-kidney transplant.[12]

Mortality/Morbidity

Thirty percent of affected newborns who present with large, echogenic kidneys die within the neonatal period owing to respiratory insufficiency[2] and presumably many of these cases have undiagnosed ARPKD. The neonates with less severe renal manifestations who survive the neonatal period have a 50% chance of developing ESRD by age 10 years. As the renal prognosis improves due to advances in renal replacement therapies, including transplantation, CHF remains the cause of death in 64% to 80% of patients. Therefore, liver-kidney transplantation is being considered a viable option in this disease, but because of its associated morbidity, it is most often reserved for the patients with ARPKD with recurrent cholangitis or complication of portal HTN.

Autosomal Dominant Polycystic Kidney Disease

ADPKD is the most common inherited kidney disease. It is a multisystem disorder characterized by progressive cystic dilation of both kidneys with variable extrarenal manifestations in the gastrointestinal tract, cardiovascular system, reproductive organs, and brain. ADPKD differs from ARPKD in a number of ways, and these differences are summarized in **Table 2**.

The genes responsible for ADPKD are localized to the short arm of chromosome 16 (*PKD1*) in 85% of the cases and the long arm of chromosome 4 (*PKD2*) in most of the remaining cases. A small number of families with ADPKD who did not demonstrate a linkage to *PKD1* or *PKD2* were thought to have an unidentified PKD3 gene. However, a subsequent study using mutational analysis suggests that increased sensitivity in genetic testing allows better identification of mutations in these 2 genes and therefore suggests against the existence of a PKD3.[13] Proteins encoded by *PKD1* and *PKD2* are polycystin 1 and polycystin 2, respectively, which are expressed in the developing kidney and have considerable overlap in their functions. The dysfunction of these proteins is thought to be pathogenetically responsible for the manifestations of ADPKD primarily by renal ciliary dysfunction.

Cystogenesis in ADPKD is believed to require an acquired somatic mutation after the inherited germline mutation. This could account for the reason only 5% of nephrons develop cysts despite the presence of an inherited mutated gene in every renal epithelial cell.[14] Modifier genes also play a role in cystogenesis, such as in patients with simultaneous mutations in the tuberous sclerosis gene (*TSC2*) and *PKD1* gene (called contiguous gene syndrome because the deletions occur in large genes adjacent to each other), where the onset of ADPKD is early and severe.[15]

Frequency

The estimated prevalence of ADPKD is 1 case in 400 to 1000 population. Because of the autosomal dominant inheritance, one parent is usually affected and each offspring has 50% chance of inheriting the gene with a penetrance of almost 100%. ADPKD is responsible for 6% to 10% of cases of ESRD in North America and Europe.

Clinical manifestations

Due to genic, allelic, and gene modifier effects, ADPKD has a wide phenotypic variability. At the time of clinical presentation, kidneys are usually enlarged with numerous, large, round nodules/cysts of varying sizes on the external surface of the kidney. The cysts are randomly distributed throughout the parenchyma involving any segment along the nephron. The cysts have thickened basement membranes with pericystic interstitial fibrosis and their epithelium maintains active secretion and reabsorption. There is an associated marked epithelial hyperplasia that some have hypothesized

Table 2
Differentiating features of ARPKD and ADPKD

Characteristic	ARPKD	ADPKD
Mode of inheritance	Autosomal recessive	Autosomal dominant
Location of cysts	Cysts are dilation of renal collecting ducts	Cysts develop anywhere along the nephron
Gross appearance	Reniform shape maintained Multiple minute cystic spaces throughout the capsular surfaces. Cut sections of the kidney show subcapsular extensions of radially oriented cylindrical or fusiform ectatic spaces from the medulla to the cortex	Loss of reniform shape of kidney Numerous, large, round nodules/ cysts of varying sizes on external surface of the kidney and randomly distributed through entire parenchyma of kidney
Age of presentation	Most often, in the neonatal period or childhood	Most often initially presents in adults aged 20 to 40 y, but increasingly there are reports of ADPKD presenting in childhood and even in utero
Frequency	1 in 20,000 live births	One case in 400–1000 population
Extrarenal features	Can occur in neonates Congenital hepatic fibrosis in *all* patients Manifestations of oligohydramnios, such as pulmonary insufficiency Potter facies, club foot, and so forth	Does NOT occur in neonates CHF and portal hypertension are very rare Manifestations of oligohydramnios are rare Includes hepatic cysts, pancreatic cysts found exclusively in patients with *PKD1*, cerebral vessel aneurysms, mitral valve prolapse, endocardial fibroelastosis, increased left ventricular mass with diastolic dysfunction even in normotensive children, ovarian cysts.
Renal prognosis	Fetuses with severe renal failure, oligohydramnios and pulmonary hypoplasia often die of pulmonary complications. Patients with less-severe renal manifestations who survive the neonatal period have a 50% chance of developing ESRD by age 10 y.	Chances of ESRD are 2% in those <40 y of age and increases to 50% by the seventh decade of life.

Abbreviations: ADPKD, autosomal dominant polycystic kidney disease; ARPKD, autosomal recessive polycystic kidney disease; CHF, congenital hepatic fibrosis; ESRD, end-stage renal disease.

may be associated a with higher rate of malignant transformation than in the general population.

ADPKD has a wide clinical spectrum. *PKD1*-associated disease is more severe with earlier development of cysts. *PKD2* associated ADPKD has a later onset and therefore a more benign course. Therefore ADPKD presenting in neonates is more likely due to a *PKD1* mutation. It may present asymptomatically as an incidental finding or it may present as severe neonatal manifestations similar to ARPKD, particularly if there is bilineal inheritance of the *PKD1* abnormality.[16] It can manifest in utero with Potter phenotype with death from pulmonary hypoplasia due to large hyperechoic kidneys with or without macrocysts with varying degrees of renal insufficiency. Prenatal ultrasound may reveal renal cysts, which with positive family history is very suggestive of ADPKD. In families with known ADPKD, routine screening ultrasound often reveals cysts in asymptomatic children. Renal involvement is often asymmetric but is usually bilateral. The initial presentation in older children includes abdominal pain, renal masses, gross or microscopic hematuria often after minor trauma, urinary tract infections, nephrolithiasis, perinephric abscess, hemorrhage, chronic pyelonephritis, sepsis and death, HTN, and abdominal or inguinal hernias. HTN can present in all age groups (even in patients with normal renal function) and rarely renal insufficiency can occur in childhood. Extrarenal manifestations are more common in adults and although they almost never occur in neonates, they can occur in those as young as 1 year of age and are summarized in **Table 2**.

Diagnostic testing

Currently, presymptomatic screening for infants or children is not recommended due to issues related to insurability and vulnerable child syndrome. In addition, ultrasonography in at-risk children is less helpful because before the age of 5 years, 50% of imaging studies are inconclusive and the negative predictive value and specificity of ultrasound is relatively low. Therefore, a normal ultrasound, MRI, or CT scan in a child does *not* rule out a diagnosis of ADPKD. Parents and pediatricians should ensure that the at-risk child has regular monitoring of blood pressure and growth as a surrogate for renal function. Presymptomatic screening may be relevant in the future when more effective therapy for the disease becomes available and as issues related to insurability continue to change.

Ultrasonography Ultrasonography is the least invasive and the most cost-effective option to diagnose ADPKD (**Fig. 2**). In a child (0–15 years of age) with family history of ADPKD, even one cyst is highly predictive of ADPKD. In infants, the presence of large echogenic kidneys without distinct macroscopic cysts may represent early ADPKD and is indistinguishable from ARPKD. Therefore, parental ultrasounds or family history are critically important in the evaluation of PKD.[17] Asymmetric development of tumorlike cysts also has been reported in children with ADPKD.[17,18] Multicystic dysplastic kidney (MCDK) differs from PKD in usually being unilateral with multiple noncommunicating macrocysts of varying size and the intervening renal tissue being nonfunctioning.

MRI and CT scans These are not diagnostic procedures of choice in ADPKD, as ultrasonography is cheaper, noninvasive, safe, and effective. However CT scan is as sensitive as ultrasonography in the detection of cystic disease and may even be more specific than ultrasonography in differentiating an obstructed renal pelvis from a parapelvic cyst, assessing for retroperitoneal cyst rupture and perinephric extension of blood or pus from an infected cyst. MRI is useful in evaluating hemorrhagic cysts and characterizing complicated cysts.

Genetic testing Genetic tests that detect mutations in the *PKD1* and *PKD2* identify ADPKD before large cysts develop, but detection of a mutation cannot predict the onset of symptoms or ultimate severity of the disease. In addition, there is no specific prevention or cure for ADPKD currently and the test is complicated by 6 PKD1 pseudogenes, large gene sizes, and allelic heterogeneity. Therefore, in most cases, ADPKD

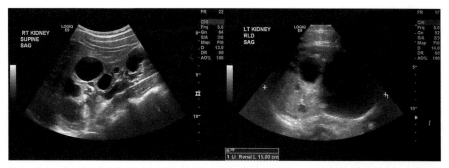

Fig. 2. Longitudinal sonogram of ADPKD. Both kidneys are enlarged. There are bilateral cysts of varying sizes with distortion of the normal reniform shape and preserved renal parenchyma between the cysts.

is a clinical diagnosis. The genetic test may be useful to determine whether an individual in an ADPKD family can donate a kidney safely to a family member with the disease or in young women of childbearing age with normal ultrasounds and a known family history who want to conclusively know whether they have the potential of passing a PKD gene to a child. Next-generation sequencing has been recently shown to be a suitable technique for genetic characterization of large ADPKD cohorts and promises to be a useful screening tool in the coming decade.[19,20]

Treatment

There is no specific therapy for ADPKD. Medications are used only to treat the complications that arise from the disease process, as in ARPKD. Management of renal insufficiency, ESRD, and HTN are similar to ARPKD. Renal insufficiency is much less common in children with ADPKD, but renal replacement therapy may be required. HTN must be treated aggressively because end-organ damage can occur in patients with untreated HTN. Because studies suggest that the HTN in ADPKD is due to intrarenal renin-angiotensin system activation,[21] ACE inhibitor is the first-line therapy if there are no contraindications.[22] In addition, ACE inhibition therapy has demonstrated structural benefit in ADPKD in association with a reduction in mean arterial blood pressure, although the mechanism of structural benefit may be simply due to lower blood pressure.[23] Although few data exist on the effect of ACE inhibitors in neonates, teratogenic effect of maternal use on fetal renal development is well documented, and there may be a risk of ACE inhibition in neonates affecting normal renal development.[24] Therefore, we typically recommend the avoidance of ACE inhibitors until the infant has reached a postconceptual age of 44 weeks.

Many studies have suggested that total kidney volume is a predictor of disease progression in ADPKD.[25] Therefore, there is much work being done into therapies such as somatostatin analogues or vasopressin 2 receptor antagonists that would slow the progression of cyst growth and renal enlargement in this disease.[26–28]

Mortality/Morbidity

Although ADPKD can present antenatally, it usually does not have the severe renal impairment seen in ARPKD. More commonly, it causes CKD in adults, which progresses with more cystic development of renal cortex into ESRD. Thus, chances of progression to ESRD are 2% in those younger than 40 years of age. ADPKD is a multisystem disorder and in some patients there may be associated intracranial aneurysms that can cause stroke and intracranial hemorrhage, but this has not been a reported complication in infants and is therefore not discussed further. Much of the morbidity of ADPKD is due to chronic HTN, and this should be aggressively addressed in all age groups.

NONHEREDITARY PKD
MCDK

MCDK is a variant of renal dysplasia, which is characterized by structural disorganization of the renal tissues with undifferentiated epithelium, primitive ducts,[29] and a spectrum that includes aplasia and hypoplasia. MCDK results in multiple noncommunicating cysts separated by dysplastic parenchyma (**Fig. 3**) and results in a grapelike cluster of cysts without preservation of normal renal architecture and function.[30] The exact mechanism of development of MCDK is unclear, but proposed theories include abnormal formation of the ureteric bud and/or aberrant interaction between the ureteric bud and metanephric mesenchyme, teratogens, including viral infections and medications, and in utero urinary tract obstruction.[31]

Frequency

MCDK occurs in 1 in 2200 to 1 in 4300 live births.[32,33] Previous to the widespread use of prenatal ultrasound, flank abdominal masses in otherwise healthy newborns was the most common presentation of unilateral MCDK,[34] but in the age of prenatal ultrasounds, the antenatal diagnosis of MCDK has dramatically increased.[35] Bilateral MCDK resulting in the absence of renal function and fetal demise due to oligohydramnios and respiratory failure has been reported to occur in 7% to 23% of all MCDK cases.[36–38] Most of the MCDK cases are sporadic, although there are reports of familial cases.[39] A meta-analysis of 3557 patients with unilateral MCDK showed a male preponderance (59.2%, $P<.0001$), and slight left-sided predominance (53.1%, $P<.02$).[33]

Clinical manifestations

Most suspected MCDK cases are now discovered by prenatal ultrasounds. Differential diagnosis of MCDK includes ADPKD, ARPKD, glomerulocystic disease, obstructive dysplasia, medullary cystic dysplasia, and hydronephrotic obstructed kidneys.[40,41] Infants with MCDK can present with flank mass but are usually otherwise asymptomatic. The contralateral kidney, however, can sometimes have anomalies, as summarized in **Table 3**, which must be investigated and appropriately managed. The most common

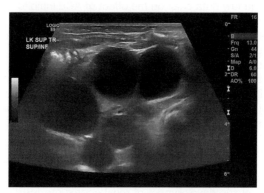

Fig. 3. Sonogram of MCDK. Gray-scale ultrasound of left kidney in a newborn shows no normal renal parenchyma and the left renal fossa filled with multiple simple-appearing cystic structures. Lack of communication between the cysts makes hydronephrosis due to a severe ureteropelvic junction obstruction less likely, but a renogram is required to rule out severe obstruction.

Table 3 Common associated anomalies of the genitourinary tract and the contralateral kidney in neonates with multicystic dysplastic kidney, frequency of the abnormality, and suggested method of investigation		
Associated Contralateral Abnormality	Frequency (%)	Suggested Investigation
Vesicoureteral reflux	4–43	Voiding cystourethrogram
Urinary tract obstruction	5–15	Mercaptoacetyltriglycine (MAG) 3 renal scan
Genital abnormalities	15	Physical examination and ultrasound

and potentially most clinically significant anomaly in the contralateral kidney is vesicoureteral reflux (VUR), which has been reported in 4% to 43% of patients with MCDK.[29,33,42,43] These patients are at a higher risk to develop pyelonephritis in the contralateral kidney, which can lead to CKD and HTN from renal scarring. Urinary obstruction, such as ureteropelvic junction obstruction and ureterovesical junction obstruction, have been reported in 5% to 15% and 6%, respectively.[33,44] In a retrospective review of 93 patients with MCDK, 14 patients (15%) were found to have ipsilateral internal genitalia: 3 cases of Gartner duct persistence, 10 cases of cystic retrovesical and laterovesical masses, and 1 blind-ending hemivagina.[45] Other rare abnormalities include ureteroceles, horseshoe kidney, and posterior urethral valves.[33]

A number of studies have shown that how MCDK tends to involute although the mechanism is unclear. Complete involution was observed in 19% to 59% and partial involution in 33% to 70% over 42 months to 10 years.[29,42,44,46] The velocity of involution tends to be fastest early in life, and the only factor associated with complete involution appears to be the initial length of MCDK less than 62 mm.[47]

One of the more important clinical indices to follow in patients with MCDK is the growth of the contralateral kidney. Compensatory hypertrophy has been defined as renal length greater than 2 SDs of the mean for age.[42] Similar to patients with congenital solitary kidney, patients with MCDK have compensatory hypertrophy of the contralateral kidney to offset the loss of functional renal tissue. Compensatory hypertrophy of the contralateral kidney is reported to occur in 24% of patients with unilateral MCDK at birth, and in 45% to 77% at a mean follow-up time of 3.5 to 4.9 years.[29,41,44] By 10 years, 81% of patients have reported compensatory hypertrophy of the contralateral kidney.[42] Absence of appropriate compensatory hypertrophy may indicate pathology in the contralateral kidney, such as hypoplasia and dysplasia.

Diagnostic testing and treatment

In countries where prenatal ultrasound is routine, postnatal renal ultrasonography should be obtained before discharge for neonates suspected to have MCDK. After confirmation of unilateral MCDK diagnosis, there is no clear consensus recommendation on initial evaluation and follow-up imaging. **Fig. 4** illustrates our recommendation based on our experience, as well as published reports.[29,31,35,42,44,46,48,49]

In cases of unilateral MCDK, we strongly recommend obtaining a diuretic renogram to confirm the absence of functioning renal tissue. If there is functioning tissue, MCDK is not the diagnosis and it is critical to evaluate for ureteral obstruction and obstructive cystic dysplasia, as is discussed later in this article. Obstruction of the contralateral kidney in MCDK cases must also be ruled out, because the patient's renal function is entirely dependent on the contralateral kidney, and prompt surgical intervention may help to preserve renal function. Whether voiding cystourethrogram (VCUG) should be obtained in every patient with unilateral MCDK is controversial, especially

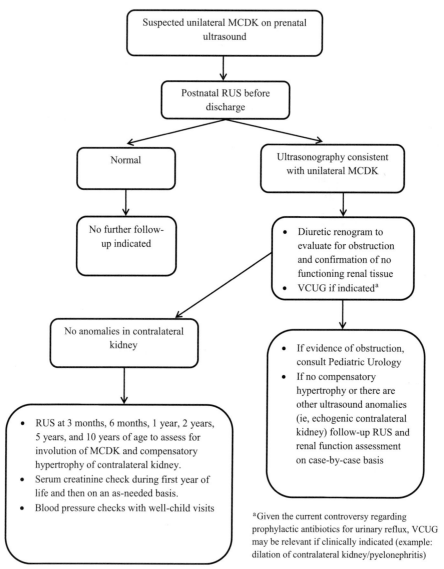

Fig. 4. Suggested initial evaluation and follow-up for unilateral MCDK. RUS, renal ultrasonography.

given that there is no clear guideline for the management of primary VUR. We currently recommend a VCUG for patients with unilateral MCDK with dilated renal pelvis in the contralateral kidney, or in patients who present with febrile urinary tract infection, because these patients are likely to have higher risk of VUR.

If no other anatomic or renal ultrasonography anomaly is identified in the unaffected kidney, then these patients should have follow-up renal ultrasonography multiple times in the first year (example: 3, 6, and 12 months), and then at 2 years, 5 years, and 10 years of age to assess involution of MCDK and compensatory hypertrophy of contralateral kidney. For patients with lack of compensatory hypertrophy or other signs of hypoplasia or dysplasia in the contralateral kidney, they need to be screened for CKD earlier and more frequently and have their follow-up managed by pediatric nephrology. These patients also should have assessment of their renal function by serum creatinine during the first year of life and then as clinically indicated. Historically, HTN had been linked with MCDK based on small case series describing higher rates of HTN in patients with MCDK and resolution of HTN with removal of the MCDK.[31] However, recent larger reports, including a systematic review, found HTN rates of 0%, 5% (with spontaneous resolution in 4 of 5 patients), and 5.4 per 1000 MCDK cases.[29,42,50] The HTN persisted even after removal of MCDK in 2 of 4 cases.[49] Therefore, even though patients with MCDK may be at a higher risk of HTN later in life from hyperfiltration and elevated renin activity, the risk is low and we merely recommend regular blood pressure checks at their regular well-child visits.

Because of previous anecdotal case reports of Wilms tumor associated with MCDK, removal of MCDKs were historically performed. Ten cases of Wilms tumor were associated with purported MCDK, but only 4 of them had known history of MCDK with all 10 cases presenting before 4 years of age without metastatic disease or death.[48] This review also found no Wilms tumor associated with involuted MCDK. However, more recent data suggest the risk of malignant transformation of MCDK to be minimal, and even if minimally higher than the general population, these cases appear to be amenable to therapy.[31] Larger case series consisting of 165 patients and 97 patients have also reported no Wilms tumor cases[29,42] and a meta-analysis of 26 retrospective and prospective studies consisting of 1041 patients with unilateral MCDK managed conservatively reported not even a single case of Wilms tumor.[51] In an editorial, the reported calculated risk of Wilms tumor with MCDK is 1 in 2000,[52] and this was confirmed subsequently by Noe and colleagues[53] who reported that 2000 MCDK nephrectomies would be needed to prevent 1 case of Wilms tumor. Other renal malignancies, such as renal cell carcinoma, have been reported with MCDK, but the accuracy of diagnosis of MCDK is debatable in these reports.[48] Thus, in summarizing more recent publications, including systematic literature reviews, routine nephrectomy of MCDK is not indicated due to low risks of malignancy and it is our opinion that more frequent ultrasonography to screen for Wilms tumor or malignancy is not indicated because of its low incidence rate and lack of evidence of improved outcome with more frequent monitoring.

Mortality/Morbidity

Renal function outcome of patients with unilateral MCDK appears to be dependent on whether they have "simple" MCDK, without any other urinary tract anomalies, versus "complex" MCDK, defined as unilateral MCDK with contralateral structural/functional anomalies or outflow obstructions. In a single-center study, patients with simple MCDK had a mean serum creatinine of 0.6 mg/dL with mean estimated glomerular filtration rate (eGFR) of 90 mL/min/1.73 m^2 with no ESRD case.[54] In contrast, patients with complex MCDK experienced higher rates of urinary tract infections, and 50% of patients with complex MCDK developed ESRD and 28% of patients had CKD with a serum creatinine ranging from 1.7 to 4.0 mg/dL and eGFR of 20 to 40 mL/min/1.73 m^2.[54] Another publication with 10 years of follow-up data reported a mean eGFR of 86 mL/min/1.73 m^2 in patients with compensatory hypertrophy of the contralateral kidney and a mean eGFR less than 60 mL/min/1.73 m^2 in those who had abnormal echogenicity of the contralateral kidney suggestive of dysplasia.[42]

Obstructive Cystic Dysplasia

Renal dysplasia is the major cause of CKD in children, and is commonly associated with urinary tract obstruction. The 2 phenotypes of renal dysplasia associated with urinary tract abnormalities are MCDK described previously and obstructive cystic dysplasia described here. Obstructive cystic dysplasia occurs from antenatal obstruction of the urinary tract secondary to posterior urethral valves, ureteropelvic junction obstruction, or atrophic moiety of duplicated ureter that is obstructed. Obstruction usually results in dilatation of the collecting system, which is often seen in prenatal ultrasounds and it has predominantly peripheral cortical cysts. Obstructive cystic dysplasia is the most common cause of neonatal hyperechoic cortex, and the affected kidney can vary in size with irregular, thinned cortex.[55] It can be unilateral or bilateral, often depending on the location of the obstruction and is often seen as part of prune belly syndrome, which consists of distended abdomen, defective abdominal wall musculature, megacystis, megaureters, hydronephrotic dysplastic kidneys, and cryptorchidism. Fetuses with bilateral cystic dysplasia and hydronephrosis warrant a VCUG to evaluate for bladder outlet obstruction, such as posterior urethral valves.

Simple Renal Cyst

Simple renal cyst is defined as a solitary, nonseptated cyst with well-defined borders, and no communication between the cyst cavity and renal pelvis in an otherwise normal-appearing kidney.[56] Twenty-eight fetuses of 29,984 consecutive pregnancies at 14 to 16 weeks of gestation were found to have simple renal cyst (0.09%). Twenty-four fetuses had resolution by 20 to 24 weeks of gestation, 1 fetus had resolution of the cyst on postnatal ultrasounds, 2 fetuses continued to have unchanged simple cysts at ages 3 and 6 years, and 1 fetus ended up having MCDK on ultrasounds later in pregnancy and postnatally.[56] The investigators of this study speculate that the mechanisms of prenatal formed simple renal cysts are reversible processes, and therefore resolve, which is in contrast with postnatal formed cysts, which have a permanent nature. In another retrospective review of simple renal cysts that included noninfant pediatric patients, 35 of 16,102 children (0.22%), aged from newborn to 18 years, were found to have simple renal cysts.[57] Of the 22 patients who had ultrasound follow-up up to 5 years, only 1 had percutaneous drainage due to its large size, and the rest were observed conservatively with no significant changes with no patient showing deterioration in renal function.[57]

Complex Renal Cyst

Complex renal cysts are rarely encountered in pediatrics. Renal tumors of infancy are usually solid but differential diagnosis of cystic renal tumors in infancy include cystic congenital mesoblastic nephroma, cystic nephroma, cystic partially differentiated nephroblastoma, adrenal hemorrhage, clear-cell sarcoma, and cystic renal cell carcinoma.[58] There has not been neonatal or infantile published data on follow-up of complex renal cyst. A case series of 39 children with complex cysts between the ages of 4 months and 14 years reported surgical resection in 5 patients due to surgeon preference and cyst characteristics. Two of these patients were found to have renal cell carcinoma with their ages being 8 and 11 years old.[59]

The Bosniak renal cyst classification system is a guide for evaluation and proper management of adult patients with renal cysts based on CT images.[60] Category I is defined as simple cyst and categories II through IV are defined as complex cysts, with category IV being a clearly malignant cystic mass requiring surgical resection. Because ultrasonography is the preferred imaging modality in children and the Bosniak renal cyst classification is based on CT images, a proposed modified Bosniak classification that includes ultrasound findings for each category and recommendations on more enhanced imaging has been suggested for children (**Table 4**). Because of concern of malignancy associated with adult complex renal cysts, historically,

Table 4 Proposed modified Bosniak classification for children with renal cysts	
Category	
I	Round, smooth thin-walled cyst. No echogenic foci and enhanced throughout transmission on ultrasound. Homogeneous content consistent with water density and absence of enhancement after intravenous contrast on computed tomography (CT) scan.
II	Cyst with thin septa with or without minimal/smooth thickening of the cyst wall or septation(s). Calcifications and/or high attenuation detected on CT scan. No evidence of enhancement after contrast administration. No detectable flow by Doppler ultrasound in septations or cyst wall.
III	Presence of thick or irregular septations. Thick/irregular calcifications detected on CT scan. Enhancement of septa or wall may be present after intravenous contrast administration. Detectable flow by Doppler ultrasound may be present in septations or cyst wall. If category III by ultrasound, contrast axial imaging study should be strongly considered.
IV	Cystic mass with thick wall, solid internal components, or nodular areas. Enhancement and marked heterogeneity after contrast administration. Detectable flow detected by Doppler ultrasound in cyst wall, septations, nodular component. If category IV by ultrasound, contrast axial imaging study should be strongly considered.

Adapted from Wallis MC, Lorenzo AJ, Farhat WA, et al. Risk assessment of incidentally detected complex renal cysts in children: potential role for a modification of the Bosniak classification. J Urol 2008;180(1):317–21; with permission.

surgical resection has been recommended in most cases.[59] On the contrary, in children, serial ultrasonography every 3 to 6 months is recommended for patients with class II cysts and contrast-enhanced axial imaging for all children with class III and IV cysts with consideration for surgical resection.[59]

REFERENCES

1. Salvador J, Borrell A, Lladonosa A. Increasing detection rates of birth defects by prenatal ultrasound leading to apparent increasing prevalence. Lessons learned from the population-based registry of birth defects of Barcelona. Prenat Diagn 2005;25(11):991–6.
2. Sweeney WE Jr, Avner ED. Diagnosis and management of childhood polycystic kidney disease. Pediatr Nephrol 2011;26(5):675–92.
3. Taneda S, Honda K, Aoki A, et al. An autopsy case of clinically un-diagnosed autosomal recessive polycystic kidney disease in 77-year-old male. Pathol Int 2012;62(12):811–6.
4. Adeva M, El-Youssef M, Rossetti S, et al. Clinical and molecular characterization defines a broadened spectrum of autosomal recessive polycystic kidney disease (ARPKD). Medicine (Baltimore) 2006;85(1):1–21.
5. Fick GM, Johnson AM, Strain JD, et al. Characteristics of very early onset autosomal dominant polycystic kidney disease. J Am Soc Nephrol 1993;3(12): 1863–70.
6. Gunay-Aygun M, Tuchman M, Font-Montgomery E, et al. PKHD1 sequence variations in 78 children and adults with autosomal recessive polycystic kidney disease and congenital hepatic fibrosis. Mol Genet Metab 2010;99(2): 160–73.

7. Zerres K, Mucher G, Becker J, et al. Prenatal diagnosis of autosomal recessive polycystic kidney disease (ARPKD): molecular genetics, clinical experience, and fetal morphology. Am J Med Genet 1998;76(2):137–44.

8. Dell KM. The spectrum of polycystic kidney disease in children. Adv Chronic Kidney Dis 2011;18(5):339–47.

9. Chapal M, Debout A, Dufay A, et al. Kidney and liver transplantation in patients with autosomal recessive polycystic kidney disease: a multicentric study. Nephrol Dial Transplant 2012;27(5):2083–8.

10. Khan K, Schwarzenberg SJ, Sharp HL, et al. Morbidity from congenital hepatic fibrosis after renal transplantation for autosomal recessive polycystic kidney disease. Am J Transplant 2002;2(4):360–5.

11. Shneider BL, Bosch J, de Franchis R, et al. Portal hypertension in children: expert pediatric opinion on the report of the Baveno v Consensus Workshop on Methodology of Diagnosis and Therapy in Portal Hypertension. Pediatr Transplant 2012;16(5):426–37.

12. Telega G, Cronin D, Avner ED. New approaches to the autosomal recessive polycystic kidney disease patient with dual kidney-liver complications. Pediatr Transplant 2013;17(4):328–35.

13. Paul BM, Consugar MB, Ryan Lee M, et al. Evidence of a third ADPKD locus is not supported by re-analysis of designated PKD3 families. Kidney Int 2014; 85(2):383–92.

14. Sutters M, Germino GG. Autosomal dominant polycystic kidney disease: molecular genetics and pathophysiology. J Lab Clin Med 2003;141(2):91–101.

15. Fain PR, McFann KK, Taylor MR, et al. Modifier genes play a significant role in the phenotypic expression of PKD1. Kidney Int 2005;67(4):1256–67.

16. Gilbert RD, Sukhtankar P, Lachlan K, et al. Bilineal inheritance of PKD1 abnormalities mimicking autosomal recessive polycystic disease. Pediatr Nephrol 2013;28(11):2217–20.

17. Verghese P, Kim Y. Unilateral localized cystic kidney. Pediatr Nephrol 2011; 26(5):713–6.

18. Shiroyanagi Y, Suzuki M, Matsuno D, et al. Asymmetric development of tumor-like cysts in a child with autosomal dominant polycystic kidney disease. J Pediatr Surg 2008;43(11):e21–3.

19. Rossetti S, Hopp K, Sikkink RA, et al. Identification of gene mutations in autosomal dominant polycystic kidney disease through targeted resequencing. J Am Soc Nephrol 2012;23(5):915–33.

20. Tan AY, Michaeel A, Liu G, et al. Molecular diagnosis of autosomal dominant polycystic kidney disease using next-generation sequencing. J Mol Diagn 2014;16(2):216–28.

21. Kocyigit I, Yilmaz MI, Unal A, et al. A link between the intrarenal renin angiotensin system and hypertension in autosomal dominant polycystic kidney disease. Am J Nephrol 2013;38(3):218–25.

22. Schrier R, McFann K, Johnson A, et al. Cardiac and renal effects of standard versus rigorous blood pressure control in autosomal-dominant polycystic kidney disease: results of a seven-year prospective randomized study. J Am Soc Nephrol 2002;13(7):1733–9.

23. Keith DS, Torres VE, Johnson CM, et al. Effect of sodium chloride, enalapril, and losartan on the development of polycystic kidney disease in Han:SPRD rats. Am J Kidney Dis 1994;24(3):491–8.

24. Guron G, Friberg P. An intact renin-angiotensin system is a prerequisite for normal renal development. J Hypertens 2000;18(2):123–37.

25. Rahbari-Oskoui F, Mittal A, Mittal P, et al. Renal relevant radiology: radiologic imaging in autosomal dominant polycystic kidney disease. Clin J Am Soc Nephrol 2014;9(2):406–15.
26. Meijer E, Drenth JP, d'Agnolo H, et al. Rationale and design of the DIPAK 1 study: a randomized controlled clinical trial assessing the efficacy of lanreotide to halt disease progression in autosomal dominant polycystic kidney disease. Am J Kidney Dis 2014;63(3):446–55.
27. Higashihara E, Torres VE, Chapman AB, et al. Tolvaptan in autosomal dominant polycystic kidney disease: three years' experience. Clin J Am Soc Nephrol 2011;6(10):2499–507.
28. Torres VE, Meijer E, Bae KT, et al. Rationale and design of the TEMPO (Tolvaptan Efficacy and Safety in Management of Autosomal Dominant Polycystic Kidney Disease and its Outcomes) 3-4 Study. Am J Kidney Dis 2011;57(5):692–9.
29. Kuwertz-Broeking E, Brinkmann OA, Von Lengerke HJ, et al. Unilateral multicystic dysplastic kidney: experience in children. BJU Int 2004;93(3):388–92.
30. Greene LF, Feinzaig W, Dahlin DC. Multicystic dysplasia of the kidney: with special reference to the contralateral kidney. J Urol 1971;105(4):482–7.
31. Hains DS, Bates CM, Ingraham S, et al. Management and etiology of the unilateral multicystic dysplastic kidney: a review. Pediatr Nephrol 2009;24(2):233–41.
32. Mallik M, Watson AR. Antenatally detected urinary tract abnormalities: more detection but less action. Pediatr Nephrol 2008;23(6):897–904.
33. Schreuder MF, Westland R, van Wijk JA. Unilateral multicystic dysplastic kidney: a meta-analysis of observational studies on the incidence, associated urinary tract malformations and the contralateral kidney. Nephrol Dial Transplant 2009;24(6):1810–8.
34. Robson WL, Leung AK, Thomason MA. Multicystic dysplasia of the kidney. Clin Pediatr (Phila) 1995;34(1):32–40.
35. Oliveira EA, Diniz JS, Vilasboas AS, et al. Multicystic dysplastic kidney detected by fetal sonography: conservative management and follow-up. Pediatr Surg Int 2001;17(1):54–7.
36. al-Khaldi N, Watson AR, Zuccollo J, et al. Outcome of antenatally detected cystic dysplastic kidney disease. Arch Dis Child 1994;70(6):520–2.
37. Heikkinen ES, Herva R, Lanning P. Multicystic kidney. A clinical and histological study of 13 patients. Ann Chir Gynaecol 1980;69(1):15–22.
38. Kleiner B, Filly RA, Mack L, et al. Multicystic dysplastic kidney: observations of contralateral disease in the fetal population. Radiology 1986;161(1):27–9.
39. Belk RA, Thomas DF, Mueller RF, et al. A family study and the natural history of prenatally detected unilateral multicystic dysplastic kidney. J Urol 2002;167(2 Pt 1):666–9.
40. Avni FE, Garel L, Cassart M, et al. Perinatal assessment of hereditary cystic renal diseases: the contribution of sonography. Pediatr Radiol 2006;36(5):405–14.
41. Singh I, Sharma D, Singh N, et al. Hydronephrotic obstructed kidney mimicking a congenital multicystic kidney: case report with review of literature. Int Urol Nephrol 2002;34(2):179–82.
42. Aslam M, Watson AR. Unilateral multicystic dysplastic kidney: long term outcomes. Arch Dis Child 2006;91(10):820–3.
43. Wacksman J, Phipps L. Report of the multicystic kidney registry—preliminary findings. J Urol 1993;150(6):1870–2.
44. John U, Rudnik-Schoneborn S, Zerres K, et al. Kidney growth and renal function in unilateral multicystic dysplastic kidney disease. Pediatr Nephrol 1998;12(7):567–71.

45. Merrot T, Lumenta DB, Tercier S, et al. Multicystic dysplastic kidney with ipsilateral abnormalities of genitourinary tract: experience in children. Urology 2006; 67(3):603–7.
46. Rabelo EA, Oliveira EA, Diniz JS, et al. Natural history of multicystic kidney conservatively managed: a prospective study. Pediatr Nephrol 2004;19(10): 1102–7.
47. Rabelo EA, Oliveira EA, Silva GS, et al. Predictive factors of ultrasonographic involution of prenatally detected multicystic dysplastic kidney. BJU Int 2005; 95(6):868–71.
48. Cambio AJ, Evans CP, Kurzrock EA. Non-surgical management of multicystic dysplastic kidney. BJU Int 2008;101(7):804–8.
49. Snodgrass WT. Hypertension associated with multicystic dysplastic kidney in children. J Urol 2000;164(2):472–3 [discussion: 3–4].
50. Narchi H. Risk of hypertension with multicystic kidney disease: a systematic review. Arch Dis Child 2005;90(9):921–4.
51. Narchi H. Risk of Wilms' tumour with multicystic kidney disease: a systematic review. Arch Dis Child 2005;90(2):147–9.
52. Homsy YL, Anderson JH, Oudjhane K, et al. Wilms tumor and multicystic dysplastic kidney disease. J Urol 1997;158(6):2256–9 [discussion: 9–60].
53. Noe HN, Marshall JH, Edwards OP. Nodular renal blastema in the multicystic kidney. J Urol 1989;142(2 Pt 2):486–8 [discussion: 9].
54. Feldenberg LR, Siegel NJ. Clinical course and outcome for children with multicystic dysplastic kidneys. Pediatr Nephrol 2000;14(12):1098–101.
55. Avni FE, Garel C, Cassart M, et al. Imaging and classification of congenital cystic renal diseases. AJR Am J Roentgenol 2012;198(5):1004–13.
56. Blazer S, Zimmer EZ, Blumenfeld Z, et al. Natural history of fetal simple renal cysts detected in early pregnancy. J Urol 1999;162(3 Pt 1):812–4.
57. McHugh K, Stringer DA, Hebert D, et al. Simple renal cysts in children: diagnosis and follow-up with US. Radiology 1991;178(2):383–5.
58. Murthi GV, Carachi R, Howatson A. Congenital cystic mesoblastic nephroma. Pediatr Surg Int 2003;19(1–2):109–11.
59. Wallis MC, Lorenzo AJ, Farhat WA, et al. Risk assessment of incidentally detected complex renal cysts in children: potential role for a modification of the Bosniak classification. J Urol 2008;180(1):317–21.
60. Israel GM, Bosniak MA. An update of the Bosniak renal cyst classification system. Urology 2005;66(3):484–8.

Long-Term Renal Consequences of Preterm Birth

 CrossMark

Megan Sutherland, BBiomedSci (Hons), PhD[a], Dana Ryan, BSc (Hons)[a],
M. Jane Black, BSc (Hons), PhD[a], Alison L. Kent, BMBS, FRACP, MD[b,c],*

KEYWORDS

- Glomeruli • Preterm • Chorioamnionitis • Diabetes • Preeclampsia
- Growth restriction • Antenatal steroids

KEY POINTS

- Several antenatal factors have the potential to impair kidney development, including fetal growth restriction, maternal hypertension, and diabetes.
- Preterm birth is associated with several postnatal risk factors for kidney development, including increased physiologic requirements related to ex utero life, nephrotoxic medications, acute kidney injury, and postnatal growth failure.
- Children and adults born preterm may have reduced kidney size and increased blood pressure (BP), which likely predispose to renal disease later in life.
- The population of individuals born preterm continues to increase worldwide; it is expected that further evidence of renal dysfunction after preterm birth will continue to emerge in the future.

CLINICAL SCENARIO 1

A woman presented to the delivery suite at 26+1 weeks' gestation with ruptured membranes and was managed with intravenous ampicillin 500 mg 6 hourly, gentamicin 120 mg daily for 48 hours and then converted to oral azithromycin 500 mg every three days. She received antenatal steroids (betamethasone 12 mg daily for 2 doses) and was admitted to the antenatal ward. Four days later, she developed a fever and tachycardia, with an associated increase in white cell count on full blood picture and increased C-reactive protein levels. Labor ensued, and she delivered a

Disclosure: None.
[a] Department of Anatomy and Developmental Biology, Monash University, Level 3, Boulevard 76, Wellington Road, Clayton, Victoria 3800, Australia; [b] Department of Neonatology, Centenary Hospital for Women and Children, Canberra Hospital, PO Box 11, Woden 2606, Australian Capital Territory, Australia; [c] Australian National University Medical School, Canberra 2601, Australian Capital Territory, Australia
* Corresponding author.
E-mail address: alison.kent@act.gov.au

Clin Perinatol 41 (2014) 561–573
http://dx.doi.org/10.1016/j.clp.2014.05.006   **perinatology.theclinics.com**
0095-5108/14/$ – see front matter Crown Copyright © 2014 Published by Elsevier Inc. All rights reserved.

26+6 week gestation male infant weighing 900 g (50th centile), who required intubation for resuscitation, received a dose of surfactant, and was extubated at 48 hours of age. Placental histology later confirmed the diagnosis of chorioamnionitis and funisitis. Certain components of this history have long-term implications on renal health (**Fig. 1**).

Chorioamnionitis

Chorioamnionitis (bacterial infection that causes inflammation of the amnion and chorion), is widely recognized as a significant contributor to preterm birth, as a cause of both spontaneous preterm labor and premature rupture of the amniotic membrane.[1,2] Chorioamnionitis also produces the fetal inflammatory response syndrome (FIRS), characterized by an inflamed umbilical cord and increased fetal serum levels of proinflammatory cytokines.[3] Consequently, FIRS can adversely influence neonatal organ development, including the lungs,[4] brain,[2,5] thymus,[6,7] and kidney.[8] In an ovine model, intrauterine exposure to chorioamnionitis (bolus intra-amniotic high dose of endotoxin [10 mg lipopolysaccharide (LPS)] at a time in gestation when nephrogenesis was near completion) was found to cause a 20% reduction in nephron endowment.[8] In response to the reduction in nephron number, there was also a significant increase in glomerular volume, most likely resulting from compensatory hypertrophy; these adverse effects on nephrogenesis occurred in the absence of fetal growth restriction.[8] This finding is clinically important, because a reduction in nephron number can lead to increased susceptibility to renal injury and disease in later life.[9–14] In a more recent ovine study,[15] it was found that exposure to a chronic low-dose intra-amniotic infusion of endotoxin (1 mg LPS), during a time when fetal nephrogenesis was still rapidly ongoing, did not lead to any observable deleterious effects on nephron endowment. Together, these findings are indicative that the extent of infection as well as the timing (acute vs chronic) may influence the impact of chorioamnionitis on renal development.

Antenatal Steroids

Besides the beneficial effects on lung function and postnatal survival, antenatal glucocorticoid treatment is also associated with increased mean arterial BP, and increased

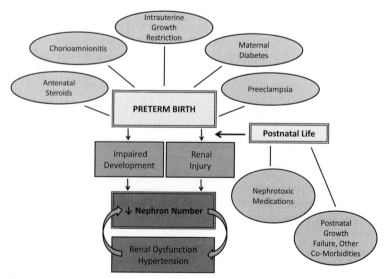

Fig. 1. Prenatal and postnatal risk factors for renal developmental injury.

renal blood flow and glomerular filtration rate (GFR),[16] indicating that accelerated functional maturation of the kidney also occurs after treatment. Similarly, in studies conducted in a baboon model of preterm birth,[17] there was evidence of accelerated renal maturation with a greater number of mature nephrons present in the glucocorticoid-exposed kidneys when examined both at the time of preterm delivery and at postnatal day 21. Although it has not been established, it is possible that this accelerated maturation results in an earlier cessation of nephrogenesis. In this regard, in other studies performed in animal models (including rodents[18–20] and sheep[21]), antenatal glucocorticoid administration was shown to lead to a significant reduction in nephron endowment of the exposed offspring. A study by de Vries and colleagues[22] similarly showed that postnatal administration of dexamethasone in the neonatal rat (at a time of ongoing postnatal nephrogenesis) leads to a reduction in glomerular density.

Preterm Birth

The transition from an intrauterine to an extrauterine environment involves a sudden increase in blood oxygen concentrations, as well as increased systemic BP and organ perfusion. The effects that this hemodynamic shift may have on the immature developing kidney (with nephrogenesis ongoing at the time of preterm birth) are poorly understood. After birth, the preterm kidney is functionally immature, with a low GFR, inability to maintain electrolyte balance,[23] and proteinuria.[24] Acute kidney injury is also common.[25] Some (but not all[26]) studies of kidney size in preterm neonates have shown significantly reduced kidney length or volume compared with neonates born at term.[27–30]

Histomorphologic studies[31] of renal tissue collected at autopsy have shown accelerated postnatal maturation of the preterm kidney, with reduced nephrogenic zone width, reduced renal vesicle formation, and increased number of glomerular generations compared with age-matched fetal controls. At the completion of nephrogenesis, a reduction in the number of glomerular generations formed (suggestive of a nephron deficit) has also been reported.[10] In addition, glomeruli that are abnormal in appearance (enlarged Bowman space and shrunken glomerular tuft) were present in the outer renal cortex of preterm kidneys[31]; in some neonates, up to 13% of glomeruli were affected. These glomeruli have scant capillarization, suggestive of impaired vascular development or injury, which is likely to render them nonfunctional.[17,32] In a baboon model of preterm birth, nephron density was found to be significantly lower in the preterm kidneys, and nephron number was at the lower end of the normal distribution,[17] and in mice delivered 1 to 2 days preterm, nephron number was significantly reduced.[33] Together, these findings suggest that preterm neonates may have both a reduced endowment of nephrons at the completion of nephrogenesis, as well a predisposition to nephron loss in the neonatal period, which may have important implications for long-term renal health.

CLINICAL SCENARIO 1 (CONTINUED)

Because of the maternal history of clinical chorioamnionitis, the preterm infant was commenced on ampicillin 25 mg/kg/dose 12 hourly and gentamicin 2.5 mg/kg/dose 24 hourly, which were ceased at 48 hours of age after a negative blood culture. On day 2 of life, an echocardiogram was performed, and the infant was found to have a large patent ductus arteriosus, with an increased left atrium/aorta ratio. He was commenced on intravenous indomethacin 0.2 mg/kg first dose, 0.1 mg/kg subsequent doses daily for 5 days; however, at the end of the third day of treatment, he developed abdominal distension, bilious aspirates, and hypotension and had an abdominal radiograph, with signs consistent with necrotizing enterocolitis. He required reintubation and inotropes, was not fed enterally for 10 days, and received 7 days of ampicillin 25 mg/kg/dose 12 hourly, gentamicin 2.5 mg/kg/dose 24 hourly, and metronidazole 7.5 mg/kg/dose 48 hourly. He was recommenced on feeds but continued to have significant feed intolerance until full feeds were achieved on day 30. He was extubated at 28 days of age, requiring dexamethasone, and continued to require continuous positive airway pressure (CPAP) until 35 weeks postconceptional age and oxygen until 38 weeks postconceptional age. His weight on discharge was 2.2 kg, which was less than the 3rd centile, having decreased from the 50th centile at birth. This relatively common series of complications of extreme prematurity have further renal implications.

Nephrotoxic Medications

The prenatal and postnatal administration of a variety of nephrotoxic medications is common practice in the setting of preterm birth.[34–38] Experimental studies have shown that antenatal exposure to the most commonly administered aminoglycoside antibiotic, gentamicin, causes significant reductions in nephron endowment.[39] Gentamicin accumulates in renal proximal tubule cells, leading to cellular necrosis[40]; postnatally, this results in increased sodium excretion, proteinuria, and reduced GFR in affected neonates.[41–43] Exposure of the developing kidney to β-lactam antibiotics (such as ampicillin) has also been shown to result in impaired nephrogenesis and cystic tubular dilation.[44]

The consequences of antenatal nonsteroidal antiinflammatory drugs (NSAIDs) (indomethacin, ibuprofen) exposure on the fetal kidney is well described both in experimental models (nephron deficits, reduced cortical renal volume,[45–47] and severe renal dysplasia[48]) and in human neonates (glomerular cysts and renal dysfunction[49,50]). However, less is known about the effects of postnatal NSAID exposure on the kidney. In general, the administration of NSAIDs causes systemic vasoconstriction, which in turn leads to significant reductions in renal blood flow and urine output.[51–53] A study in human preterm neonates[54] recently showed significantly increased number of podocytes in the urine, and increased urine albumin excretion in those treated with indomethacin after birth, which indicates glomerular injury. Furthermore, an experimental study conducted in a neonatal rodent model[55] showed that postnatal administration of NSAIDs or gentamicin led to proximal tubule vacuolization, interstitial edema, and podocyte foot process effacement; the most severe effects were observed in animals that received combined NSAID and gentamicin treatment. In a nonhuman primate (baboon) model,[56] animals administered ibuprofen after preterm birth had a significantly reduced nephrogenic zone width. This finding suggests that prostaglandin inhibition may impair nephrogenesis. Kent and colleagues[57] in their early study reported that there was no effect of early postnatal NSAID and gentamicin exposure on nephron endowment in a rat model at 14 days but have now shown that the adult rat has a significantly reduced nephron number after early administration of indomethacin but not ibuprofen (Kent AL, Koina M, Gubhaju L, et al: Indomethacin administered early in the postnatal period results in reduced glomeruli in the adult rat. Submitted for publication).

Growth Restriction

Over the past decade, it has been well established that intrauterine growth restriction (IUGR) results in a reduced nephron endowment[58–62] and is linked to subsequent renal dysfunction.[9,58,63–66] The number of nephrons formed during nephrogenesis in early life determines the lifelong functional capacity of the kidney; there have been a multitude of experimental studies (in many species) showing that the number of nephrons formed within the kidney is directly proportional to kidney size at birth but may not be consistent in fetuses that have been growth-restricted late in gestation (when nephrogenesis is completed).[17,62,67,68] IUGR is often a comorbidity of preterm birth; it is linked to the cause of spontaneous preterm birth, and is also a common cause of interventional preterm delivery, which is required to facilitate infant survival.[69] Of greatest concern, newborns who are born both prematurely and IUGR are at a high risk of infant morbidity and mortality.[70–73] Long-term studies in children and adults have found that individuals born both preterm and IUGR have an increased propensity for impaired kidney growth[28,59,74] and renal dysfunction,[75,76] compared with preterm individuals who were non-IUGR at birth. Besides impaired growth in utero, extrauterine growth restriction is a common sequela of preterm birth and has been shown to have a similarly adverse effect on renal function.[76]

CLINICAL SCENARIO 2

A woman presented to the antenatal clinic at 26+0 weeks' gestation and was found to have preeclampsia with BP of 140/95, an increased urate level, but at this stage, normal renal function and normal umbilical arterial Doppler results. She had a body mass index (calculated as weight in kilograms divided by the square of height in meters) of 40 and had insulin-requiring gestational diabetes. The estimated fetal weight was 660 g, which is on the 5th centile, with the fetal size at her 20-week morphology scan being on the 78th centile. She was admitted to the antenatal ward and commenced on oral antihypertensives (Labetalol 200 mg 8 hourly) and received antenatal steroids. Over the next 2 weeks, her BP became more difficult to control and she was on 2 antihypertensive medications on maximal doses (Labetalol, Methyldopa 250 mg 6 hourly). Her renal function began to deteriorate, and the umbilical arterial Doppler results were increased. At 28+4 weeks, she was given magnesium sulfate for fetal neuroprotection, and the female neonate was delivered by cesarean section with a birth weight of 720 g (10th centile). The placental histology confirmed uteroplacental insufficiency, with accelerated maturation, increased syncytial knot formation, and areas of infarction and chorangiosis.

Maternal Disease

Diabetes

This clinical scenario has become increasingly more frequent in infants born to mothers with maternal diseases.[77,78] With the increasing prevalence of obesity and associated type 2 diabetes in the United States and other developed countries, the incidence of maternal diabetes is increasing.[79] Intrauterine exposure to maternal diabetes can lead to either macrosomia or microsomia of the fetus.[80] Fetal macrosomia, specifically asymmetric macrosomia, results in exaggerated fetal growth in response to the increased supply of glucose and other nutrients across the placenta.[81] However, conversely, in the case of severe maternal diabetes, maternal complications such as vasculopathy and nephropathy may occur, which subsequently lead to IUGR of the developing fetus.

In addition, maternal diabetes has been shown to have other adverse effects on embryogenesis, which may further increase the risk of IUGR[82] and consequently increase the susceptibility of impaired nephrogenesis and renal injury in the neonatal period. For example, in a study of Pima Indians with type 2 diabetes,[83] there was found to be a strong association with renal dysfunction after birth; 58% of infants who were exposed to diabetes in utero showed 4 times higher urinary albumin excretion (albumin/creatinine ratio >30 mg/g), compared with unexposed infants. Other studies[84] have clearly shown a risk of renal malformations in infants born to diabetic mothers;

the estimated risk of delivering a child with renal agenesis/dysgenesis is more than 3 times greater for mothers with diabetes compared with nondiabetic mothers. Animal studies have further highlighted the adverse effects of intrauterine exposure to maternal diabetes on kidney development and function. In the mouse model,[82] a high-glucose intrauterine milieu led to significantly smaller body length, kidney size, and glomerular size, and a 40% reduction in nephron endowment compared with control offspring; the level of maternal hyperglycemia predicted the severity of the adverse effects on kidney size and on glomerular endowment. There was also evidence of glomerular collapse as a result of an increase in glomerular and tubular apoptotic events.[82] In follow-up studies,[85] 20-week-old mice offspring exposed to maternal diabetes were 20% lighter, with significantly increased urinary albumin excretion, glomerular hypertrophy, renal fibrosis, and an increased propensity for the development of hypertension.

Preeclampsia

Preeclampsia is known to be a major risk factor for fetal and neonatal mortality, IUGR, and preterm birth; maternal hypertension alone also increases risk, but to a lesser extent than preeclampsia.[86] Besides inducing growth restriction via impaired uteroplacental perfusion, preeclampsia also stimulates a proinflammatory, prooxidant and antiangiogenic intrauterine environment.[87] In animal models, this setting is known to lead to IUGR, decreased kidney size, hypertension, and impaired vascularization of the developing lung[88,89]; however, potential effects on the vascular development of other organs are unknown. Among children born preterm, maternal preeclampsia is an independent risk factor for the development of hypertension.[90]

CLINICAL SCENARIO 2 (CONTINUED)

This 28-week gestation baby required CPAP for 3 weeks, took 3 weeks to achieve full feeds, and went home at 40 weeks postconceptional age formula feeding weighing 3.1 kg (10th centile). Over the next 12 months, her weight gain increased significantly, such that her weight at 12 months of age was 11.4 kg (95th centile).

Obesity After Growth Restriction

The increasing epidemic of obesity worldwide has also seen a resultant increase in chronic renal failure,[91] and there is mounting evidence of the adverse effects of obesity on renal hemodynamics and structure.[92] The preterm infant has several early renal hits, which may compromise long-term renal function, and this is further compounded later in life by insults such as the induction of obesity; this supports the multihit nature of chronic renal disease.[93] Preterm birth and the associated renal risk factors outlined so far have the potential to significantly reduce nephron number. With the increased functional demands (as seen with obesity), there is likely to be accelerated onset and increased severity of renal disease when glomerular number (functional reserve) is low as a result of growth restriction early in life. A reduced nephron endowment subsequently leads to glomerular hypertrophy, and this is likely to be greatly accentuated when the functional demands on the kidneys are increased. Furthermore, the sustained glomerular hyperfiltration may lead to glomerular dysfunction and subsequent glomerular demise.[93] Supporting this theory, Abitbol and colleagues[94] have shown that obesity and preterm birth are additive risks in the progression of kidney disease in children.

Long-Term Consequences of Preterm Birth on the Kidney

As described, there are a multitude of factors associated with preterm birth that have the potential to impair renal development in the fetus or neonate. Impaired growth and a reduced nephron endowment are strongly linked to the later development of hypertension, glomerular injury, and renal dysfunction.[95,96] In this regard, there is now an increasing body of evidence supporting the hypothesis that preterm birth has long-term consequences for health; in particular, preterm birth has been strongly linked to increased hypertension risk in both children and adults.[97] In children born preterm, most studies have reported a reduction in kidney size compared with age-matched individuals born at term.[98–100] Zaffanello and colleagues[99] further reported a significantly decreased kidney size in children born at 26 to 28 weeks' gestation, compared with those born at 30 to 31 weeks' gestation, indicating that the severity of prematurity has an important effect on kidney growth. Only 1 study has examined the effect of preterm birth on kidney size in adulthood. In this study, Keijzer-Veen and colleagues[101] found that at 20 years of age, after preterm birth at less than 32 weeks' gestation, female adults had a significantly decreased kidney length and volume (both absolute and relative) compared with individuals born at term.

However, findings from the few studies to have examined long-term renal function after preterm birth are less conclusive. Rodriguez-Soriano and colleagues[102] and Iacobelli and colleagues[103] showed that GFR was significantly reduced in preterm-born children compared with term controls, with impairments in electrolyte excretion

Table 1
Potential causes of renal impairment in preterm neonates and potential minimization strategies

	Potential Minimization Strategies
Prenatal Factors	
FGR	Use of aspirin, clexane in early pregnancy for past history of FGR in previous pregnancies to improve placentation and reduce risk of FGR
Maternal disease (hypertension, diabetes)	Close monitoring, evidence still to be determined as to ideal target ranges for BP and blood glucose levels for optimal fetal growth
Antenatal steroids	Antenatal steroids for women at high risk of preterm delivery, not to be used just in case (ie, twin pregnancy, judicious use of multiple courses)
Chorioamnionitis	None apparent at this time
Postnatal Factors	
Increased functional demand because of premature delivery	Physiologic change which must occur for ex utero life, careful fluid balance, and BP observation
Nephrotoxic drugs	Minimize use of gentamicin, vancomycin, indomethacin. Ensure staff are aware of total gentamicin days, and use other antibiotics if further septic episodes occur
Postnatal growth failure	Careful attention to nutritional requirements, ensure adequate caloric and protein content
Acute kidney injury	Careful attention to aseptic techniques with central lines and feeding regimens to minimize sepsis/necrotizing enterocolitis, which may result in acute kidney injury with early diagnosis and initiation of management strategies

Abbreviation: FGR, fetal growth restriction.

also evident. In children examined at 6 to 8 years of age, Iacobelli and colleagues[103] also found microalbuminuria in 8.3% of the preterm children. In contrast, other studies in children[98,105] and young adults[104,106] born preterm reported no difference in renal function compared with term controls. However, survival after extremely preterm birth is a relatively recent phenomenon. Hence, it is likely that as the increasing population worldwide of survivors of very and extremely preterm birth reach middle and older age, the adverse long-term consequences of preterm birth will become increasingly evident. We need to continue to look carefully at the evidence available and try to minimize known potential adverse effects on the developing kidney (**Table 1**) as well as pursuing further research in this arena to prevent long-term health sequelae.

SUMMARY

The early life environment, as first postulated by Barker,[107] has the potential to influence future cardiovascular health risks. The developing kidney of the preterm infant may be affected by several in utero and neonatal insults that may influence nephrogenesis, resulting in reduced functional nephron number at the beginning of life. This reduction in nephron number may lead to vulnerability to hypertension in adulthood, increasing cardiovascular risks for myocardial infarction and stroke, as well as impaired renal function. Ongoing research is required into the potential risks to nephrogenesis, along with ways to minimize harm and maximize nephron number and function in preterm neonates to reduce the risk of long-term renal and cardiovascular sequelae.

REFERENCES

1. Mueller-Heubach E, Rubinstein DN, Schwarz SS. Histologic chorioamnionitis and preterm delivery in different patient populations. Obstet Gynecol 1990; 75(4):622–6.
2. Goldenberg RL, Hauth JC, Andrews WW. Intrauterine infection and preterm delivery. N Engl J Med 2000;342(20):1500–7.
3. Gantert M, Been JV, Gavilanes AW, et al. Chorioamnionitis: a multiorgan disease of the fetus. J Perinatol 2010;30(Suppl 1):s21–30.
4. Kallapur SJ, Jobe AH. Contribution of inflammation to lung injury and development. Arch Dis Child Fetal Neonatal Ed 2006;91:F132–5.
5. De Felice C, Toti P, Laurini RN, et al. Early neonatal brain injury in histologic chorioamnionitis. J Pediatr 2001;138(1):101–4.
6. Toti P, De Felice C, Stumpo M, et al. Acute thymic involution in fetuses and neonates with chorioamnionitis. Hum Pathol 2000;31(9):1121–8.
7. Kunzmann S, Glogger K, Been JV, et al. Thymic changes after chorioamnionitis induced by intraamniotic lipopolysaccharide in fetal sheep. Am J Obstet Gynecol 2010;190:e471–9.
8. Galinsky R, Moss TJ, Gubhaju L, et al. Effect of intra-amniotic lipopolysaccharide on nephron number in preterm fetal sheep. Am J Physiol Renal Physiol 2011;301(2):F280–5.
9. Brenner B, Garcia D, Anderson S. Glomeruli and blood pressure. Less of one, more the other? Am J Hypertens 1988;1(4 Pt 1):335–47.
10. Rodríguez MM, Gómez AH, Abitbol CL, et al. Histomorphometric analysis of postnatal glomerulogenesis in extremely preterm infants. Pediatr Dev Pathol 2004;7(1):17–25.
11. Hoy WE, Hughson MD, Bertram JF, et al. Nephron number, hypertension, renal disease, and renal failure. J Am Soc Nephrol 2005;16(9):2557–64.

12. Zandi-Nejad K, Luyckx V, Brenner B. Adult hypertension and kidney disease: the role of fetal programming. Hypertension 2006;47(3):502–8.
13. Nehiri T, Duong Van Huyen JP, Viltard M, et al. Exposure to maternal diabetes induces salt-sensitive hypertension and impairs renal function in adult rat offspring. Diabetes 2008;57(8):2167–75.
14. Gray IP, Cooper PA, Cory BJ, et al. The intrauterine environment is a strong determinant of glucose tolerance during the neonatal period, even in prematurity. J Clin Endocrinol Metab 2002;87(9):4252–6.
15. Ryan D, Atik A, De Matteo R, et al. Chronic intrauterine exposure to endotoxin does not alter fetal nephron number or glomerular size. Clin Exp Pharmacol Physiol 2013;40(11):789–94.
16. Jahnukainen T, Chen M, Berg U, et al. Antenatal glucocorticoids and renal function after birth. Semin Neonatol 2001;6(4):351–5.
17. Gubhaju L, Sutherland MR, Yoder BA, et al. Is nephrogenesis affected by preterm birth? Studies in a non-human primate model. Am J Physiol Renal Physiol 2009;297(6):F1668–77.
18. Celsi G, Kistner A, Aizman R, et al. Prenatal dexamethasone causes oligonephronia, sodium retention, and higher blood pressure in offspring. Pediatr Res 1998;44:317–22.
19. Ortiz LA, Quan A, Weinberg A, et al. Effect of prenatal dexamethasone on rat renal development. Kidney Int 2001;59(5):1663–9.
20. Ortiz LA, Quan A, Zarzar F, et al. Prenatal dexamethasone programs hypertension and renal injury in the rat. Hypertension 2003;41(2):328–34.
21. Wintour EM, Moritz KM, Johnson K, et al. Reduced nephron number in adult sheep, hypertensive as a result of prenatal glucocorticoid treatment. J Physiol 2003;549(Pt 3):929–35.
22. de Vries WB, van den Borne P, Goldschmeding R, et al. Neonatal dexamethasone treatment in the rat leads to kidney damage in adulthood. Pediatr Res 2010;67(1):72–6.
23. Aperia A, Broberger O, Elinder G, et al. Postnatal development of renal function in pre-term and full-term infants. Acta Paediatr Scand 1981;70(2):183–7.
24. Tsukahara H, Fujii Y, Tsuchida S, et al. Renal handling of albumin and beta-2-microglobulin in neonates. Nephron 1994;68(2):212–6.
25. Walker MW, Clark RH, Spitzer AR. Elevation in plasma creatinine and renal failure in premature neonates without major anomalies: terminology, occurrence and factors associated with increased risk. J Perinatol 2011;31(3):199–205.
26. Kent AL, Jyoti R, Robertson C, et al. Does extreme prematurity affect kidney volume at term corrected age? J Matern Fetal Neonatal Med 2009;22(5):435–8.
27. Schmidt IM, Chellakooty M, Boisen KA, et al. Impaired kidney growth in low-birth-weight children: distinct effects of maturity and weight for gestational age. Kidney Int 2005;68(2):731–40.
28. Drougia A, Giapros V, Hotoura E, et al. The effects of gestational age and growth restriction on compensatory kidney growth. Nephrol Dial Transplant 2009;24(1):142–8.
29. Huang HP, Tsai IJ, Lai YC, et al. Early postnatal renal growth in premature infants. Nephrology (Carlton) 2007;12(6):572–5.
30. Kandasamy Y, Smith R, Wright IM, et al. Extra-uterine renal growth in preterm infants: oligonephropathy and prematurity. Pediatr Nephrol 2013;28(9):1791–6.
31. Sutherland MR, Gubhaju L, Moore L, et al. Accelerated maturation and abnormal morphology in the preterm neonatal kidney. J Am Soc Nephrol 2011;22(7):1365–74.

32. Gubhaju L, Sutherland MR, Black MJ. Preterm birth and the kidney: implications for long-term renal health. Reprod Sci 2011;18(4):322–33.

33. Stelloh C, Allen KP, Mattson DL, et al. Prematurity in mice leads to reduction in nephron number, hypertension, and proteinuria. Transl Res 2012;159(2): 80–9.

34. Schreuder MF, Bueters RR, Huigen MC, et al. Effect of drugs on renal development. Clin J Am Soc Nephrol 2011;6(1):212–7.

35. Cullen L, Young R, Bertram J. Studies on the effects of gentamicin on rat metanephric development in vitro. Nephrology 2000;5:115–23.

36. Gilbert T, Gaonach S, Moreau E, et al. Defect of nephrogenesis induced by gentamicin in rat metanephric organ culture. Lab Invest 1994;70:656–66.

37. Gilbert T, Lelievre-Pegorier M, Merlet-Benichou C. Immediate and long-term renal effects of fetal exposure to gentamicin. Pediatr Nephrol 1990;4:445–50.

38. Gilbert T, Lelievre-Pegorier M, Malienou R, et al. Effects of prenatal and postnatal exposure to gentamicin on renal differentiation in the rat. Toxicology 1987;43(3):301–13.

39. Mallie JP, Gerard H, Gerard A. In-utero gentamicin-induced nephrotoxicity in rats. Pediatr Pharmacol (New York) 1986;5(4):229–39.

40. Nagai J, Takano M. Molecular aspects of renal handling of aminoglycosides and strategies for preventing the nephrotoxicity. Drug Metab Pharmacokinet 2004; 19(3):159–70.

41. Giapros V, Andronikou SK, Cholevas VI, et al. Renal function and effect of aminoglycoside therapy during the first ten days of life. Pediatr Nephrol 2003;18: 46–52.

42. Giapros VI, Andronikou SK, Cholevas VI, et al. Acute effects of gentamicin on glomerular and tubular functions in preterm neonates. Pediatr Nephrol 2006; 21(10):1389–92.

43. Langhendries JP, Battisti O, Bertrand J. Aminoglycoside nephrotoxicity and urinary excretion of N-acetyl-beta-D-glucosaminidase. Biol Neonate 1988;53: 253–9.

44. Nathanson S, Moreau E, Merlet-Benichou C, et al. In utero and in vitro exposure to beta-lactams impair kidney development in the rat. J Am Soc Nephrol 2000; 11(5):874–84.

45. Sáez F, Reverte V, Salazar F, et al. Hypertension and sex differences in the age-related renal changes when cyclooxygenase-2 activity is reduced during nephrogenesis. Hypertension 2009;53(2):331–7.

46. Kömhoff M, Wang JL, Cheng HF, et al. Cyclooxygenase-2-selective inhibitors impair glomerulogenesis and renal cortical development. Kidney Int 2000; 57(2):414–22.

47. Olliges A, Wimmer S, Nusing RM. Defects in mouse nephrogenesis induced by selective and non-selective cyclooxygenase-2 inhibitors. Br J Pharmacol 2011; 163(5):927–36.

48. Norwood VF, Morham SG, Smithies O. Postnatal development and progression of renal dysplasia in cyclooxygenase-2 null mice. Kidney Int 2000;58(6): 2291–300.

49. Kaplan BS, Restaino I, Raval DS, et al. Renal failure in the neonate associated with in utero exposure to non-steroidal anti-inflammatory agents. Pediatr Nephrol 1994;8(6):700–4.

50. van der Heijden BJ, Carlus C, Narcy F, et al. Persistent anuria, neonatal death, and renal microcystic lesions after prenatal exposure to indomethacin. Am J Obstet Gynecol 1994;171(3):617–23.

51. Sener A, Smith FG. Glomerular and tubular responses to N(G)-nitro-L-arginine methyl ester are age dependent in conscious lambs. Am J Physiol Regul Integr Comp Physiol 2002;282(5):R1512–20.
52. Keller RL, Tacy TA, Fields S, et al. Combined treatment with a nonselective nitric oxide synthase inhibitor (l-NMMA) and indomethacin increases ductus constriction in extremely premature newborns. Pediatr Res 2005;58(6): 1216–21.
53. Kang NS, Yoo KH, Cheon H, et al. Indomethacin treatment decreases renal blood flow velocity in human neonates. Biol Neonate 1999;76(5):261–5.
54. Kent AL, Brown L, Broom M, et al. Increased urinary podocytes following indomethacin suggests drug-induced glomerular injury. Pediatr Nephrol 2012;27(7): 1111–7.
55. Kent AL, Maxwell LE, Koina ME, et al. Renal glomeruli and tubular injury following indomethacin, ibuprofen, and gentamicin exposure in a neonatal rat model. Pediatr Res 2007;62(3):307–12.
56. Sutherland MR, Yoder BA, McCurnin D, et al. Effects of ibuprofen treatment on the developing preterm baboon kidney. Am J Physiol Renal Physiol 2012; 302(10):F1286–92.
57. Kent AL, Douglas-Denton R, Shadbolt B, et al. Indomethacin, ibuprofen and gentamicin administered during late stages of glomerulogenesis do not reduce glomerular number at 14 days of age in the neonatal rat. Pediatr Nephrol 2009; 24(6):1143–9.
58. Hinchliffe SA, Lynch MR, Sargent PH, et al. The effect of intrauterine growth retardation on the development of renal nephrons. Br J Obstet Gynaecol 1992;99:296–301.
59. Mañalich R, Reyes L, Herrera M, et al. Relationship between weight at birth and the number and size of renal glomeruli in humans: a histomorphometric study. Kidney Int 2000;58:770–3.
60. Zimanyi MA, Denton KM, Forbes JM, et al. A developmental nephron deficit in rats is associated with increased susceptibility to a secondary renal injury due to advanced glycation end-products. Diabetologia 2006;49(4):801–10.
61. Makrakis J, Zimanyi MA, Black MJ. Retinoic acid enhances nephron endowment in rats exposed to maternal protein restriction. Pediatr Nephrol 2007;22(11): 1861–7.
62. Zohdi V, Moritz KM, Bubb KJ, et al. Nephrogenesis and the renal renin-angiotensin system in fetal sheep: effects of intrauterine growth restriction during late gestation. Am J Physiol Regul Integr Comp Physiol 2007;293(3): R1267–73.
63. Brenner BM, Chertow GM. Congenital oligonephropathy and the etiology of adult hypertension and progressive renal injury. Am J Kidney Dis 1994;23(2): 171–5.
64. Merlet-Bénichou C, Gilbert T, Muffat-Joly M, et al. Intrauterine growth retardation leads to a permanent nephron deficit in the rat. Pediatr Nephrol 1994;8(2): 175–80.
65. Bassan H, Trejo LL, Kariv N, et al. Experimental intrauterine growth retardation alters renal development. Pediatr Nephrol 2000;15:192–5.
66. White SL, Perkovic V, Cass A, et al. Is low birth weight an antecedent of CKD in later life? A systematic review of observational studies. Am J Kidney Dis 2009; 54(2):248–61.
67. Gubhaju L, Black MJ. The baboon as a good model for studies of human kidney development. Pediatr Res 2005;58(3):505–9.

68. Sutherland MR, Gubhaju L, Yoder BA, et al. The effects of postnatal retinoic acid administration on nephron endowment in the preterm baboon kidney. Pediatr Res 2009;65(4):397–402.

69. Diderholm B. Perinatal energy metabolism with reference to IUGR and SGA: studies in pregnant women and newborn infants. Indian J Med Res 2009;130: 612–7.

70. Behrman RE, Lees MH, Peterson EN, et al. Distribution of the circulation in the normal and asphyxiated fetal primate. Am J Obstet Gynecol 1970;108(6): 956–69.

71. Lang U, Baker RS, Braems G, et al. Uterine blood flow–a determinant of fetal growth. Eur J Obstet Gynecol Reprod Biol 2003;110(Suppl 1):S55–61.

72. Kiserud T. Physiology of the fetal circulation. Semin Fetal Neonatal Med 2005; 10(6):493–503.

73. Cox B, Kotlyar M, Evangelou AI, et al. Comparative systems biology of human and mouse as a tool to guide the modeling of human placental pathology. Mol Syst Biol 2009;5:279.

74. Woods L, Weeks D, Rasch R. Programming of adult blood pressure by maternal protein restriction: role of nephrogenesis. Kidney Int 2004;65(4):1339–48.

75. Keijzer-Veen MG, Schrevel M, Finken MJ, et al, Dutch POPS-19 Collaborative Study Group. Microalbuminuria and lower glomerular filtration rate at young adult age in subjects born very premature and after intrauterine growth retardation. J Am Soc Nephrol 2005;16(9):2762–8.

76. Bacchetta J, Harambat J, Dubourg L, et al. Both extrauterine and intrauterine growth restriction impair renal function in children born very preterm. Kidney Int 2009;76(4):445–52.

77. Poston L. Intergenerational transmission of insulin resistance and type 2 diabetes. Prog Biophys Mol Biol 2011;106(1):315–22.

78. Boney CM, Verma A, Tucker R, et al. Metabolic syndrome in childhood: association with birth weight, maternal obesity, and gestational diabetes mellitus. Pediatrics 2005;115(3):e290–6.

79. Kim SY, England JL, Sharma JA, et al. Gestational diabetes mellitus and risk of childhood overweight and obesity in offspring: a systematic review. Exp Diabetes Res 2011;2011:541308.

80. Aerts L, Holemans K, Van Assche FA. Maternal diabetes during pregnancy: consequences for the offspring. Diabetes Metab Rev 1990;6(3):147–67.

81. Van Assche FA, Holemans K, Aerts L. Long-term consequences for offspring of diabetes during pregnancy. Br Med Bull 2001;60:173–82.

82. Tran S, Chen YW, Chenier I, et al. Maternal diabetes modulates renal morphogenesis in offspring. J Am Soc Nephrol 2008;19(5):943–52.

83. Nelson RG, Morgenstern H, Bennet PH. Intrauterine diabetes exposure and the risk of renal disease in diabetic Pima Indians. Diabetes 1998;47:1489–93.

84. Davis EM, Peck JD, Thompson D, et al. Maternal diabetes and renal agenesis/dysgenesis. Birth Defects Res 2010;88:722–7.

85. Chen YW, Chenier I, Tran S, et al. Maternal diabetes programs hypertension and kidney injury in offspring. Pediatr Nephrol 2010;25(7):1319–29.

86. Villar J, Carroli G, Wojdyla D, et al, World Health Organization Antenatal Care Trial Research Group. Preeclampsia, gestational hypertension and intrauterine growth restriction, related or independent conditions? Am J Obstet Gynecol 2006;194(4):921–31.

87. Suppo de Souza Rugolo LM, Bentlin MR, Trindade CE. Preeclampsia: effect on the fetus and newborn. Neo Reviews 2011;12:e198–206.

88. Alexander BT. Placental insufficiency leads to development of hypertension in growth-restricted offspring. Hypertension 2003;41(3):457–62.
89. Tang JR, Karumanchi SA, Seedorf G, et al. Excess soluble vascular endothelial growth factor receptor-1 in amniotic fluid impairs lung growth in rats: linking pre-eclampsia with bronchopulmonary dysplasia. Am J Physiol Lung Cell Mol Physiol 2012;302(1):L36–46.
90. Vohr BR, Allan W, Katz KH, et al. Early predictors of hypertension in prematurely born adolescents. Acta Paediatr 2010;99(12):1812–8.
91. Ejerblad E, Fored CM, Lindblad P, et al. Obesity and risk for chronic renal failure. J Am Soc Nephrol 2006;17:1695–702.
92. Mallamaci F, Tripepi G. Obesity and CKD progression: hard facts on fat CKD patients. Nephrol Dial Transplant 2013;28(Suppl 4):iv105–8.
93. Nenov VD, Taal MW, Sakharova OV, et al. Multi-hit nature of chronic renal disease. Curr Opin Nephrol Hypertens 2000;9:85–97.
94. Abitbol CL, Chandar J, Rodriguez MM, et al. Obesity and preterm birth: additive risks in the progression of kidney disease in children. Pediatr Nephrol 2009; 24(7):1363–70.
95. Hoy WE, Bertram JF, Denton RD, et al. Nephron number, glomerular volume, renal disease and hypertension. Curr Opin Nephrol Hypertens 2008;17(3): 258–65.
96. Luyckx VA, Bertram JF, Brenner BM, et al. Effect of fetal and child health on kidney development and long-term risk of hypertension and kidney disease. Lancet 2013;382(9888):273–83.
97. Sutherland MR, Bertagnolli M, Lukaszewski MA, et al. Preterm birth and hypertension risk: the oxidative stress paradigm. Hypertension 2014;63(1):12–8.
98. Rakow A, Johansson S, Legnevall L, et al. Renal volume and function in school-age children born preterm or small for gestational age. Pediatr Nephrol 2008; 23(8):1309–15.
99. Zaffanello M, Brugnara M, Bruno C, et al. Renal function and volume of infants born with a very low birth-weight: a preliminary cross-sectional study. Acta Paediatr 2010;99(8):1192–8.
100. Kwinta P, Klimek M, Drozdz D, et al. Assessment of long-term renal complications in extremely low birth weight children. Pediatr Nephrol 2011;26(7): 1095–103.
101. Keijzer-Veen MG, Devos AS, Meradji M, et al. Reduced renal length and volume 20 years after very preterm birth. Pediatr Nephrol 2010;25:499–507.
102. Rodríguez-Soriano J, Aguirre M, Oliveros R, et al. Long-term renal follow-up of extremely low birth weight infants. Pediatr Nephrol 2005;20:579–84.
103. Iacobelli S, Loprieno S, Bonsante F, et al. Renal function in early childhood in very low birthweight infants. Am J Perinatol 2007;24(10):587–92.
104. Keijzer-Veen MG, Kleinveld HA, Lequin MH, et al. Renal function and size at young adult age after intrauterine growth restriction and very premature birth. Am J Kidney Dis 2007;50(4):542–51.
105. Vanpée M, Blennow M, Linné T, et al. Renal function in very low birth weight infants: normal maturity reached during early childhood. J Pediatr 1992; 121(5 Pt 1):784–8.
106. Kistner A, Celsi G, Vanpee M, et al. Increased blood pressure but normal renal function in adult women born preterm. Pediatr Nephrol 2000;15(3–4):215–20.
107. Barker DJP, Osmond C. Infant mortality, childhood, nutrition, and ischaemic heart disease in England and Wales. Lancet 1986;1(8489):1077–81.

Electrolyte Disorders

Detlef Bockenhauer, MD, PhD[a],*, Jakub Zieg, MD, PhD[b]

KEYWORDS

- Electrolyte disorders • Hyponatremia • Hypernatremia • Hypokalemia
- Hyperkalemia • Newborn • Renal physiology

KEY POINTS

- Electrolyte homoeostasis is maintained by the kidneys.
- Disorders of plasma sodium commonly reflect disorders of water.
- Sodium handling by the kidneys is determined by volume homeostasis rather than plasma sodium.
- Volume (ie, sodium) homeostasis and potassium homeostasis are interdependent.
- Low glomerular filtration rate and tubular immaturity contribute to an increased frequency of electrolyte abnormalities in the neonatal period.

INTRODUCTION

The evolution of life started in the sea, which contained a steady concentration of salts. The function of living cells is thus critically dependent on a constant electrolyte composition, and the evolution of life on land was only possible because of the development of kidneys, which provided this constant "internal milieu."[1] Disorders in the electrolyte composition of this milieu thus can have serious consequences and are associated with morbidity and mortality.[2] Abnormalities of plasma sodium and potassium are a frequent occurrence in neonates, especially in the neonatal intensive care unit (NICU). To provide adequate treatment, it is important to understand the underlying problem and physiology.[3] For instance, a common response to hyponatremia is to increase sodium supplementation. Yet most patients with hyponatremia do not have a sodium deficiency, but water excess. Increasing sodium administration in these patients may correct the hyponatremia but will result in volume overload, which has serious risks in the neonatal period, such as patent ductus arteriosus, bronchopulmonary dysplasia, and necrotizing enterocolitis.[4–6]

Disclosures: None.
[a] UCL Institute of Child Health, Great Ormond Street Hospital for Children NHS Foundation Trust, Nephrology Unit, 30 Guilford Street, London WC1 3EH, UK; [b] Department of Pediatrics, 2nd Faculty of Medicine, Charles University in Prague and Motol University Hospital, V Úvalu 84, 15006 Praha 5, Czech Republic
* Corresponding author.
E-mail address: d.bockenhauer@ucl.ac.uk

This article reviews the physiology of renal water and electrolyte handling with respect to dysnatremias and dyskalemias in the context of the special circumstances of the transition from intrauterine to extrauterine life. In addition, some rare inherited disorders associated with neonatal electrolyte abnormalities are discussed.

Basics of Renal Water and Electrolyte Handling

In an average adult (surface area 1.73 m^2) with a glomerular filtration rate (GFR) of 100 mL/min, the kidneys produce 144 L of primary filtrate a day. Assuming a sodium and potassium concentration of 140 and 4 mmol/L, respectively, these 144 L contain approximately 20,000 mmol of sodium and 500 mmol of potassium. While most (60%–80%) of this is reabsorbed isotonically in the proximal tubule, there is still a large volume of water, sodium, and potassium delivered to the distal tubule, where decisions can then be made about either reabsorption or excretion. Urine osmolality can range from less than 50 to greater than 1000 mOsm/kg, so that, depending on intake and extrarenal losses, urine output can vary roughly between 500 mL and 20 L per day. Similarly, tubular sodium reabsorption can be adjusted so that sodium excretion may range from less than 10 to greater than 1000 mmol per day.[7] Potassium can even be secreted, so that potassium excretion may exceed the filtered amount.[8] Thus with normal kidney function renal water, sodium, and potassium excretion can be adjusted over a very wide range to provide homeostasis even under extreme circumstances. However, with decreased GFR the ability of the kidneys to maintain volume and electrolyte homeostasis diminishes, so that abnormalities can occur more easily.

The Special Circumstances of the Neonatal Kidney

Although the same physiologic principles apply to neonatal and adult kidneys, there are some important differences in the ability to maintain water and electrolyte homeostasis.

- *Neonatal kidneys have a low GFR.* GFR measured by creatinine clearance in preterm infants from 27 to 31 weeks of gestation without apparent kidney disease can be lower than 10 mL/min/1.73 m^2 in the first week of life, only increasing to greater than 15.5 mL/min/1.73 m^2 by 4 weeks of life.[9]
- *Urinary concentrating ability is not fully developed until about 1 year of age.* In fact, all neonates have a degree of physiologic nephrogenic diabetes insipidus, so that maximal urine concentration may not exceed 300 mOsm/kg, even in a term neonate.[10,11] It is because of this decreased urinary concentrating capacity that normal saline, which is commonly recommended as the basic intravenous fluid solution in older children,[12] is not suitable in the NICU, as it typically will be hypertonic in comparison with the baby's urine and thus may lead to hypernatremia.

The impaired ability of the neonatal, and especially premature kidneys to maintain electrolyte homeostasis is also reflected in the wider reference range for plasma electrolytes. For instance, plasma sodium levels between 125 and 150 mmol/L are usually considered normal in this age group.[13] This relative instability is further compounded by some factors specific to the transition from intrauterine to extrauterine life and the early neonatal period:

- *Extrarenal water losses are increased* because of the greater ratio of surface area to body mass, and will be further increased by the use of radiant heaters and ultraviolet therapy. Moreover, immature skin is more permeable to water, probably because of higher expression of water channels (aquaporins).[14,15]

- *The composition and distribution of body water changes with gestation.* At 23 weeks, water makes up 90% of body weight, with two-thirds in the extracellular fluid (ECF) and one-third in the intracellular fluid (ICF). At term 75% of body weight is water, and this is now roughly equally distributed between ECF and ICF, whereas in an adult, water makes up approximately 60% of body weight with one-third in ECF and two-thirds in ICF.[16,17] Thus there is a marked contraction of the ECF in the third trimester and the neonatal period, which is reflected in the physiologic weight loss that newborns normally experience.

Considering all of these circumstances, it is easy to understand that electrolyte abnormalities can easily occur in the NICU.

DYSNATREMIAS

Abnormalities of plasma sodium are probably the most common electrolyte disorder encountered in neonates. Nevertheless they are associated with serious morbidity, including a poorer long-term neurologic outcome.[13]

There are technical obstacles to accurate measurement of the serum sodium. Most laboratories measure sodium using a so-called indirect ion-selective electrode.[3] Using this method, the sample is diluted to maximize sample volume and minimize interference from plasma proteins. The formula used to calculate plasma sodium concentration from the activity of sodium ions in the sample assumes that water comprises 93% of plasma volume, but this assumption fails in plasma samples with abnormal protein or lipid content, the so-called ion-exclusion effect.[18] This process leads to the well-recognized phenomenon of pseudohyponatremia in lipemic samples or those with excess protein content. However, the converse is also true: in samples with low protein content, the sodium concentration is overestimated, leading to pseudonormonatremia or pseudohypernatremia.[19] In one study, hypoproteinemia was present in almost 60% of plasma samples obtained in the NICU and led to an overestimation of the sodium concentration by greater than 3 mmol/L in about one-third of all samples, and on some occasions by more than 10 mmol/L, when compared with the measurement with a direct ion-selective electrode, which is not susceptible to this ion-exclusion effect.[20] This finding needs to be considered when assessing a plasma sodium result from a hypoproteinemic neonate, and it is important to remember that the point-of-care analyzers often present in the NICU do not use the indirect method. Thus, results from these analyzers are likely to be more accurate in samples with abnormal protein content than in those obtained in the main laboratory.[20]

HYPONATREMIA

When faced with a low plasma sodium result, the first consideration should be the patient: if the patient is seizing and the sodium is substantially lower than in previous results, the result is likely real and emergency treatment with hypertonic saline should be instigated. If the patient is stable, there is time for a careful assessment:

- Is this true or pseudohyponatremia? (See ion-exclusion effect)
- What is the cause of the hyponatremia?

How to Assess the Cause of True Hyponatremia

The immediate first question should be: Is hyponatremia due to an excess of water or a deficiency of sodium?

Excess water is the most common cause (**Fig. 1**). In this case, weight and blood pressure are either stable or increased, and there is normal skin turgor and peripheral perfusion. Of course, owing to the special circumstances of the perinatal period, the weight is more difficult to interpret. A weight loss of 5% to 10% of body weight is physiologic and is expected in the first postnatal days. Thus, hyponatremia associated with this expected weight loss, and otherwise clinically normal volume status does not indicate hypovolemia and salt loss. Once the assessment of water excess versus salt loss has been made, biochemical evaluation of the urine can help delineate the etiology.

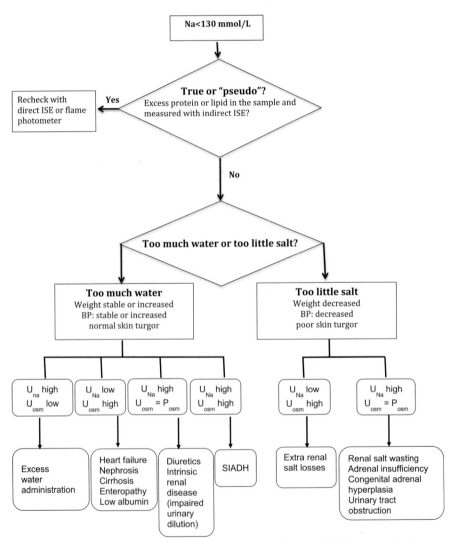

Fig. 1. Algorithm for the assessment of hyponatremia. After establishing that the hyponatremia is true and not a measurement artifact, the most important step is to determine whether the cause is an excess of water or a deficiency of salt. Once this distinction is made, urinary indices can help delineate the etiology. BP, blood pressure; ISE, ion-selective electrode; SIADH, syndrome of inappropriate diuretic hormone.

A key point to remember is that kidneys regulate sodium reabsorption to maintain volume homeostasis, but not to maintain a normal sodium concentration. There are no sodium sensors or osmosensors in the kidneys. Therefore, with excess water the kidneys will excrete sodium to restore euvolemia. For this reason, weight and blood pressure can be stable and not increased with water excess. Thus, an elevated urine sodium level does not necessarily indicate primary renal salt loss, but may be the appropriate physiologic response to water overload.

Interpretation of biochemical urinary indices is again more difficult in the NICU. The physiologic contraction of the extracellular fluid volume in the first days of life is associated with excretion of sodium. Moreover, as already discussed, maximal urinary concentration is impaired in neonates. A urine osmolality isotonic to plasma thus may reflect appropriate maximal concentration of immature kidneys, or may be pathologic. Therefore, making clear-cut isolated interpretations of urine biochemistries is difficult and sometimes impossible. Biochemical and clinical data (**Box 1**) need to be integrated to generate a reasonable diagnosis.

Treatment of Hyponatremia

Emergency treatment of hyponatremia in an acutely symptomatic child involves administration of salt, irrespective of the underlying cause. A commonly used protocol is a bolus of 2 mL/kg 3% NaCl, repeated as necessary.[21]

In the asymptomatic child, several options are available. In the case of water excess, the simplest treatment is to reduce the volume of water administered. The excess volume can be calculated: assuming a total body water content of 75% (this may be higher in premature babies, see earlier discussion), the excess volume is weight (kg) $\times$ 0.75 $\times$ (130 − observed Na)/130. Thus, a euvolemic 3-kg neonate with a sodium level of 120 mmol/L would be estimated to have 3 $\times$ 0.75 $\times$ 10/130 = 0.173 L excess water, and reduction of water administration by this amount over the next 24 to 48 hours would be expected to normalize plasma sodium to 130 mmol/L over the same time period, assuming that other factors, such as insensible water losses and urine output, remain unchanged. It is clear from this last statement that close observation is important for successful management.

Recently, antagonists for the type 2 vasopressin receptor AVPR2 have been introduced for the treatment of patients with hyponatremia caused by vasopressin excess.[22] However, no efficacy or toxicity data in neonates currently exist and, given the ease of control over fluid administration in the NICU and the impaired concentrating capacity of neonates, these drugs are unlikely to be used commonly in this setting.

Box 1
Clinical parameters for the assessment of dysnatremias

- Weight
- Blood pressure
- Skin turgor
- Peripheral perfusion
- Type and volume of administered fluids
- Insensible water losses (radiant warmer? Ultraviolet therapy?)
- Urine output
- Renal ultrasonography

For those patients presumed to have a sodium deficit, sodium supplementation is the correct treatment, and the sodium deficit can be calculated in similar fashion to water excess: weight [kg] $\times$ 0.75 $\times$ (130 $-$ observed Na). Thus, a hypovolemic 3-kg neonate with a sodium level of 120 mmol/L would be estimated to have 3 $\times$ 0.75 $\times$ 10 = 7.5 mmol sodium deficit, and administration of this amount over the next 24 to 48 hours would be expected to normalize plasma sodium to 130 mmol/L over the same time period, assuming that the other factors remain unchanged. In an asymptomatic child, slow correction of the plasma sodium concentration is generally advised because of concerns over osmotic demyelination, especially in chronic hyponatremia. An increase by not more than 10 mmol/L per day is generally considered safe.[23]

HYPERNATREMIA

The basic considerations in hypernatremia are the same as for hyponatremia. The sodium can be falsely high owing to low protein content of the plasma, and this can be verified by checking with a different method that is not prone to the ion-exclusion effect (see earlier discussion). If true, the next question is whether the high sodium reflects a deficiency in water or an excess of salt, and based on the clinical and biochemical data an underlying diagnosis can be made (**Fig. 2**). As with hyponatremia, the most common explanation for abnormal plasma sodium is a disorder of water, rather than sodium, but there are many hidden sources of sodium, mostly from line flushes and bronchial lavage with normal saline, or from medications, which may add up sufficiently to exceed renal excretory capacity and thus cause hypernatremia.[24]

A deficiency in water can occur, for instance, when insensible water losses are underestimated.

Treatment

The main concern in the treatment of hypernatremia is the development of cell swelling as plasma sodium decreases, resulting in cerebral edema. For this reason a slow correction, not exceeding 10 mmol/L per day, is generally advised. The same formulas listed under hyponatremia (see earlier discussion) can be used to estimate the water deficit or sodium excess, and water administration can be increased or sodium administration decreased accordingly.

DYSKALEMIAS

A few key facts on potassium are:

- It is the most abundant intracellular ion, and intracellular potassium concentration is usually between 100 and 150 mmol/L.
- It is a critical component for many cellular functions, including cell growth and division, DNA and protein synthesis, and many enzyme and transport processes.[25]
- Approximately 98% of total body potassium is in the ICF, especially in skeletal muscle, and thus only 2% is in the ECF, where it is accessible to routine clinical measurements.[26]
- The usual normal range in neonates is 4.0 to 6.5 mmol/L, and thus somewhat higher than in older children and adults.[27,28]
- The kidneys maintain potassium homeostasis by adjusting potassium excretion to intake. Approximately 90% of ingested potassium is absorbed and only about 5% to 10% of this is excreted via extrarenal pathways, mainly the gut, although this can increase substantially in renal failure.[29]

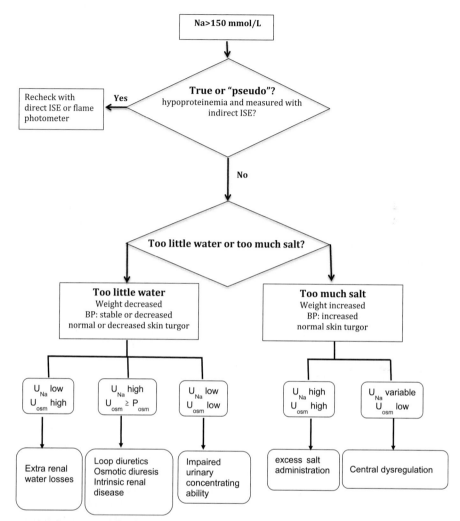

Fig. 2. Algorithm for the assessment of hypernatremia. After establishing that the hyperna-tremia is true and not a measurement artifact, the most important step is to determine whether the cause is a deficiency of water or an excess of salt. Once this distinction is made, urinary indices can help delineate the etiology.

- Neonates and infants maintain positive potassium balance to allow incorporation into cells newly formed during the period of somatic growth.[30]

Internal Potassium Balance

An important concept for the understanding and management of dyskalemia is the so-called internal potassium balance, which describes the ability of potassium to shift between the ICF and ECF.[31] Several factors affect this balance, including:

- Acid-base status, as acidosis leads to a shift out of the cells and vice versa in alkalosis.[32] A wide range of different transport processes is involved in this shift, which results in buffering of the acid-base abnormality by the cells.[33] In one study, a pH shift by 0.1 led to a change in plasma potassium by approximately 0.6 mmol (range 0.2–1.7).[34]

- Hormones and medications affect the activity of the cellular Na,K-ATPase, such as insulin, adrenalin, and drugs affecting the sympathetic nervous system and digitalis derivatives.[35]

Consequently, an important first assessment of dyskalemia is whether it is due to a disturbed internal balance (potassium shift) or external balance (imbalance between intake and output).

HYPOKALEMIA
Clinical Manifestations

Patients with mild hypokalemia are usually asymptomatic, but symptoms may occur with potassium levels less than 3 mmol/L. Symptoms may include muscle weakness, constipation, and ileus. With severe hypokalemia rhabdomyolysis, arrhythmias, and even cardiac or respiratory arrest have been reported.[36,37]

Clinical Assessment

As already discussed, an important consideration is whether the derangement reflects a change in the internal balance (and total body potassium is unaffected) or the external balance (altered intake or excretion). Clinical factors taken into this consideration are listed in **Box 2**.

An important initial consideration is the medication list. Many drugs commonly used in the NICU affect the internal potassium balance (eg, xanthines [theophylline, caffeine] and bronchodilators [β2-sympathomimetics]). Others increase urinary losses (eg, loop diuretics, amphotericin). A list of commonly used medications affecting potassium levels is given in **Table 1**.

In addition, there are some rare inherited disorders that can cause hypokalemia in the newborn, including neonatal Bartter syndrome (see later discussion), congenital adrenal hyperplasia (with salt retention), apparent mineralocorticoid excess, and congenital chloride-losing diarrhea.

In cases with disturbed external potassium balance (potassium loss), biochemical analysis of plasma and urine can help distinguish between renal and extrarenal potassium loss. Commonly used is the fractional excretion of potassium (FEK), with an FEK of greater than 15% usually considered suggestive of renal losses.[38] A more specific

---

Box 2
Clinical parameters for the assessment of dyskalemias

- Electrocardiography (T waves, U waves, QT interval)
- Acid-base status
- Plasma biochemistries (associated other electrolyte abnormality, kidney function, muscle enzymes in suspected rhabdomyolysis)
- Potassium intake (concentration in administered fluids and nutrition)
- Urinary potassium excretion (volume of urine and urinary potassium concentration)
- Extrarenal potassium losses (stool, nasogastric or other drainage)
- Medications
- Renal ultrasonography (nephrocalcinosis, obstruction)

| Table 1 |
| Medications associated with hypokalemia |

Internal Balance	Renal Excretion	Extrarenal Excretion
Insulin	Loop diuretics (eg, furosemide)	Laxatives
Xanthines (eg, caffeine, theophylline)	Thiazide diuretics	Exchange resins (eg, sodium or calcium polystyrene sulfate)
β2-Agonists (eg, adrenalin, salbutamol)	Carbonic anhydrase inhibitors (eg, acetazolamide)	
	Amphotericin	
	Foscarnet	
	Cisplatin	
	Aminoglycosides	
	Mineralocorticoids	

Data from Gennari FJ. Hypokalemia. N Engl J Med 1998;339(7):453.

way to assess potassium secretion in the collecting duct (see **Fig. 4** for the molecular basis) is the transtubular potassium gradient TTKG (**Box 3**).[39]

Treatment

Treatment of hypokalemia depends on the symptoms and the underlying etiology. In patients with disturbed internal balance, removal of the underlying cause (eg, discontinuation of medications causing potassium shift) will usually result in normalization of the plasma levels within hours.

In cases with disturbed external potassium balance and a true potassium deficit, potassium supplementation is usually commenced, ideally with removal of the underlying cause (eg, discontinuation of medications causing potassium wasting).

Urgent supplementation, such as infusion of 0.3 mmol/kg of potassium chloride over 1 hour, is usually only given in cases of severe symptomatic hypokalemia (eg, serious cardiac arrhythmias, respiratory depression). As rapid changes of plasma potassium concentration can lead to cardiac arrhythmia in itself, these patients should be monitored carefully. It is also important to recognize that potassium supplementation

---

Box 3
The transtubular potassium gradient TTKG

Calculating the TTKG is based on the idea that potassium concentration in the collecting duct can change primarily because of 2 factors:

1. Secretion of potassium

2. Extraction of water

It is calculated as follows: $(U_K/U_{osm})/(P_K/P_{osm})$

where U_K and P_K are urinary and plasma potassium concentration, respectively, and U_{osm} and P_{osm} are urinary and plasma osmolality.

The higher the TTKG, the more potassium is secreted in the collecting duct. A value of less than 2 is consistent with little to no secretion. Normal range for term newborns in one study was 5.65 to 18.22. TTKG in preterm neonates is usually lower, reflecting tubular immaturity.[40]

The TTKG is valid only during antidiuresis. Thus, if U_{osm} is less than P_{osm}, the TTKG is not useful, limiting its applicability in the NICU, given the physiologic concentrating defect of neonates.

in a patient with hypokalemia attributable to a shift in the internal balance can experience rebound hyperkalemia once the cause of the shift resolves.

HYPERKALEMIA

Hyperkalemia in newborns is defined as a plasma potassium concentration greater than 6.5 mmol/L. As with hypokalemia, a key concern is cardiac arrhythmia. In an asymptomatic patient, a first consideration should be whether this is true hyperkalemia or an artifact from hemolysis caused by traumatic phlebotomy (ie, from squeezing or prolonged application of a tourniquet).[41] An electrocardiogram can help assess the severity, with peaked T waves indicating true hyperkalemia.

Otherwise, the same considerations apply as in hypokalemia: is it a disturbance of the internal or external potassium balance? Presence of a metabolic acidosis or administration of medications such as digitalis would suggest disturbance of the internal balance. If the external balance is affected, assessment of urinary potassium excretion (see **Box 3**) can help distinguish between excess administration (FEK and TTKG high) and impaired elimination (FEK and TTKG low). An increased potassium load can also result from cellular lysis (eg, after an internal bleed, such as gastrointestinal or intraventricular hemorrhage). Premature babies are especially at risk of hyperkalemia because of their impaired potassium secretory ability reflecting tubular immaturity. Indeed, hyperkalemia is seen in more than 50% of extremely premature babies with a birth weight of less than 1000 g.[42]

Impaired kidney function is, of course, another important consideration in any patient with hyperkalemia. In addition, there are a few rare inherited diseases that can cause hyperkalemia, including pseudohypoaldosteronism type 1 (PHA1; see later discussion) and congenital adrenal hyperplasia (salt-wasting forms).

Treatment

Hyperkalemia-induced arrhythmias are a medical emergency. Treatment usually includes intravenous calcium salts to decrease myocyte excitability. In nonoliguric neonates, medications affecting internal potassium balance, including glucose with insulin and β-adrenergic agonists, seem preferable to rectal exchange resins for the treatment of acute hyperkalemia.[28] However, these resins are the only choice in oliguric neonates for long-term potassium removal apart from dialysis, although obstruction and intestinal necrosis have been reported.[43,44]

Nonacute treatment depends on the underlying etiology. Correction of an underlying acidosis or discontinuation of the causative medication (**Table 2**) is the obvious solution in many cases. Administration of loop diuretics can increase renal potassium excretion to help eliminate an acute potassium load.

INHERITED DISORDERS ASSOCIATED WITH ELECTROLYTE ABNORMALITIES

There are several inherited disorders that can affect electrolytes in the neonatal period, but 2 (Bartter syndrome and PHA1) are briefly discussed here, as they illuminate the underlying renal physiology of renal electrolyte handling, the understanding of which is important for any electrolyte disorder. For a more detailed discussion of these disorders, the interested reader is referred to more specific reviews.[38,45,46]

Bartter Syndrome

Bartter syndrome is primarily a disorder of salt reabsorption in the thick ascending loop of Henle.[38] Several genes have been associated with Bartter syndrome, but 3 are typically associated with antenatal presentation (**Fig. 3**): SLC12A1, encoding the

Table 2		
Medications associated with hyperkalemia		
Internal Balance	**Impaired Renal Excretion**	**Increased Potassium Load**
Digitalis	Angiotensin-converting enzyme inhibitors and angiotensin receptor blockers	Penicillin K
β2-Antagonists	Nonsteroidal anti-inflammatory drugs (indomethacin)	Stored packed red blood cells
ε-Aminocaproic acid	ENaC blocker (amiloride, triamterene)	
	Spironolactone	
	Antifungals (eg, ketoconazole)	
	Calcineurin inhibitors (eg, cyclosporine, tacrolimus)	
	Trimethoprim	
	Heparin	
	Pentamidine	

Data from Perazella MA. Drug-induced hyperkalemia: old culprits and new offenders. Am J Med 2000;109(4):308.

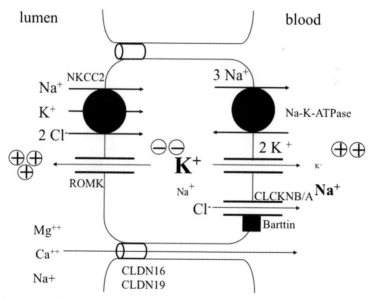

Fig. 3. An epithelial cell in the thick ascending limb. Sodium is reabsorbed together with potassium and chloride via the apical transporter NKCC2, the target of loop diuretics. Transport is facilitated by the action of the basolateral Na,K-ATPase, which creates the electrochemical gradient favoring sodium movement into the cell and also provides a basolateral exit for sodium. Chloride exits the cell via the basolateral chloride channels CLCKNA and CLCKNB. The function of NKCC2 is critically dependent on the availability of potassium, which is ensured through recycling of potassium via the potassium channel ROMK. This recycling of potassium across the apical membrane contributes to a lumen-positive transepithelial voltage, which enables reabsorption of calcium, magnesium, and sodium through a paracellular pathway lined by CLDN16 and CLDN19. ATPase, adenosine triphosphatase. (*Modified from* Kleta R, Bockenhauer D. Bartter syndromes and other salt-losing tubulopathies. Nephron Physiol 2006;104(2):75.)

target of loop diuretics, the $N^+-K^+-2Cl^-$ cotransporter NKCC2 (Bartter syndrome type 1), *KCNJ1*, encoding the potassium channel ROMK (Bartter syndrome type 2), and *BSND*, encoding the chloride channel subunit Barttin (Bartter syndrome type 4). Although there is a huge spectrum of clinical severity with each of these types, typical antenatal presentation manifests in utero with polyhydramnios, often requiring multiple amniocentesis to relieve the fluid load. The polyhydramnios reflects the polyuria of the fetus, the high salt content of which can be used diagnostically.[47] These salt and water losses continue immediately postnatally, and may necessitate supplementation of fluid of greater than 250 mL/kg/d and sodium chloride level of greater than 15 mmol/kg/d.[48] Typically associated with the polyuria is a hypokalemic metabolic alkalosis, which is due to highly elevated renin and aldosterone levels, reflecting the kidneys' attempt to salvage the salt not reabsorbed in the thick ascending limb by upregulating sodium reabsorption in the collecting duct. As sodium uptake in this segment is balanced by potassium and proton secretion (**Fig. 4**), the patient develops hypokalemia and metabolic alkalosis. Hypernatremia can also be present because of an often associated urinary concentrating defect.[49,50] Without adequate supplementation, affected neonates may develop severe dehydration and acute kidney injury, resulting in hyperkalemia and acidosis, and confusing the diagnostic picture. A history of polyhydramnios, although rarely due to Bartter syndrome, should nevertheless alert the clinician to this diagnostic possibility so that severe dehydration can be avoided.

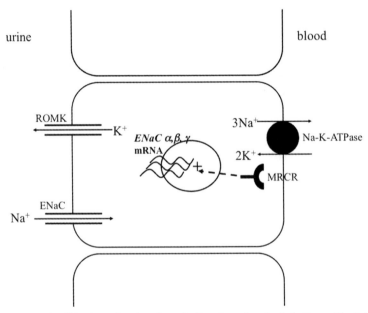

Fig. 4. A principal cell in the collecting duct. Sodium is reabsorbed via the epithelial sodium channel ENaC, expressed on the apical side. Uptake is facilitated by the action of the basolateral Na,K-ATPase, which creates the electrochemical gradient favoring sodium movement into the cell and also provides a basolateral exit for sodium. Electrical balance for sodium uptake can be provided by potassium secretion through the apical potassium channel ROMK or by proton secretion from neighboring intercalated cells (not shown). Thus, sodium (ie, volume) homeostasis is molecularly linked with potassium and acid-base homeostasis in this nephron segment. (*Adapted from* Kleta R, Bockenhauer D. Bartter syndromes and other salt-losing tubulopathies. Nephron Physiol 2006;104(2):78; with permission.)

Besides fluid and electrolyte supplementation, treatment of Bartter syndrome involves nonsteroidal anti-inflammatory drugs, such as indomethacin.[51] Although in some cases this has even been given antenatally, most neonatologists are hesitant to use this drug in the neonatal period owing to concerns of serious side effects, such as intestinal perforation and bleeding.[52,53]

Bartter syndrome type 2 can be an especially challenging diagnosis in the neonatal period, as the underlying protein, the potassium channel ROMK, is important not only for salt reabsorption in the thick ascending limb but also for potassium secretion in the collecting duct (see **Figs. 3** and **4**). Thus, these patients typically experience hyperkalemia in the first weeks of life, which slowly converts to hypokalemia, as other potassium channels start compensating for the lack of ROMK in the collecting duct.[54] In some cases, patients initially resemble the phenotype of PHA1 (see later discussion), with severe hyperkalemia, hyponatremia, and acidosis.[55]

Pseudohypoaldosteronism Type 1

PHA1 is primarily a disorder of salt reabsorption in the collecting duct, characterized by an inability of this segment to respond to aldosterone. One must distinguish a recessive form, due to loss-of-function mutations in genes encoding the epithelial sodium channel ENaC (see **Fig. 4**) from a dominant form, due to loss-of-function mutations in the gene encoding the mineralocorticoid receptor. The recessive form is more severe and can include extrarenal manifestation, such as cystic fibrosis-like lung disease, in addition to skin problems caused by expression of ENaC in these organs. The dominant form is milder, restricted to the kidney, and often improves spontaneously over time.[56] For this review, the renal features are of relevance: patients present with severe volume depletion, potentially life-threatening hyperkalemia (sometimes >10 mmol/L), moderate hyponatremia, and acidosis. This electrolyte constellation can be easily explained by the molecular characteristics of salt transport in the collecting duct (see **Fig. 4**): reabsorption of sodium occurs via ENaC, expressed in the principal cells of the collecting duct, but needs to be electrically balanced. This balance can occur by potassium secretion through ROMK, or by proton secretion from the neighboring intercalated cells. Thus sodium (ie, volume) homeostasis is molecularly coupled to potassium and acid-base homeostasis, and disturbance of one pathway automatically affects the others as well. Hyponatremia results from a combination of sodium loss and water retention, as hypovolemia leads to vasopressin-mediated urinary concentration.

REFERENCES

1. Smith HW. From fish to philosopher: the story of our internal environment. Summit (NJ): CIBA Pharmaceutical Products Inc; 1959.
2. Verbalis JG, Goldsmith SR, Greenberg A, et al. Diagnosis, evaluation, and treatment of hyponatremia: expert panel recommendations. Am J Med 2013; 126(10 Suppl 1):S1–42.
3. Bockenhauer D, Aitkenhead H. The kidney speaks: interpreting urinary sodium and osmolality. Arch Dis Child Educ Pract Ed 2011;96(6):223–7.
4. Bell EF, Warburton D, Stonestreet BS, et al. Effect of fluid administration on the development of symptomatic patent ductus arteriosus and congestive heart failure in premature infants. N Engl J Med 1980;302(11):598–604.
5. Bell EF, Warburton D, Stonestreet BS, et al. High-volume fluid intake predisposes premature infants to necrotising enterocolitis. Lancet 1979;2(8133):90.

6. Van Marter LJ, Pagano M, Allred EN, et al. Rate of bronchopulmonary dysplasia as a function of neonatal intensive care practices. J Pediatr 1992;120(6):938–46.
7. Weinstein AM. Sodium and chloride transport: proximal nephron. In: Alpern R, Caplan MJ, Moe OW, editors. Seldin and Giebisch's the kidney physiology & pathophysiology. 5th edition. London: Elsevier; 2012. p. 1081–142.
8. Giebisch G, Satlin LM. Regulation of potassium excretion. In: Alpern R, Caplan MJ, Moe OW, editors. Seldin and Giebisch's the kidney physiology & pathophysiology. 5th edition. London: Elsevier; 2012. p. 1659–716.
9. Vieux R, Hascoet JM, Merdariu D, et al. Glomerular filtration rate reference values in very preterm infants. Pediatrics 2010;125(5):e1186–92.
10. McCance RA. Renal function in early life. Physiol Rev 1948;28(3):331–48.
11. Winberg J. Determination of renal concentration capacity in infants and children without renal disease. Acta Paediatr 1958;48:318–28.
12. Moritz ML, Ayus JC. Prevention of hospital-acquired hyponatremia: a case for using isotonic saline. Pediatrics 2003;111(2):227–30.
13. Baraton L, Ancel PY, Flamant C, et al. Impact of changes in serum sodium levels on 2-year neurologic outcomes for very preterm neonates. Pediatrics 2009; 124(4):e655–61.
14. Agren J, Zelenin S, Hakansson M, et al. Transepidermal water loss in developing rats: role of aquaporins in the immature skin. Pediatr Res 2003;53(4):558–65.
15. Chiou YB, Blume-Peytavi U. Stratum corneum maturation. A review of neonatal skin function. Skin Pharmacol Physiol 2004;17(2):57–66.
16. Modi N, Betremieux P, Midgley J, et al. Postnatal weight loss and contraction of the extracellular compartment is triggered by atrial natriuretic peptide. Early Hum Dev 2000;59(3):201–8.
17. Hartnoll G, Betremieux P, Modi N. Body water content of extremely preterm infants at birth. Arch Dis Child Fetal Neonatal Ed 2000;83(1):F56–9.
18. Ladenson JH, Apple FS, Aguanno JJ, et al. Sodium measurements in multiple myeloma: two techniques compared. Clin Chem 1982;28(12):2383–6.
19. Lang T, Prinsloo P, Broughton AF, et al. Effect of low protein concentration on serum sodium measurement: pseudohypernatraemia and pseudonormonatraemia! Ann Clin Biochem 2002;39(Pt 1):66–7.
20. King RI, Mackay RJ, Florkowski CM, et al. Electrolytes in sick neonates - which sodium is the right answer? Arch Dis Child Fetal Neonatal Ed 2013;98(1):F74–6.
21. Moritz ML, Ayus JC. 100 cc 3% sodium chloride bolus: a novel treatment for hyponatremic encephalopathy. Metab Brain Dis 2010;25(1):91–6.
22. Lemmens-Gruber R, Kamyar M. Vasopressin antagonists. Cell Mol Life Sci 2006;63(15):1766–79.
23. Moritz ML, Ayus JC. Preventing neurological complications from dysnatremias in children. Pediatr Nephrol 2005;20(12):1687–700.
24. Noble-Jamieson CM, Kuzmin P, Airede KI. Hidden sources of fluid and sodium intake in ill newborns. Arch Dis Child 1986;61(7):695–6.
25. Bygrave FL. The ionic environment and metabolic control. Nature 1967; 214(5089):667–71.
26. Youn JH, McDonough AA. Recent advances in understanding integrative control of potassium homeostasis. Annu Rev Physiol 2009;71:381–401.
27. Chevalier RL. What are normal potassium concentrations in the neonate? What is a reasonable approach to hyperkalemia in the newborn with normal renal function? Semin Nephrol 1998;18(3):360–1.
28. Vemgal P, Ohlsson A. Interventions for non-oliguric hyperkalaemia in preterm neonates. Cochrane Database Syst Rev 2012;(5):CD005257.

29. Hayslett JP, Binder HJ. Mechanism of potassium adaptation. Am J Phys 1982; 243(2):F103–12.
30. Zhou H, Satlin LM. Renal potassium handling in healthy and sick newborns. Semin Perinatol 2004;28(2):103–11.
31. Sterns RH, Cox M, Feig PU, et al. Internal potassium balance and the control of the plasma potassium concentration. Medicine (Baltimore) 1981;60(5):339–54.
32. Burnell JM, Scribner BH, Uyeno BT, et al. The effect in humans of extracellular pH change on the relationship between serum potassium concentration and intracellular potassium. J Clin Invest 1956;35(9):935–9.
33. Aronson PS, Giebisch G. Effects of pH on potassium: new explanations for old observations. J Am Soc Nephrol 2011;22(11):1981–9.
34. Adrogue HJ, Madias NE. Changes in plasma potassium concentration during acute acid-base disturbances. Am J Med 1981;71(3):456–67.
35. Sarici D, Sarici S. Neonatal hypokalemia. Res Rep Neonatol 2012;2:15–9.
36. Gennari FJ. Hypokalemia. N Engl J Med 1998;339(7):451–8.
37. Wedenoja S, Hoglund P, Holmberg C. Review article: the clinical management of congenital chloride diarrhoea. Aliment Pharmacol Ther 2010;31(4):477–85.
38. Kleta R, Bockenhauer D. Bartter syndromes and other salt-losing tubulopathies. Nephron Physiol 2006;104(2):73–80.
39. Gomella TL. Neonatology: management, procedures, on-call problems, diseases and drugs. 5th edition. New York; London: Lange Medical Books; 2004.
40. Nako Y, Ohki Y, Harigaya A, et al. Transtubular potassium concentration gradient in preterm neonates. Pediatr Nephrol 1999;13(9):880–5.
41. Davis PJ, Cladis FP, Motoyama EK. Smith's anesthesia for infants and children. 8th edition. St Louis (MO): Mosby; 2011. Available at: http://www.sciencedirect.com/science/book/9780323066129.
42. Mildenberger E, Versmold HT. Pathogenesis and therapy of non-oliguric hyperkalaemia of the premature infant. Eur J Pediatr 2002;161(8):415–22.
43. Chlumska A, Boudova L, Pavlovsky M, et al. Intestinal necrosis following Calcium Resonium-sorbitol administration in a premature uraemic infant. Cesk Patol 2002;38(4):169–72.
44. British Medical Association, Royal Pharmaceutical Society of Great Britain, Royal College of Paediatrics, et al. BNF for children 2012–2013. London: BMJ; 2012.
45. Chadha V, Alon US. Hereditary renal tubular disorders. Semin Nephrol 2009; 29(4):399–411.
46. Landau D. Potassium-related inherited tubulopathies. Cell Mol Life Sci 2006; 63(17):1962–8.
47. Marek S, Tekesin I, Hellmeyer L, et al. Differential diagnosis of a polyhydramnion in hyperprostaglandin E syndrome: a case report. Z Geburtshilfe Neonatol 2004; 208(6):232–5 [in German].
48. Bockenhauer D, Cruwys M, Kleta R, et al. Antenatal Bartter's syndrome: why is this not a lethal condition? QJM 2008;101(12):927–42.
49. Bockenhauer D, van't Hoff W, Dattani M, et al. Secondary nephrogenic diabetes insipidus as a complication of inherited renal diseases. Nephron Physiol 2010; 116(4):23–9.
50. Bockenhauer D, Bichet DG. Inherited secondary nephrogenic diabetes insipidus: concentrating on humans. Am J Physiol Renal Physiol 2013;304:F1037–42.
51. Seyberth HW, Schlingmann KP. Bartter- and Gitelman-like syndromes: salt-losing tubulopathies with loop or DCT defects. Pediatr Nephrol 2011;26: 1789–802.

52. Konrad M, Leonhardt A, Hensen P, et al. Prenatal and postnatal management of hyperprostaglandin E syndrome after genetic diagnosis from amniocytes. Pediatrics 1999;103(3):678–83.

53. Ataoglu E, Civilibal M, Ozkul AA, et al. Indomethacin-induced colon perforation in Bartter's syndrome. Indian J Pediatr 2009;76(3):322–3.

54. Gurkan S, Estilo GK, Wei Y, et al. Potassium transport in the maturing kidney. Pediatr Nephrol 2007;22(7):915–25.

55. Finer G, Shalev H, Birk OS, et al. Transient neonatal hyperkalemia in the antenatal (ROMK defective) Bartter syndrome. J Pediatr 2003;142(3):318–23.

56. Riepe FG. Clinical and molecular features of type 1 pseudohypoaldosteronism. Horm Res 2009;72(1):1–9.

Hematuria in the Newborn

Stephanie M. Jernigan, MD

KEYWORDS

- Hematuria • Neonate • Renal function • Thrombosis

KEY POINTS

- Hematuria is uncommon in the healthy newborn, but is more common in premature infants, with incidence increasing as birth weight and gestation decrease.
- The causes of hematuria in the newborn differ from those seen in older children.
- Most causes of microscopic hematuria in the newborn are transient, require no intervention, and have no long-term sequelae.
- Newborn hematuria with concurrent hypertension, flank mass, changes in urine output, or decreased renal function often indicates more significant disease.

INTRODUCTION

Hematuria in the newborn is uncommon, and information about the true incidence of hematuria in infants is scarce. Microscopic and gross hematuria, while rare in healthy newborns, is more common in premature infants, particularly those cared for in the neonatal intensive care unit. Hematuria may be transient, but may require evaluation, investigation, and intervention in a timely manner.

Incidence

Recent studies of the incidence of newborn hematuria do not exist. A retrospective study of infants with gross hematuria over a 17-year period between 1950 and 1967 describes an incidence of 0.21 per 1000 admissions in infants younger than 1 month.[1] Studies of premature infants have shown microscopic hematuria to be more common. The incidence of microscopic hematuria increases with lower birth weight and gestation.[2,3] Though often transient, microscopic hematuria of longer duration is a cause for concern.

Definition

Gross hematuria is visible blood. Microscopic hematuria is generally defined as greater than 5 red blood cells per high-power field on a spun urine sample. A fresh

Disclosures: None.
Division of Pediatric Nephrology, Emory University School of Medicine and Children's Healthcare of Atlanta, 2015 Uppergate Drive Northeast, Atlanta, GA 30322, USA
E-mail address: smjerni@emory.edu

Clin Perinatol 41 (2014) 591–603
http://dx.doi.org/10.1016/j.clp.2014.05.008
0095-5108/14/$ – see front matter © 2014 Elsevier Inc. All rights reserved.

perinatology.theclinics.com

sample is recommended, as a delay increases the risk of red cell hemolysis and, thus, a false-negative result. Urine screening for hematuria is accomplished by dipstick evaluation, and a positive reading suggests the presence of red blood cells, free hemoglobin, or myoglobin. Positive urine dipstick readings for hematuria are based on a peroxidase-like activity of hemoglobin, which catalyzes a reaction resulting in a color change on the reagent strips. Urine dipsticks are exquisitely sensitive and can detect as little as 150 µg/L of free hemoglobin.[4] A positive dipstick necessitates a microscopic examination to evaluate for the presence of red blood cells.

The microscopic examination of urinary red blood cells can provide a clue to the origin of the hematuria. Red blood cells that maintain normal morphology suggest a lower tract origin. By contrast, red blood cells that transition through the glomerulus are more likely to be dysmorphic because of shearing stresses. Red blood cell casts are highly suggestive of glomerulonephritis.

Gross hematuria in the newborn requires careful evaluation, but the initial assessment focuses on whether the patient truly has hematuria. Urate crystals are common in newborns and give the urine a pink tinge. Such crystals are more common in dehydrated infants and thus are often seen in breast-fed infants. Less commonly in newborns, urine may appear pink, red, or brown as a result of porphyrins or medications (rifampin, chloroquine, and nitrofurantoin). The dipstick will be negative for blood. Vaginal bleeding in newborn females can also be confused for hematuria. Skin breakdown from diaper dermatitis can cause urine to appear red in the diaper, as can rectal bleeding and blood from a recent circumcision.

Etiology

There are a variety of different causes of hematuria in children (**Box 1**). True gross hematuria in a newborn should be evaluated promptly because several causes are associated with renal injury, including thrombotic events, infections, acute tubular or cortical necrosis, and glomerulonephritis.

History

The history in the newborn with hematuria should include prenatal history, family and maternal health history, birth events, and postnatal medical events and interventions. **Box 2** summarizes important inquiries. Hematuria is more common in premature, small for gestational age, and hospitalized infants.[2,3] In the hospitalized infant it is important to review the medical record for risk factors such as procedures (umbilical lines or bladder catheterization), acute events (sepsis, necrotizing enterocolitis, or hypotensive episodes), recent medications, and nutrition.

Physical Examination

The physical examination should investigate other possible sources of bleeding, including the perineum, rectum, vagina, and circumcision. Elevated temperature suggests infection such as urinary tract infection (UTI). Elevated blood pressure suggests kidney involvement and is particularly worrisome, as it can be due to thrombosis, cortical necrosis, and mass effect, all of which require urgent intervention. Infants with autosomal recessive polycystic kidney disease (ARPKD) are particularly prone to hypertension. Hypotension may indicate infection or cardiac dysfunction.

Edema and hematuria are seen in patients with glomerulonephritis. A murmur may indicate glomerulonephritis secondary to endocarditis. Flank masses or a distended abdomen may be secondary to enlarged kidneys from obstructive uropathy, ARPKD, or renal artery or vein thrombosis. Findings in a patient with a bleeding disorder may include petechiae, bruising, or bleeding from the umbilical stump.

> **Box 1**
> **Causes of hematuria in the newborn**
>
> Trauma
> - Bladder catheterization/suprapubic bladder tap
>
> Cortical Necrosis/Acute Tubular Necrosis
>
> Structural Abnormalities
> - Genetic
>   - Autosomal recessive polycystic kidney disease (ARPKD)
>   - Autosomal dominant polycystic kidney disease (ADPKD)
>   - Medullary sponge kidney
> - Obstructive uropathy
>   - Posterior urethral valves
>   - Ureteropelvic junction obstruction
> - Tumor
>   - Wilms
>   - Mesoblastic nephroma
> - Vascular malformation
>
> Glomerulonephritis
>
> Nephrocalcinosis/Nephrolithiasis
>
> Thrombotic Events
> - Renal vein thrombosis
> - Renal artery thrombosis
>
> Bleeding Disorder
> - Vitamin K deficiency bleeding/hemorrhagic disease of the newborn
> - Thrombocytopenia
>
> Infection
>
> Medications

Laboratory

A urinalysis, including microscopy, is important to demonstrate that the patient has hematuria, given other potential causes of red or brown urine. In addition, other findings may suggest a specific diagnosis. White blood cells (WBCs) in the urine occur with UTIs. Proteinuria and red blood cell casts support a diagnosis of glomerulonephritis. Most patients should have a urine culture, because UTIs are a relatively common cause of hematuria and require urgent treatment. A complete blood cell count may demonstrate an elevated WBC count suggesting a UTI, anemia or polycythemia, or thrombocytopenia, which may cause hematuria or be a consequence of a renal vein thrombosis (RVT) or cortical necrosis. Other potentially useful tests include a creatinine, urine calcium/creatinine ratio, prothrombin time, and partial thromboplastin time.

Imaging

Imaging should begin with renal bladder ultrasonography (RBUS). Renal Doppler is important for examining vascular flow. Depending on the results of ultrasonography,

> **Box 2**
> **History in the newborn with hematuria**
>
> Prenatal History
> - Prenatal ultrasonography
>   - Renal abnormalities
>   - Abdominal mass
>   - Amniotic fluid volume
> - Maternal History
>   - Medications (angiotensin-converting enzyme inhibitor, warfarin, isoniazid, antiepileptics)
>   - Kidney disease (glomerulonephritis, autoimmune disorders)
>   - Diabetes
>   - Previous pregnancies
> - Family History
>   - Genetic kidney disease (ARPKD, ADPKD)
>   - Kidney stones
>   - Bleeding disorders
>
> Birth History
> - Prematurity or small for gestational age
> - Traumatic, difficult or home delivery
> - Apgar scores
> - Vitamin K administration
>
> Postnatal History
> - Feeding history
> - Urine output/urinary stream
> - Weight gain or loss

a voiding cystourethrogram or computed tomography (CT) scan are useful for evaluation of bladder outlet obstruction or tumors, respectively. A CT scan may be more sensitive than RBUS for the evaluation of thrombosis and renal calcification. Nuclear imaging studies are rarely required.

DISORDERS ASSOCIATED WITH NEWBORN HEMATURIA

Many of the disorders associated with newborn hematuria are discussed in detail in other articles elsewhere in this issue. These disorders are addressed briefly here, with more information provided for those causes not addressed elsewhere.

Trauma

Trauma leading to hematuria is most commonly derived from bladder catheterization or suprapubic bladder tap. Trauma to the urethral mucosa commonly leads to microscopic hematuria. A catheter passing through a narrowed or obstructed urethra can produce gross hematuria. Trauma to the bladder from catheterization is uncommon, but may occur with a suprapubic tap. Rare complications of a bladder tap include bladder wall hematoma and lacerated vessel on the anterior bladder wall. Gross hematuria occurs transiently in up to 3.4% of bladder taps.[5] Hematuria following either procedure is usually self-limited and resolves quickly. Intervention is rarely needed.[6] Birth trauma is another rare cause of gross hematuria.[7]

Acute Tubular Necrosis and Cortical Necrosis

Acute tubular necrosis (ATN) rarely causes gross hematuria. However, microscopic or gross hematuria is more common if a newborn develops cortical necrosis, which is more common in neonates than in older children. ATN and cortical necrosis are secondary to 1 or more insults to the kidneys (eg, nephrotoxic medications, infection, hypovolemia, ischemia), but the injury is more severe in patients with cortical necrosis. Risk factors for cortical necrosis include necrotizing enterocolitis, sepsis, perinatal anoxia, placental abruption, twin-twin transfusion, and other causes of neonatal hemorrhage leading to decreased blood volume and blood pressure.[8]

Patients with cortical necrosis have decreased urine output and uremia. Hypertension is common because of renal vascular injury and microthrombi, which may also lead to thrombocytopenia.[9] Radiographic studies are often nonspecific, with renal ultrasonography (RUS) demonstrating increased echogenicity and loss of cortical medullary differentiation, particularly in the outer rim of the kidney. At the area of necrosis, a hypoechoic band or zone may be seen on ultrasonography and CT scan.[10] Doppler may reveal decreased perfusion with patent renal vessels. Unlike ATN, which shows delayed uptake on nuclear studies, cortical necrosis results in little or no perfusion and delayed or absent function of the affected kidney. Patients with cortical necrosis may require acute dialysis, along with other interventions needed in acute kidney injury. There is a significant lifetime risk of kidney failure, even in those who do not require dialysis as newborns.[8]

Structural Abnormalities

Cystic kidney disease may present with gross hematuria in a newborn.[1] Most cases of ARPKD and some cases of autosomal dominant polycystic kidney disease (ADPKD) are diagnosed by prenatal imaging. In ARPKD, flank masses are often present on physical examination, in addition to respiratory symptoms from the enlarged renal size and pulmonary hypoplasia.

Medullary sponge kidney is a rare but reported cause of hematuria in the newborn period.[1] In medullary sponge kidney, there is cystic dilation of the terminal collecting ducts of the renal medulla. The dilation of the ducts leads to diffuse small and large cysts that do not involve the renal cortex. In general a benign condition, patients with medullary sponge disease have a higher incidence of nephrolithiasis and UTIs.[11] There is an association of medullary sponge kidney with hemihypertrophy and Beckwith-Wiedemann syndrome.[12]

Obstructive uropathies are usually diagnosed by prenatal ultrasonography, but may present postnatally, often in the first week.[1,13] The most common cause of lower urinary tract obstruction is posterior urethral valves (PUVs). If not diagnosed by prenatal imaging, PUVs often present with a UTI; however, gross hematuria may be the presenting complaint.[13–15]

Ureteropelvic junction obstruction may present with gross hematuria.[1] Even mild birth trauma may precipitate bleeding in the kidney with hydronephrosis. This susceptibility to renal injury may be due to decreased perirenal fat, decreased protection from less ossified ribs, and the relatively larger size of kidneys in the newborn.[15]

Newborn tumors are uncommon, with very few presenting in infants younger than 6 months.[16] Tumors are often detected by prenatal ultrasonography, but may present as an abdominal mass or with gross hematuria. Congenital mesoblastic nephroma (CMN) is the most common, followed by Wilms tumor. If not diagnosed prenatally, CMN usually presents in the first 3 months after birth. Only approximately 2% of Wilms tumors are found this early. Ossifying renal tumor of infancy is a very rare benign tumor, but it typically presents with hematuria. Imaging reveals a noninvasive calcified mass in the renal pelvis.[17,18] Treatment is with resection. Vascular abnormalities are a rare cause of hematuria.[19,20]

Glomerulonephritis

Glomerulonephritis is extremely rare in the newborn,[21–28] and always includes microscopic or gross hematuria. Proteinuria is usually present, and renal function may be decreased. The differential diagnosis includes acquired maternal antibodies, infections, and atypical hemolytic uremic syndrome.

Nephrocalcinosis and Nephrolithiasis

Nephrocalcinosis and nephrolithiasis are uncommon in healthy newborns, but occur in premature infants.[29–35] One recent study reported these findings in 41% of preterm neonates, but there is wide variation between studies as a result of different screening protocols and imaging equipment.[33] Nephrolithiasis is more likely than nephrocalcinosis to cause hematuria. Premature infants are at increased risk for these complications, owing to the immaturity of the tubular handling of electrolytes in the neonatal kidney and medical interventions that are more common in premature neonates (eg, loop diuretics).

Calcium deposits in the kidneys are composed of calcium oxalate and, less commonly, calcium phosphate. Renal calcification can be identified by radiography, RUS (**Fig. 1**), and CT. Ultrasonography is more sensitive than radiography and CT.[33] CT scans are more specific, but require radiation and are more difficult to perform in the ill premature infant.

Laboratory evaluation should include electrolytes, calcium, and phosphorus. The presence of hypercalcemia should prompt measurement of levels of parathyroid

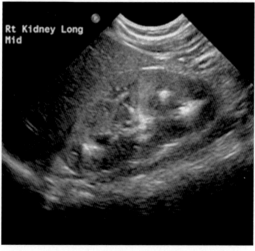

Fig. 1. A renal ultrasonogram showing hyperechoic renal pyramids in a patient with medullary nephrocalcinosis.

hormone, 25-vitamin D, and 1,25-vitamin D. A spot urine calcium/creatinine ratio is the simplest method for detecting hypercalciuria. In term newborns and those up to 6 months of age, a normal ratio is less than 0.8 mg/mg creatinine. Unfortunately, ratios in premature infants are not well established; the ratio is inversely related to postnatal age. Many other factors affect calcium excretion.[36]

The type of nutrition an infant receives alters the risk of renal calcification. Premature infants often receive feedings higher in calcium to prevent bone disease and rickets, but this increases the risk of nephrocalcinosis. Infants receiving total parenteral nutrition (TPN) are at higher risk for nephrocalcinosis. Patients receiving TPN have higher calcium-to-citrate ratios in the urine, which decrease calcium solubility. TPN contains more ascorbic acid and glycine, precursors to oxalate. Premature infants have higher oxalate excretion at baseline, and TPN may increase it further. Infants consuming breast milk have lower calcium/creatinine ratios than infants receiving TPN, and lower oxalate/creatinine ratios than formula-fed infants.[37]

Hypercalcemia is observed in infants with subcutaneous fat necrosis. Hypercalcemia can occur as a result of perinatal hypoxic stress or total-body cooling treatments for hypoxic ischemic encephalopathy.[38,39]

Furosemide, by causing hypercalciuria, increases the risk of renal calcification.[40,41] Use of dexamethasone has also been associated with nephrocalcinosis. Glucocorticoids have effects on both bone and kidney tubules, which result in hypercalcemia and hypercalciuria.[42] Methylxanthines, such as caffeine and theophylline, may also cause hypercalciuria.[33,43]

In older patients with renal calcification, hydrochlorothiazide diuretics and citrate have been used to decrease calcium excretion and increase calcium solubility, respectively. Studies in infants looking at the relationship between urinary citrate concentrations and nephrocalcinosis are inconclusive.[44] In a study of premature infants, sodium citrate did not prevent nephrocalcinosis.[45]

Treatment of renal calcification focuses on increasing urine flow by increasing fluid intake while balancing restrictions attributable to underlying pulmonary or cardiac disease. It is also helpful to minimize, when possible, the use of medications that cause hypercalciuria. Replacing a loop diuretic with a thiazide diuretic may be possible in some patients.

The long-term outlook for newborn renal calcification is excellent, with most infants experiencing resolution of nephrocalcinosis. Intervention is rarely needed for renal stones. There are small reports suggesting the possibility of an increased risk of hypertension and lowered glomerular filtration rate, but these are small samples, and most patients seem to suffer no long-term consequences.[33]

Thrombotic Event

Thrombosis of either a renal artery or a renal vein is an important consideration in the neonate with hematuria. Neonates may be particularly susceptible to thrombosis because of an imbalance of prothrombotic and anticoagulant proteins. Newborns have decreased levels of clotting inhibitors such as protein C, protein S, and antithrombin III, and lower levels of plasminogen, a fibrinolytic.[46] In addition, newborn kidneys have a lower perfusion pressure, which further increases the risk of thrombosis.

The classic triad of RVT is gross hematuria (50%), flank mass (41%), and thrombocytopenia (29%). One of these presenting features occurs in most cases, but all 3 in only 13% to 22%.[46] Other findings include hypertension, oliguria, and renal insufficiency. RVT is the most common thrombosis in the newborn period not associated with an indwelling catheter. RVT has a male predominance and is usually unilateral, with the left renal vein more commonly involved.[46,47]

Risk factors for RVT include prematurity, maternal diabetes (either type 1 or gestational), umbilical venous catheterization, asphyxia, infections, and polycythemia. Inherited disorders of clotting have also been described in patients with RVT.[46–48] Most cases have an associated risk identified (**Box 3**). The mean presentation time of RVT in neonates is the second day of life, with many occurring within 24 hours of birth. Given the high association with prematurity and the knowledge that RVT can occur in utero, there is the possibility that RVT is the cause of fetal distress and premature birth rather than the result of a stressful birth.[47]

Though not definitively proven, it is suspected that thrombosis starts in the smaller interlobular or arcuate veins and then progresses to the larger renal veins and, occasionally, the inferior vena cava (IVC). As a result, RUS findings of RVT vary depending on the timing.[46] Scans done soon after the event show an enlarged kidney with increased echogenicity and loss of corticomedullary differentiation. More specific early signs are perivascular echogenic streaks, which represent intralobular and interlobar thrombus. Echogenic streaks disappear quickly, limiting the specificity of a later RUS. In the second week after RVT, the kidneys remain large and hyperechoic, and hypoechoic areas, if seen, represent areas of hemorrhage and edema, respectively. It may be possible to visualize a thrombosis in the renal vein and IVC. Later ultrasonograms may demonstrate decreasing renal size, with small kidneys suggesting renal atrophy. The thrombus may later calcify, making it more visible on ultrasonography. Doppler ultrasonography in RVT reveals decreased flow in the main renal vein or abnormal flow patterns in renal vein branches (**Fig. 2**).

There are a variety of different acute treatment strategies for RVT, including supportive care, thrombolytic agents, and unfractionated or low molecular weight heparin. Guidelines suggest that more severe cases be treated, including patients with bilateral RVT, renal insufficiency, or thrombus extending into the IVC.[46,49]

Mortality from RVT is low but morbidity is high, with complications of adrenal hemorrhage, thromboemboli to other areas, hypertension, and short-term and long-term renal insufficiency. Hypertension is reported in 34%.[48] Patients with bilateral RVT are more likely to have persistent hypertension. Seventy percent of patients with RVT sustain permanent damage to the affected kidney documented by atrophy on imaging. Treatment does not seem to affect the likelihood of chronic renal damage.[49] Renal dysfunction is reported in 29% and end-stage renal disease requiring renal replacement therapy in 3%.[48]

Box 3
Risk factors for renal vein thrombosis

Prematurity

Umbilical vein catheter

Infant of a diabetic mother

Sepsis/shock

Dehydration

Perinatal asphyxia

Cyanotic congenital heart disease

Conjoined twin

Polycythemia

Prothrombotic conditions (activated protein C resistance, Factor V Leiden mutation)

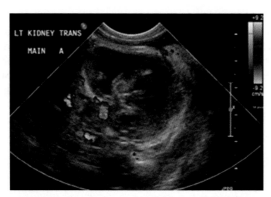

Fig. 2. A renal ultrasonogram showing an enlarged hypoechoic kidney with no flow in the renal vein.

Renal artery thrombosis (RAT) is much less common than RVT. It is often associated with an aortic thrombus, and in the neonate is almost always associated with umbilical arterial catheters. A review of catheter complications suggests that high-placed umbilical catheters with the tip above the diaphragm may have a lower incidence of vascular complications.[50] There are case reports of non–catheter-related RAT; however, these infants were all critically ill.[51]

Symptoms of RAT include microscopic or gross hematuria, hypertension, thrombocytopenia, and, if there is bilateral involvement, acute kidney injury with oliguria. With associated aortic involvement, decreased peripheral pulses and cyanotic skin findings of decreased perfusion may be present.

Diagnosis requires a high index of suspicion, as initial RUS evaluation may not demonstrate early thrombus or abnormalities of the affected kidney. CT, magnetic resonance imaging, and aortography may also reveal thrombi, but are often less readily available than RUS.[52,53] A renal scan will show little to no renal blood flow or renal perfusion. Prognosis for the affected kidney is poor, and serial sonograms will show diminishing renal size. Hypertension may be chronic.[54]

The arterial catheter should be removed in all patients with RAT. Treatment of the thrombus may include thrombolytic therapy, such as tissue plasminogen activator, and low molecular weight heparin.[52,55] Newer therapies are on the horizon.[56]

Bleeding Disorders

Severe thrombocytopenia, defined as a platelet count of less than 60,000, is commonly associated with microscopic hematuria. Thrombocytopenia is uncommon in healthy newborns, but is more common in premature infants and babies admitted to the intensive care unit.[57] A complete blood count quickly identifies a low platelet count as a possible cause of hematuria. There are numerous causes of thrombocytopenia in this population, with treatment aimed at the specific determinant. Microscopic hematuria requires no intervention, but platelet transfusion should be considered if gross hematuria occurs.

Bleeding caused by vitamin K deficiency, formally known as hemorrhagic disease of the newborn, is rare in developed countries. It is more common in developing nations where prophylactic vitamin K is not as readily available and breast feeding is often exclusive, as breast milk is low in vitamin K. Hematuria is a rare complication.[58,59] Most infants present with bleeding of the skin, gastrointestinal tract, or umbilical stump. The newborn and maternal histories are useful in identifying the risk factors for this condition. Maternal use of certain medications such as anticonvulsants, warfarin, rifampin, and isoniazid can result in decreased vitamin K storage and function in the newborn, which can lead to very early presentation in the first 24 hours of life. Classic onset at 2 to 7 days occurs more often in infants who are exclusively breast-fed, although lack of prophylaxis may also play a role. Late-onset disease occurs in infants who do not receive prophylactic vitamin K. These infants often present with more devastating bleeds, including intracranial hemorrhage.

Administration of vitamin K to correct coagulopathy is the primary treatment. Fresh frozen plasma may also be indicated.[60]

Infectious

UTIs occur more frequently in infants than in older children, and the incidence is higher in preterm infants.[61] Common symptoms include fever, lethargy, poor feeding, and jaundice.[62] Hematuria in the newborn is an uncommon presentation of UTI, but a urine culture should be obtained to investigate this treatable cause of hematuria. The morbidity associated with infant UTIs is high. These infants are much more likely to have bacteremia[62] and urosepsis,[61] making early diagnosis and treatment crucial.

Infectious endocarditis is a rare and often fatal disease in newborn infants. It is more common in infants who have congenital heart disease or invasive intensive care monitoring, or who have positive blood cultures or clinical sepsis. Common presenting signs in this age group are a new or changing heart murmur and hematuria.[63,64] Other signs include skin pustules and thrombocytopenia. The Duke Criteria of major and minor signs can be used to assist with diagnosis; however, if there is suspicion, an echocardiogram is warranted to evaluate for cardiac vegetations. Hematuria in the setting of endocarditis results from embolic injury or, more commonly, glomerulonephritis from circulating immune complexes.[65] Complement C3 may be low. Antibiotic treatment should result in resolution of the hematuria as the infection clears.

Medications

The most common medications associated with hematuria in infants are nonsteroidal anti-inflammatory drugs (NSAIDs), particularly indomethacin. NSAIDs inhibit prostaglandin E and thromboxane A_2, and have the potential to cause vaso-occlusive injury, interstitial nephritis, and hematuria. NSAID-related episodes of hematuria are usually microscopic and self-resolving.

SUMMARY

There are multiple causes of hematuria in newborn infants. A thorough history and physical examination can usually quickly identify the cause and allow for focused evaluation. Some causes necessitate little to no intervention; however, there are causes that require quick investigation and intervention to preserve renal health and prevent long-term complications.

REFERENCES

1. Emanuel B, Aronson N. Neonatal hematuria. Am J Dis Child 1974;128:204–6.
2. Cramer A, Steele A, Wishnie P, et al. Transient hematuria in premature and sick neonates. Pediatr Res 1981;15:692.
3. Delgado MM, Khan S, Satlin LM, et al. Incidence and duration of microscopic hematuria (MH) in the premature infant. Pediatr Res 1999;45:194a.

4. Barratt T, Niaudet P. Clinical evaluation. In: Avner E, Harmon W, Niaudet P, editors. Pediatric nephrology. Philadelphia: Lippincott, Williams and Wilkins; 2004. p. 397.
5. Akierman AR. Suprapubic bladder aspiration in neonates. Can Fam Physician 1987;33:2099–100.
6. Pollack CV Jr, Pollack ES, Andrew ME. Suprapubic bladder aspiration versus urethral catheterization in ill infants: success, efficiency and complication rates. Ann Emerg Med 1994;23:225–30.
7. Newman B, Smith S. Unusual renal mass in a newborn infant. Radiology 1987; 163:193–4.
8. Andreoli S. Clinical evaluation and management. In: Avner E, Harmon W, Niaudet P, editors. Pediatric nephrology. 5th edition. Philadelphia: Lippincott, Williams and Wilkins; 2004. p. 1240.
9. Lerner GR, Kurnetz R, Bernstein J, et al. Renal cortical and renal medullary necrosis in the first 3 months of life. Pediatr Nephrol 1992;6:516–8.
10. Sefczek RJ, Beckman I, Lupetin AR, et al. Sonography of acute renal cortical necrosis. Am J Roentgenol 1984;142:553–4.
11. Potter EL, Osathanondh V. Medullary sponge kidney. Two cases in young infants. J Pediatr 1963;62:901–7.
12. Beetz R, Schofer O, Riedmiller H, et al. Medullary sponge kidneys and unilateral Wilms tumour in a child with Beckwith-Wiedemann syndrome. Eur J Pediatr 1991;150:489–92.
13. Bensman A, Baudon JJ, Jablonski JP, et al. Uropathies diagnosed in the neonatal period: symptomatology and course. Acta Paediatr Scand 1980;69:499–503.
14. Hodges SJ, Patel B, McLorie G, et al. Posterior urethral valves. TheScientificWorldJournal 2009;9:1119–26.
15. Diamond DA, Ford C. Neonatal gross hematuria as a presenting sign of posterior urethral valves. Urology 1992;40:267–9.
16. Glick RD, Hicks MJ, Nuchtern JG, et al. Renal tumors in infants less than 6 months of age. J Pediatr Surg 2004;39:522–5.
17. Lee SH, Choi YH, Kim WS, et al. Ossifying renal tumor of infancy: findings at ultrasound, CT and MRI. Pediatr Radiol 2014;44(5):625–8.
18. Schelling J, Schroder A, Stein R, et al. Ossifying renal tumor of infancy. J Pediatr Urol 2007;3:258–61.
19. Fernandes ET, Manivel JC, Reinberg Y. Hematuria in a newborn infant caused by bladder hemangioma. Urology 1996;47:412–5.
20. Guthrie SO, Rhodes M, Janco R, et al. An infant with Kasabach-Merritt syndrome with associated renal hematoma and intussusception. J Perinatol 2005; 25:143–5.
21. Lam C, Imundo L, Hirsch D, et al. Glomerulonephritis in a neonate with atypical congenital lupus and toxoplasmosis. Pediatr Nephrol 1999;13:850–3.
22. Linshaw MA, Stapleton FB, Cuppage FE, et al. Hypocomplementemic glomerulonephritis in an infant and mother. Evidence for an abnormal form of C3. Am J Nephrol 1987;7:470–7.
23. Besbas N, Gulhan B, Karpman D, et al. Neonatal onset atypical hemolytic uremic syndrome successfully treated with eculizumab. Pediatr Nephrol 2013;28:155–8.
24. DeFranco PE, Shook LA, Goebel J, et al. Solitary hepatic abscess with associated glomerulonephritis in a neonate. J Perinatol 2000;20:384–6.
25. Nortier JL, Debiec H, Tournay Y, et al. Neonatal disease in neutral endopeptidase alloimmunization: lessons for immunological monitoring. Pediatr Nephrol 2006;21:1399–405.

26. Schlieben DJ, Korbet SM, Kimura RE, et al. Pulmonary-renal syndrome in a newborn with placental transmission of ANCAs. Am J Kidney Dis 2005;45: 758–61.
27. Dolfin T, Pomeranz A, Korzets Z, et al. Acute renal failure in a neonate caused by the transplacental transfer of a nephrotoxic paraprotein: successful resolution by exchange transfusion. Am J Kidney Dis 1999;34:1129–31.
28. Bansal PJ, Tobin MC. Neonatal microscopic polyangiitis secondary to transfer of maternal myeloperoxidase-antineutrophil cytoplasmic antibody resulting in neonatal pulmonary hemorrhage and renal involvement. Ann Allergy Asthma Immunol 2004;93:398–401.
29. Chandra S, Verma R. Idiopathic congenital nonobstructive nephrolithiasis: a case report and review. J Perinatol 2004;24:196–9.
30. Hein G, Richter D, Manz F, et al. Development of nephrocalcinosis in very low birth weight infants. Pediatr Nephrol 2004;19:616–20.
31. Gilsanz V, Fernal W, Reid BS, et al. Nephrolithiasis in premature infants. Radiology 1985;154:107–10.
32. Cranefield DJ, Odd DE, Harding JE, et al. High incidence of nephrocalcinosis in extremely preterm infants treated with dexamethasone. Pediatr Radiol 2004;34: 138–42.
33. Schell-Feith EA, Kist-van Holthe JE, van der Heijden AJ. Nephrocalcinosis in preterm neonates. Pediatr Nephrol 2010;25:221–30.
34. Schell-Feith EA, Kist-van Holthe JE, Conneman N, et al. Etiology of nephrocalcinosis in preterm neonates: association of nutritional intake and urinary parameters. Kidney Int 2000;58:2102–10.
35. Chang HY, Hsu CH, Tsai JD, et al. Renal calcification in very low birth weight infants. Pediatr Neonatol 2011;52:145–9.
36. Aladangady N, Coen PG, White MP, et al. Urinary excretion of calcium and phosphate in preterm infants. Pediatr Nephrol 2004;19:1225–31.
37. Hoppe B, Hesse A, Neuhaus T, et al. Influence of nutrition on urinary oxalate and calcium in preterm and term infants. Pediatr Nephrol 1997;11:687–90.
38. Akcay A, Akar M, Oncel MY, et al. Hypercalcemia due to subcutaneous fat necrosis in a newborn after total body cooling. Pediatr Dermatol 2013;30: 120–3.
39. Fumagalli M, Ramenghi LA, Pisoni S, et al. Total body cooling: skin and renal complications. Arch Dis Child Fetal Neonatal Ed 2011;96:F377.
40. Downing GJ, Egelhoff JC, Daily DK, et al. Furosemide-related renal calcifications in the premature infant. A longitudinal ultrasonographic study. Pediatr Radiol 1991;21:563–5.
41. Gimpel C, Krause A, Franck P, et al. Exposure to furosemide as the strongest risk factor for nephrocalcinosis in preterm infants. Pediatr Int 2010;52:51–6.
42. Canalis E, Mazziotti G, Giustina A, et al. Glucocorticoid-induced osteoporosis: pathophysiology and therapy. Osteoporos Int 2007;18:1319–28.
43. Zanardo V, Dani C, Trevisanuto D, et al. Methylxanthines increase renal calcium excretion in preterm infants. Biol Neonate 1995;68:169–74.
44. Sikora P, Roth B, Kribs A, et al. Hypocitraturia is one of the major risk factors for nephrocalcinosis in very low birth weight (VLBW) infants. Kidney Int 2003;63: 2194–9.
45. Schell-Feith EA, Moerdijk A, van Zwieten PH, et al. Does citrate prevent nephrocalcinosis in preterm neonates? Pediatr Nephrol 2006;21:1830–6.
46. Brandao LR, Simpson EA, Lau KK. Neonatal renal vein thrombosis. Semin Fetal Neonatal Med 2011;16:323–8.

47. Kuhle S, Massicotte P, Chan A, et al. A case series of 72 neonates with renal vein thrombosis. Data from the 1-800-NO-CLOTS Registry. Thromb Haemost 2004; 92:729–33.
48. Marks SD, Massicotte MP, Steele BT, et al. Neonatal renal venous thrombosis: clinical outcomes and prevalence of prothrombotic disorders. J Pediatr 2005; 146:811–6.
49. Lau KK, Stoffman JM, Williams S, et al. Neonatal renal vein thrombosis: review of the English-language literature between 1992 and 2006. Pediatrics 2007;120: e1278–84.
50. Barrington KJ. Umbilical artery catheters in the newborn: effects of catheter materials. Cochrane Database Syst Rev 2000;(2):CD000949.
51. Kavaler E, Hensle TW. Renal artery thrombosis in the newborn infant. Urology 1997;50:282–4.
52. Ellis D, Kaye RD, Bontempo FA. Aortic and renal artery thrombosis in a neonate: recovery with thrombolytic therapy. Pediatr Nephrol 1997;11:641–4.
53. Ergaz Z, Simanovsky N, Rozovsky K, et al. Clinical outcome of umbilical artery catheter-related thrombosis - a cohort study. J Perinatol 2012;32:933–40.
54. Proesmans W, van de Wijdeven P, Van Geet C. Thrombophilia in neonatal renal venous and arterial thrombosis. Pediatr Nephrol 2005;20:241–2.
55. Revel-Vilk S, Ergaz Z. Diagnosis and management of central-line-associated thrombosis in newborns and infants. Semin Fetal Neonatal Med 2011;16:340–4.
56. Young G. Old and new antithrombotic drugs in neonates and infants. Semin Fetal Neonatal Med 2011;16:349–54.
57. Muthukumar P, Venkatesh V, Curley A, et al. Severe thrombocytopenia and patterns of bleeding in neonates: results from a prospective observational study and implications for use of platelet transfusions. Transfus Med 2012;22:338–43.
58. McNinch AW, Tripp JH. Haemorrhagic disease of the newborn in the British Isles: two year prospective study. BMJ 1991;303:1105–9.
59. Rana MT, Noureen N, Iqbal I. Risk factors, presentations and outcome of the haemorrhagic disease of newborn. J Coll Physicians Surg Pak 2009;19:371–4.
60. Burke CW. Vitamin K deficiency bleeding: overview and considerations. J Pediatr Health Care 2013;27:215–21.
61. Biyikli NK, Alpay H, Ozek E, et al. Neonatal urinary tract infections: analysis of the patients and recurrences. Pediatr Int 2004;46:21–5.
62. Beetz R. Evaluation and management of urinary tract infections in the neonate. Curr Opin Pediatr 2012;24:205–11.
63. Oelberg DG, Fisher DJ, Gross DM, et al. Endocarditis in high-risk neonates. Pediatrics 1983;71:392–7.
64. O'Callaghan C, McDougall P. Infective endocarditis in neonates. Arch Dis Child Fetal Neonatal Ed 1988;63:53–7.
65. Ferrieri P, Gewitz MH, Gerber MA, et al. Unique features of infective endocarditis in childhood. Pediatrics 2002;109:931–43.

Nephrotic and Nephritic Syndrome in the Newborn

Michelle N. Rheault, MD

KEYWORDS

- Proteinuria • Hematuria • Congenital nephrotic syndrome
- Diffuse mesangial sclerosis • Nephritis • Hemolytic uremic syndrome
- Neonatal lupus

KEY POINTS

- Congenital nephrotic syndrome (CNS) presents within the first 3 months of life with massive proteinuria, hypoalbuminemia, and edema.
- Elevated maternal serum α-fetoprotein, enlarged placenta (>25% of birth weight), and prematurity are suggestive of CNS.
- CNS is most often caused by single gene mutations affecting kidney podocyte structural or signaling proteins.
- Infants with CNS are at risk for infection and thromboembolism, which may be the initial clinical manifestation.
- Nephritic syndrome in the newborn is rare, and presenting features may include hematuria, proteinuria, hypertension, acute kidney injury, oliguria, and edema.

INTRODUCTION

Glomerular disorders in infancy are rare, and can include both nephrotic and nephritic syndromes. These syndromes can be idiopathic, or due to primary genetic disorders, congenital infections, or maternal antibody transfer. Regardless of etiology, dysfunction of the glomerular filtration barrier is evident in these conditions. The kidney glomerular filtration barrier is a size-selective and charge-selective filter that prevents the passage of red blood cells and plasma proteins into the urine while allowing the passage of water and small solutes. It is composed of 3 layers: an endothelium, a glomerular basement membrane (GBM), and epithelial cells, also known as podocytes. Podocytes are highly differentiated cells that have a complex cellular architecture consisting of a cell body, major processes, and foot processes. Adjacent foot processes are connected by a slit diaphragm, which comprises the main size-selective filtration

Disclosure: None.

Division of Pediatric Nephrology, University of Minnesota Children's Hospital, 2450 Riverside Avenue, MB680, Minneapolis, MN 55454, USA

E-mail address: rheau002@umn.edu

Clin Perinatol 41 (2014) 605–618

http://dx.doi.org/10.1016/j.clp.2014.05.009   **perinatology.theclinics.com** barrier in the kidney (**Fig. 1**).[1–3] Dysfunction in any of the 3 components of the glomerular filtration barrier can lead to loss of red blood cells and plasma proteins in the urine, and clinical nephrotic or nephritic syndromes. The presence of these syndromes in the neonate can cause significant morbidity and mortality; therefore, urgent diagnosis and treatment are necessary.

DIAGNOSIS OF CONGENITAL NEPHROTIC SYNDROME

Nephrotic syndrome (NS) is defined as massive leakage of plasma proteins into the urine caused by dysfunction of the glomerular filtration barrier, leading to hypoalbuminemia and edema. NS can be further classified by age at presentation as congenital NS (CNS, age at presentation <3 months), infantile NS (age at presentation 3–12 months), or childhood NS (age at presentation >1 year). As the genetics of NS have started to be unraveled over the past 15 years, it has become clear that different mutations in the same gene can manifest at various ages, making the classification by age somewhat arbitrary (*NPHS1*- and *NPHS2*-related disease can present in infancy, childhood, or rarely in adulthood, for example).[4,5] Nonetheless, the designation of "congenital nephrotic syndrome" still guides diagnosis, management, and prognosis, and this terminology has been retained by the pediatric nephrology community.

Prenatal diagnosis of CNS is suggested by elevated maternal serum α-fetoprotein (MSAFP) obtained in routine second-trimester screening. Fetal serum contains high concentrations of α-fetoprotein (AFP) that is lost into the urine/amniotic fluid during the nephrotic state. Elevated MSAFP is common and is found in approximately 1% of all pregnancies using a cutoff of greater than 2.5 multiples of the mean (MoM). Elevated MSAFP can be seen in pregnancies complicated by neural tube defects, gastroschisis, or chromosomal abnormalities as well as CNS.[6,7] CNS is a rare cause of elevated MSAFP, with one retrospective study identifying only 5 infants with CNS among 658 women with elevated MSAFP (<1%).[7] Most patients with pregnancies affected by CNS have persistently elevated MSAFP on follow up screens in addition to elevated AFP in amniotic fluid obtained by amniocentesis.[7] Median MSAFP concentrations were 8.3 MoM in pregnancies affected with CNS attributable to *NPHS1*

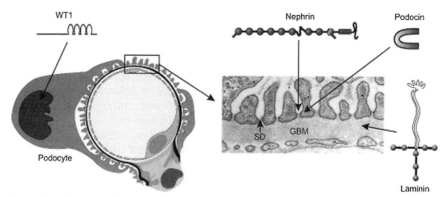

Fig. 1. The glomerular filtration barrier. Cross section of a glomerular capillary (*left*) and electron microscopy image of a normal capillary wall (*right*). WT1 is a transcription factor important for podocyte function. Nephrin is a major component of the slit diaphragm (SD) connecting podocyte foot processes. Podocin is an adapter protein located intracellularly in the SD area. Laminin is a major structural protein of the glomerular basement membrane (GBM). Genetic mutations in these proteins lead to congenital nephrotic syndrome. (*From* Jalanko H. Congenital nephrotic syndrome. Pediatr Nephrol 2009; 24(11):2121–8.)

mutations while median AFP concentrations in amniotic fluid were even higher, at 33.4 MoM.[8] Of importance, heterozygous carriers of *NPHS1* mutations also demonstrate elevated MSAFP and amniotic fluid AFP levels that overlap with values in homozygous affected infants.[8] This situation is hypothesized to be due to temporary dysfunction in the glomerular filtration barrier during glomerulogenesis in *NPHS1* heterozygotes that improves with time.[9] Thus, elevated MSAFP cannot be used to distinguish CNS carriers from affected infants.

A universal finding in children with CNS is elevated urine protein excretion. Normal urine protein excretion varies by age, with the highest values in preterm infants and decreasing values throughout childhood. In one study, healthy premature infants in the first month of life demonstrated urine protein concentration of 88 to 845 mg/L (mean 182 mg/m²/d) in a 24-hour urine collection, whereas term infants excreted slightly less, between 95 and 455 mg/L (mean 145 mg/m²/d).[10] By contrast, children aged 10 to 16 years excreted between 45 and 391 mg/L (mean 63 mg/m²/d). Urine protein-to-creatinine ratios have also been used to estimate protein excretion, owing to the technical difficulties in obtaining a 24-hour urine collection in a neonate. For children younger than 2 years, a normal urine protein-to-creatinine ratio is less than 0.5 mg/mg, but normal values in neonates have not been well described.[11]

Urine protein excretion in children with CNS is generally massive, and greater than 2000 mg/L in most affected infants.[12,13] Urine protein loss leads to low serum albumin levels less than 2.5 g/dL, with presenting values often less than 1.5 g/dL. In infants with extremely low serum albumin levels, the magnitude of proteinuria may not be apparent until serum albumin levels are restored with albumin infusions. Hematuria and leukocyturia are often present as well.[12] In addition to albumin, several other proteins are lost in the urine, including immunoglobulins, transferrin, antithrombin III, ceruloplasmin, vitamin D–binding protein, and thyroid-binding protein.[14] Hypoalbuminemia and the resultant decreased plasma oncotic pressure leads to leakage of fluid from the intravascular to the interstitial space, causing hypovolemia, renal hypoperfusion, and secondary renal sodium and fluid retention with clinical edema.[15] Massive edema (ie, anasarca) can lead to serious complications, including respiratory distress from pulmonary edema and/or pleural effusions in addition to severe ascites and scrotal edema.

The differential diagnosis of CNS is broad, and includes several primary genetic disorders and congenital infections (**Table 1**). Most children with CNS have a monogenic cause for their disease with mutations in proteins that regulate the glomerular filtration barrier, particularly proteins important in formation of and signaling from the podocyte slit diaphragm. Two large studies have demonstrated that more than 80% of infants with CNS have a mutation identified in 1 of 5 genes: *NPHS1* (39%–61%), *NPHS2* (15%–39%), *LAMB2* (2%–4%), *WT1* (~2%), or *PLCE1* (~2%).[16,17]

CONGENITAL NEPHROTIC SYNDROME OF THE FINNISH TYPE (*NPHS1*)

CNS of the Finnish Type (CNF) is the most common cause of CNS and is named because of its high incidence in Finland of 1:8200 live births, owing to the effect of founder mutations.[18] There is also a very high concentration of disease among Old Order Mennonites in Lancaster County, Pennsylvania, with an incidence of 1 in 500 live births.[19] CNF is inherited in an autosomal recessive manner and is caused by mutations in nephrin (*NPHS1*), the major structural component of the glomerular slit diaphragm (see **Fig. 1**).[20] Absence of the slit diaphragm and its size-selective barrier properties leads to massive loss of plasma proteins into the urine that begins in utero. Infants with CNF do not have associated major extrarenal findings, as *NPHS1* is expressed almost exclusively in the kidney podocyte.[21]

Table 1
Causes of congenital nephrotic syndrome

	Protein Function	Syndrome Association
Monogenic Causes		
NPHS1 (Nephrin)	Podocyte slit-diaphragm protein	Congenital nephrotic syndrome of the Finnish type
NPHS2 (Podocin)	Podocyte slit-diaphragm protein	
PLCE1 (Phospholipase C ε1)	Podocyte signaling protein	
WT1 (Wilms tumor suppressor 1)	Podocyte transcription factor	Isolated DMS or Denys-Drash syndrome
LAMB2 (Laminin β2)	GBM protein	Pierson syndrome
LAMB3 (Laminin β3)	GBM protein	Herlitz junctional epidermolysis bullosa
LMXB1 (Lim homeobox transcription factor 1β)	Podocyte transcription factor	Nail-patella syndrome
ITGA3 (integrin α3)	Adhesion molecule between podocytes and the GBM	NS with interstitial lung disease
ARHGDIA (Rho GDP dissociation inhibitor α)	Podocyte cytoskeletal regulation	
PMM2 (phosphomannomutase)	Enzyme necessary for synthesis of GDP-mannose	Congenital disorder of glycosylation, type I
SLC17A5 (sodium-phosphate cotransporter)	Vesicular amino acid transporter	Sialic acid storage disease
OCRL1	Enzyme involved in cytoskeletal regulation	Lowe syndrome
Mitochondrial mutations		
Unknown		Galloway-Mowat syndrome
Infectious Causes		
Cytomegalovirus		
Congenital syphilis		
Toxoplasmosis		
Malaria		
Rubella		
Hepatitis B		
HIV		
Other Causes		
Maternal SLE		
Maternal autoantibodies against neutral endopeptidase		

Abbreviations: DMS, diffuse mesangial sclerosis; GBM, glomerular basement membrane; GDP, guanosine diphosphate; HIV, human immunodeficiency virus; NS, nephrotic syndrome; SLE, systemic lupus erythematosus.

The diagnosis of CNF can often be made on a clinical basis (**Table 2**). More than 80% of infants with CNF are born prematurely, and most are appropriate for gestational age.[12] The placenta is typically larger than normal, weighing more than 25% of the infant's birth weight. Approximately 80% of affected infants present with edema and NS within the first week of life, with the remainder presenting within 3 months.[12] The initial urinalysis demonstrates proteinuria, hematuria, and leukocyturia with a negative urine culture.[12] Severe hypoalbuminemia is present with the serum albumin concentration generally less than 1.5 mg/dL. Renal function is initially normal, with decline in kidney function observed over several years. Over the first several months of life, hypothyroidism develops from loss of thyroid-binding globulin in the urine, and responds to thyroxine therapy.[22] In the first 2 months of life, kidneys are enlarged (+2 standard deviations above the mean) and hyperechoic on ultrasonography with preserved corticomedullary differentiation.[23] By 12 months of age, corticomedullary differentiation is lost and kidneys remain hyperechoic.

Kidney biopsy in CNF is rarely necessary for diagnosis. When performed, light microscopy demonstrates a mild increase in mesangial matrix and increased mesangial hypercellularity at early stages, with glomerular sclerosis and interstitial fibrosis evident with advancing age.[24] Microcystic dilatation of proximal and distal tubules can be observed.[12] On electron microscopy there is retraction and broadening of podocyte foot processes, classically described as effacement. In infants with severe NPHS1 mutations, slit diaphragms may be completely absent.[12]

Diagnosis of CNF can be confirmed by detection of mutations in NPHS1. Genetic testing is commercially available. More than 100 mutations in NPHS1 have been identified in affected patients. Mutations have been found throughout all 29 exons.[25,26] In Finland, greater than 90% of affected individuals have 1 of 2 mutations (nt121delCT or R1109X) that lead to premature stop codons and the absence of detectable protein at the slit diaphragm.[12]

CONGENITAL NEPHROTIC SYNDROME RESULTING FROM PODOCIN MUTATIONS (NPHS2)

Podocin, encoded by NPHS2, is a transmembrane protein localized to glomerular slit diaphragms that is required for targeting of nephrin to slit diaphragms (see **Fig. 1**).[27] Mutations in NPHS2 typically lead to childhood-onset steroid-resistant NS; however, the most severe mutations can present in the neonatal period.[28] CNS caused by

Table 2	
Diagnosis of congenital nephrotic syndrome of the Finnish type (NPHS1)	
Symptom/Sign	**Frequency (%)**
Proteinuria (>2000 mg/L)	100
Hypoalbuminemia (<2.5 mg/dL)	100
Edema	100
Elevated MSAFP (>2.5 MoM)	Unknown
Premature birth (<38 wk)	~80
Large placenta (placental weight/birth weight ratio >25%)	~95
Enlarged kidneys by renal ultrasonography (> +2 SD)	Unknown
Nephrotic syndrome in first week of life	~80

Abbreviations: MoM, multiples of the median; MSAFP, maternal serum α-fetoprotein; SD, standard deviation.

NPHS2 mutations is an autosomal recessive disorder. Clinical findings in infants with *NPHS2*-associated CNS are not well described; however, extrarenal manifestations are not observed. Disease onset is later on average in infants with *NPHS2* mutations than in those with *NPHS1* mutations. In a cohort of 63 European infants with CNS, 37% of those presenting with NS after 1 month of age had detectable *NPHS2* mutations, whereas mutations in *NPHS1* presenting after 1 month of age were less common, at 16%.[17] Children with *NPHS2*-associated CNS have a slower deterioration of renal function than children with CNF.[4]

Renal pathology in infants with *NPHS2*-associated CNS is variable. Most demonstrate either normal appearance of the kidney by light microscopy or evidence of focal segmental glomerulosclerosis (FSGS).[17] However, some infants with *NPHS2*-associated CNS demonstrate findings more typically associated with CNF, such as microcystic tubular dilatation or mesangial sclerosis, making these disorders difficult to distinguish definitively by biopsy alone.

DIFFUSE MESANGIAL SCLEROSIS CAUSED BY *WT1* MUTATIONS

WT1 encodes a zinc-finger transcription factor involved in kidney and gonadal development. The WT1 protein is highly expressed in podocytes, and controls the expression of slit diaphragm proteins such as nephrin as well as several growth factors and transcription factors (see **Fig. 1**).[29] Heterozygous mutations in *WT1* can cause either isolated diffuse mesangial sclerosis (DMS) or Denys-Drash syndrome. DMS is a distinct pathologic appearance of the kidney with diffuse increase in mesangial matrix with no mesangial cellular proliferation by light microscopy, with eventual contraction and obliteration of the glomerular tuft. Denys-Drash syndrome is characterized by early onset of NS, male pseudohermaphroditism, DMS on renal biopsy, rapid progression to end-stage kidney disease, and Wilms tumor, although incomplete forms of the syndrome have been described (**Box 1**).[30] NS typically begins at a few months of age, but Wilms tumor may be the first manifestation of the disease.[31] Genotypic male patients (46XY) display either ambiguous genitalia or female phenotype. Genotypic female patients (46XX) have normal female genitalia and normal puberty. *WT1* mutations are also found in older children causing Frasier syndrome, WAGR syndrome, or isolated NS.[30,32]

Children with *WT1* mutations require close ultrasonographic surveillance for development of Wilms tumor. Removal of native kidneys should be performed to prevent the development of Wilms tumor. Phenotypic females with DMS should have karyotypes performed.

PIERSON SYNDROME (*LAMB2*)

Pierson syndrome was originally described as CNS with DMS on renal biopsy and complex ocular anomalies.[33,34] The most common ocular finding is microcoria, but abnormalities of the lens, cornea, and retina have also been reported.[35] Pierson syndrome is caused by mutations in *LAMB2* encoding laminin-β2, a component of the

---

Box 1
Diagnosis of Denys-Drash syndrome

Congenital nephrotic syndrome (CNS) with diffuse mesangial sclerosis on kidney biopsy

Male pseudohermaphroditism or ambiguous genitalia

Wilms tumor

GBM responsible for cell adhesion (see **Fig. 1**). Laminin-β2 is also expressed in the nervous system, leading to neurologic deficits in affected children.[36]

OTHER GENETIC CAUSES OF CNS

Mutations in *PLCE1* lead to autosomal recessive nonsyndromic CNS with DMS on renal biopsy[37]; this has been found to be a common cause of isolated DMS, with one study demonstrating mutations in *PLCE1* in 28.6% of affected families.[38] *PLCE1* encodes a phospholipase enzyme that is involved in slit-diaphragm signaling in the podocyte.[39] Most affected children demonstrate rapidly progressive chronic kidney disease, and require dialysis or transplantation by the age of 5 years.[37,38] Of interest, there have been reports of affected infants who have remission of proteinuria with immune suppression.[37]

Galloway-Mowat syndrome is an autosomal recessive disorder caused by mutations in an unidentified gene. Affected infants present with CNS in association with central nervous system anomalies such as microcephaly, psychomotor retardation, and structural brain abnormalities.[40,41] Kidney biopsy may demonstrate minimal changes, FSGS, or DMS. Finally, several reports of infants with CNS caused by autosomal recessive mutations in *LAMB3, LMXB1, ITGA3,* or *ARGDIA* have been published.[42–45] CNS has also been described in rare association with Lowe syndrome, sialic acid storage disease, type 1 carbohydrate-deficient glycoprotein syndrome, and mitochondrial disease.[46–49]

NONGENETIC CAUSES OF CNS

Several congenital infections have been reported to cause CNS, particularly in developing countries.[50] The observed proteinuria and hypoalbuminemia is generally less severe than in genetic forms of CNS. Congenital syphilis may manifest in the newborn, but most often presents between 1 and 4 months of age. Early treatment with penicillin can be curative.[51] Renal pathology commonly demonstrates a membranous nephropathy. Cytomegalovirus (CMV)-associated CNS has also been described, and responds to treatment with gancyclovir.[52,53] Renal pathology in CMV-associated CNS usually shows DMS. Rare infants with CNS associated with congenital rubella and toxoplasmosis have also been described.[54,55] NS arising from infections with hepatitis B or human immunodeficiency virus have been reported in older children but not infants; nevertheless, this remains a diagnostic consideration in this population.[56,57]

EVALUATION OF AN INFANT WITH NEPHROTIC SYNDROME

All infants diagnosed with CNS should undergo a thorough family and birth history (**Table 3**). In addition, a complete physical examination including formal eye examination should be performed to uncover any associated syndromes. Renal ultrasonography should be performed to exclude other congenital anomalies of the kidney and urinary tract. Confirmation of NS is made through urine and blood testing. Screening examinations for congenital infections should be performed by either TORCH titer or polymerase chain reaction if available. Finally, genetic testing should be performed as indicated.

MANAGEMENT OF AN INFANT WITH NEPHROTIC SYNDROME

Other than 2 children reported in the literature with *PLCE1* mutations, immunosuppressive medications are not useful in the treatment of CNS. Treatment is generally

Table 3	
Evaluation of an infant with suspected congenital nephrotic syndrome	
Family history	Finnish ancestry
	Nephrotic syndrome
	Wilms tumor
	SLE
Birth history	MSAFP levels
	Placental size
	Maternal SLE
	Maternal infections
Physical examination	OFC
	Blood pressure
	Eye examination
	Genitalia
Imaging	Renal ultrasonography
Laboratory examinations	Urinalysis
	Urine protein-to-creatinine ratio
	Serum electrolytes
	BUN and creatinine
	Serum albumin
	Karyotype
	TORCH titers or PCR if available for congenital infections
	Genetic testing as indicated

Abbreviations: BUN, blood urea nitrogen; MSAFP, maternal serum α-fetoprotein; OFC, occipital-frontal circumference; PCR, polymerase chain reaction; SLE, systemic lupus erythematosus.

supportive, with the ultimate goal of kidney transplantation. Intravenous albumin infusions with loop diuretics are required on a chronic basis to manage edema, and may require placement of an indwelling catheter. Infants with CNS require close monitoring of growth and need a hypercaloric diet ($\sim$130 kcal/kg/d) with added protein ($\sim$4 g/kg/d). Nasogastric or gastrostomy tubes are often required to ensure adequate nutrition. Some infants will demonstrate an improvement in proteinuria with treatment with captopril or indomethacin, but infants with severe nephrin (*NPHS1*) mutations often do not respond.[58] Bilateral nephrectomies are performed when children are nearing end-stage kidney disease or if the NS cannot be managed by medical means. Kidney transplantation often takes place between 1 and 3 years of age.

COMPLICATIONS OF NEPHROTIC SYNDROME

Children with NS are at risk for infection, owing to losses of components of the alternative complement pathway into their urine.[59] This process results in increased susceptibility to infection with encapsulated organisms such as *Streptococcus pneumoniae, Haemophilus influenzae,* and *Escherichia coli.* Common infections include pneumonia, cellulitis, peritonitis, urinary tract infection, and sepsis.[60] A high degree of suspicion for infection is warranted in infants with CNS and fever, and broad-spectrum antibiotics should be initiated pending culture results. Prophylactic antibiotics or intravenous immunoglobulin infusions do not seem to influence the incidence of infection in this population, and are not recommended.[61]

Thromboembolism is a potentially serious complication of NS, and may be the presenting sign. The most common types of thrombosis include deep vein thrombosis, pulmonary embolism, renal vein thrombosis, and central sinus thrombosis.[62]

Nephrotic infants are at risk for thromboembolism for several reasons. First, there is urinary loss of factors that inhibit clot formation, such as antithrombin III. Second, there is increased production of procoagulant factors by the liver. Intravascular volume depletion attributable to NS itself or diuretic therapy can also increase the risk of thromboembolism. Some centers treat all infants with CNS prophylactically with warfarin to prevent thrombosis, particularly if there is an indwelling catheter.[63]

DIAGNOSIS OF NEPHRITIC SYNDROME

Nephritic syndrome in the newborn is rare and presents with hematuria, proteinuria, hypertension, acute kidney injury, oliguria, and edema (**Box 2**). Causes may overlap with those of congenital NS and include primary glomerulonephritis in addition to systemic disease, infections, and passive transplacental transfer of certain maternal antibodies (**Table 4**).

HEMOLYTIC UREMIC SYNDROME IN THE NEONATE

Hemolytic uremic syndrome (HUS) is a rare disease characterized by microangiopathic hemolytic anemia, thrombocytopenia, and renal dysfunction. Affected children demonstrate hematuria, oliguria, acute kidney injury, and hypertension along with schistocytes on peripheral smear, hemoglobin less than 10 g/dL, and platelet count less than 150×10^9/L.[64] HUS is caused by mutations in genes encoding complement regulatory proteins or by the effect of shiga-toxin released by *E coli* O157:H7 or related bacteria. Children with familial complement factor mutations can present in the first weeks of life.[64] Neonates with maternal to child transmission of shiga-toxin–producing *E coli* O157:H7 have also been reported.[65]

ANTENATAL MEMBRANOUS GLOMERULONEPHRITIS RESULTING FROM MATERNAL ANTIBODY TRANSFER

Neutral endopeptidase (NEP) is a widely distributed enzyme that is present on podocytes. Women with genetic mutations leading to complete absence of NEP may develop anti-NEP antibodies that cross the placenta and cause a pathologic form of glomerulonephritis known as membranous nephropathy.[66] Affected infants present at birth with proteinuria, oliguria, and acute kidney injury.[66,67] Anti-NEP antibodies can be detected in the maternal and infant serum, and disappear in the first weeks to months of life. Kidney disease resolves in most cases, although chronic kidney disease has been reported.[67]

Box 2
Diagnosis of nephritic syndrome in the neonate

Hematuria

Proteinuria

Acute kidney injury

Oliguria

Hypertension

Edema

Table 4 Causes of nephritic syndrome in the neonate	
Primary glomerulonephritis	Postinfectious glomerulonephritis Diffuse mesangial sclerosis
Systemic disease	Atypical hemolytic uremic syndrome Hemolytic uremic syndrome due to *Escherichia coli* O157:H7 Primary lupus nephritis
Infection	Syphilis Hepatitis B
Maternal antibody transfer	Neutral endopeptidase antibodies Maternal SLE

Abbreviation: SLE, systemic lupus erythematosus.

LUPUS NEPHRITIS

Lupus in neonates can be caused by either maternal transfer of autoantibodies or primary development of lupus. Neonatal lupus caused by passive transplacental transfer of maternal autoantibodies against Ro (SS-A) or La (SS-B) is typically characterized by cutaneous lesions and congenital heart block.[68] Nephritis in infants with maternally acquired neonatal lupus has rarely been described.[69,70] Primary lupus with nephritis can also develop in infants.[71] Affected infants have typical features of lupus nephritis, with hematuria, proteinuria, edema, hypertension, hypocomplementemia, anti–double-stranded DNA antibodies, and acute kidney injury.

EVALUATION OF AN INFANT WITH NEPHRITIC SYNDROME

Infants with nephritic syndromes should have an evaluation similar to that for infants with CNS (see **Table 3**). Maternal and family history of lupus should be explored. In addition, a complete blood count should be performed to evaluate for anemia or thrombocytopenia. Hypocomplementemia and elevated double-stranded DNA antibodies may suggest primary lupus. Kidney biopsy may be required to make a definitive diagnosis.

MANAGEMENT OF NEONATAL NEPHRITIC SYNDROME

Treatment of glomerulonephritis in the newborn is tailored to the primary cause. Infants with HUS resulting from complement mutations may benefit from treatment with eculizumab, a monoclonal antibody that targets the terminal component of the complement cascade.[64] Infants with hemolytic uremic syndrome may require frequent blood transfusions. Primary lupus nephritis is treated with immunosuppression. General supportive management includes diuretics, antihypertensive therapy, and dialysis if necessary.

REFERENCES

1. Reiser J, Kriz W, Kretzler M, et al. The glomerular slit diaphragm is a modified adherens junction. J Am Soc Nephrol 2000;11(1):1–8.
2. Mundel P, Shankland SJ. Podocyte biology and response to injury. J Am Soc Nephrol 2002;13(12):3005–15.
3. Oh J, Reiser J, Mundel P. Dynamic (re)organization of the podocyte actin cytoskeleton in the nephrotic syndrome. Pediatr Nephrol 2004;19(2):130–7.

4. Hinkes B, Vlangos C, Heeringa S, et al. Specific podocin mutations correlate with age of onset in steroid-resistant nephrotic syndrome. J Am Soc Nephrol 2008;19(2):365–71.

5. Santin S, Garcia-Maset R, Ruiz P, et al. Nephrin mutations cause childhood- and adult-onset focal segmental glomerulosclerosis. Kidney Int 2009;76(12): 1268–76.

6. Muller F, Forestier F, Dingeon B, ABA Study Group. Second trimester trisomy 21 maternal serum marker screening. Results of a countrywide study of 854,902 patients. Prenat Diagn 2002;22(10):925–9.

7. Spaggiari E, Ruas M, Dreux S, et al. Management strategy in pregnancies with elevated second-trimester maternal serum alpha-fetoprotein based on a second assay. Am J Obstet Gynecol 2013;208(4):303.e1–7.

8. Patrakka J, Martin P, Salonen R, et al. Proteinuria and prenatal diagnosis of congenital nephrosis in fetal carriers of nephrin gene mutations. Lancet 2002; 359(9317):1575–7.

9. Kestila M, Jarvela I. Prenatal diagnosis of congenital nephrotic syndrome (CNF, NPHS1). Prenat Diagn 2003;23(4):323–4.

10. Miltenyi M. Urinary protein excretion in healthy children. Clin Nephrol 1979; 12(5):216–21.

11. Houser M. Assessment of proteinuria using random urine samples. J Pediatr 1984;104(6):845–8.

12. Patrakka J, Kestila M, Wartiovaara J, et al. Congenital nephrotic syndrome (NPHS1): features resulting from different mutations in Finnish patients. Kidney Int 2000;58(3):972–80.

13. Holmberg C, Antikainen M, Ronnholm K, et al. Management of congenital nephrotic syndrome of the Finnish type. Pediatr Nephrol 1995;9(1):87–93.

14. Antikainen M, Holmberg C, Taskinen MR. Growth, serum lipoproteins and apo-proteins in infants with congenital nephrosis. Clin Nephrol 1992;38(5):254–63.

15. Siddall EC, Radhakrishnan J. The pathophysiology of edema formation in the nephrotic syndrome. Kidney Int 2012;82(6):635–42.

16. Hinkes BG, Mucha B, Vlangos CN, et al. Nephrotic syndrome in the first year of life: two thirds of cases are caused by mutations in 4 genes (NPHS1, NPHS2, WT1, and LAMB2). Pediatrics 2007;119(4):e907–19.

17. Machuca E, Benoit G, Nevo F, et al. Genotype-phenotype correlations in non-Finnish congenital nephrotic syndrome. J Am Soc Nephrol 2010;21(7): 1209–17.

18. Huttunen NP. Congenital nephrotic syndrome of Finnish type. Study of 75 patients. Arch Dis Child 1976;51(5):344–8.

19. Bolk S, Puffenberger EG, Hudson J, et al. Elevated frequency and allelic hetero-geneity of congenital nephrotic syndrome, Finnish type, in the old order Menno-nites. Am J Hum Genet 1999;65(6):1785–90.

20. Kestila M, Lenkkeri U, Mannikko M, et al. Positionally cloned gene for a novel glomerular protein–nephrin–is mutated in congenital nephrotic syndrome. Mol Cell 1998;1(4):575–82.

21. Kuusniemi AM, Kestila M, Patrakka J, et al. Tissue expression of nephrin in human and pig. Pediatr Res 2004;55(5):774–81.

22. McLean RH, Kennedy TL, Rosoulpour M, et al. Hypothyroidism in the congenital nephrotic syndrome. J Pediatr 1982;101(1):72–5.

23. Saraga M, Jaaskelainen J, Koskimies O. Diagnostic sonographic changes in the kidneys of 20 infants with congenital nephrotic syndrome of the Finnish type. Eur Radiol 1995;5:49–54.

24. Kuusniemi AM, Merenmies J, Lahdenkari AT, et al. Glomerular sclerosis in kidneys with congenital nephrotic syndrome (NPHS1). Kidney Int 2006;70(8): 1423–31.

25. Heeringa SF, Vlangos CN, Chernin G, et al. Thirteen novel NPHS1 mutations in a large cohort of children with congenital nephrotic syndrome. Nephrol Dial Transplant 2008;23(11):3527–33.

26. Beltcheva O, Martin P, Lenkkeri U, et al. Mutation spectrum in the nephrin gene (NPHS1) in congenital nephrotic syndrome. Hum Mutat 2001;17(5): 368–73.

27. Boute N, Gribouval O, Roselli S, et al. NPHS2, encoding the glomerular protein podocin, is mutated in autosomal recessive steroid-resistant nephrotic syndrome. Nat Genet 2000;24(4):349–54.

28. Weber S, Gribouval O, Esquivel EL, et al. NPHS2 mutation analysis shows genetic heterogeneity of steroid-resistant nephrotic syndrome and low post-transplant recurrence. Kidney Int 2004;66(2):571–9.

29. Stoll R, Lee BM, Debler EW, et al. Structure of the Wilms tumor suppressor protein zinc finger domain bound to DNA. J Mol Biol 2007;372(5):1227–45.

30. Niaudet P, Gubler MC. WT1 and glomerular diseases. Pediatr Nephrol 2006; 21(11):1653–60.

31. Habib R, Gubler MC, Antignac C, et al. Diffuse mesangial sclerosis: a congenital glomerulopathy with nephrotic syndrome. Adv Nephrol Necker Hosp 1993;22: 43–57.

32. Moorthy AV, Chesney RW, Lubinsky M. Chronic renal failure and XY gonadal dysgenesis: "Frasier" syndrome–a commentary on reported cases. Am J Med Genet Suppl 1987;3:297–302.

33. Zenker M, Aigner T, Wendler O, et al. Human laminin beta2 deficiency causes congenital nephrosis with mesangial sclerosis and distinct eye abnormalities. Hum Mol Genet 2004;13(21):2625–32.

34. Pierson M, Cordier J, Hervouuet F, et al. An unusual congenital and familial congenital malformative combination involving the eye and kidney. J Genet Hum 1963;12:184–213 [in French].

35. Matejas V, Hinkes B, Alkandari F, et al. Mutations in the human laminin beta2 (LAMB2) gene and the associated phenotypic spectrum. Hum Mutat 2010; 31(9):992–1002.

36. Wuhl E, Kogan J, Zurowska A, et al. Neurodevelopmental deficits in Pierson (microcoria-congenital nephrosis) syndrome. Am J Med Genet A 2007;143(4): 311–9.

37. Hinkes B, Wiggins RC, Gbadegesin R, et al. Positional cloning uncovers mutations in PLCE1 responsible for a nephrotic syndrome variant that may be reversible. Nat Genet 2006;38(12):1397–405.

38. Gbadegesin R, Hinkes BG, Hoskins BE, et al. Mutations in PLCE1 are a major cause of isolated diffuse mesangial sclerosis (IDMS). Nephrol Dial Transplant 2008;23(4):1291–7.

39. Chaib H, Hoskins BE, Ashraf S, et al. Identification of BRAF as a new interactor of PLCepsilon1, the protein mutated in nephrotic syndrome type 3. Am J Physiol Renal Physiol 2008;294(1):F93–9.

40. Galloway WH, Mowat AP. Congenital microcephaly with hiatus hernia and nephrotic syndrome in two sibs. J Med Genet 1968;5(4):319–21.

41. Meyers KE, Kaplan P, Kaplan BS. Nephrotic syndrome, microcephaly, and developmental delay: three separate syndromes. Am J Med Genet 1999; 82(3):257–60.

42. Hata D, Miyazaki M, Seto S, et al. Nephrotic syndrome and aberrant expression of laminin isoforms in glomerular basement membranes for an infant with Herlitz junctional epidermolysis bullosa. Pediatrics 2005;116(4):e601–7.
43. Lemley KV. Kidney disease in nail-patella syndrome. Pediatr Nephrol 2009; 24(12):2345–54.
44. Nicolaou N, Margadant C, Kevelam SH, et al. Gain of glycosylation in integrin alpha3 causes lung disease and nephrotic syndrome. J Clin Invest 2012; 122(12):4375–87.
45. Gupta IR, Baldwin C, Auguste D, et al. ARHGDIA: a novel gene implicated in nephrotic syndrome. J Med Genet 2013;50(5):330–8.
46. Nielsen KF, Steffensen GK. Congenital nephrotic syndrome associated with Lowe's syndrome. Child Nephrol Urol 1990;10(2):92–5.
47. Lemyre E, Russo P, Melancon SB, et al. Clinical spectrum of infantile free sialic acid storage disease. Am J Med Genet 1999;82(5):385–91.
48. van der Knaap MS, Wevers RA, Monnens L, et al. Congenital nephrotic syndrome: a novel phenotype of type I carbohydrate-deficient glycoprotein syndrome. J Inherit Metab Dis 1996;19(6):787–91.
49. Goldenberg A, Ngoc LH, Thouret MC, et al. Respiratory chain deficiency presenting as congenital nephrotic syndrome. Pediatr Nephrol 2005;20(4):465–9.
50. Vachvanichsanong P, Mitarnun W, Tungsinmunkong K, et al. Congenital and infantile nephrotic syndrome in Thai infants. Clin Pediatr 2005;44(2):169–74.
51. Basker M, Agarwal I, Bendon KS. Congenital nephrotic syndrome - a treatable cause. Ann Trop Paediatr 2007;27(1):87–90.
52. Besbas N, Bayrakci US, Kale G, et al. Cytomegalovirus-related congenital nephrotic syndrome with diffuse mesangial sclerosis. Pediatr Nephrol 2006;21(5):740–2.
53. Batisky DL, Roy S 3rd, Gaber LW. Congenital nephrosis and neonatal cytomegalovirus infection: a clinical association. Pediatr Nephrol 1993;7(6):741–3.
54. Esterly JR, Oppenheimer EH. Pathological lesions due to congenital rubella. Arch Pathol 1969;87(4):380–8.
55. Shahin B, Papadopoulou ZL, Jenis EH. Congenital nephrotic syndrome associated with congenital toxoplasmosis. J Pediatr 1974;85(3):366–70.
56. Gilbert RD, Wiggelinkhuizen J. The clinical course of hepatitis B virus-associated nephropathy. Pediatr Nephrol 1994;8(1):11–4.
57. Chaparro AI, Mitchell CD, Abitbol CL, et al. Proteinuria in children infected with the human immunodeficiency virus. J Pediatr 2008;152(6):844–9.
58. Licht C, Eifinger F, Gharib M, et al. A stepwise approach to the treatment of early onset nephrotic syndrome. Pediatr Nephrol 2000;14(12):1077–82.
59. Matsell DG, Wyatt RJ. The role of I and B in peritonitis associated with the nephrotic syndrome of childhood. Pediatr Res 1993;34(1):84–8.
60. Rheault MN, Wei CC, Hains DS, et al. Increasing frequency of acute kidney injury amongst children hospitalized with nephrotic syndrome. Pediatr Nephrol 2014;29(1):139–47.
61. Ljungberg P, Holmberg C, Jalanko H. Infections in infants with congenital nephrosis of the Finnish type. Pediatr Nephrol 1997;11(2):148–52.
62. Kerlin BA, Ayoob R, Smoyer WE. Epidemiology and pathophysiology of nephrotic syndrome-associated thromboembolic disease. Clin J Am Soc Nephrol 2012; 7(3):513–20.
63. Jalanko H. Congenital nephrotic syndrome. Pediatr Nephrol 2009;24(11):2121–8.
64. Besbas N, Gulhan B, Karpman D, et al. Neonatal onset atypical hemolytic uremic syndrome successfully treated with eculizumab. Pediatr Nephrol 2013; 28(1):155–8.

65. Ulinski T, Lervat C, Ranchin B, et al. Neonatal hemolytic uremic syndrome after mother-to-child transmission of *Escherichia coli* O157. Pediatr Nephrol 2005; 20(9):1334–5.

66. Debiec H, Guigonis V, Mougenot B, et al. Antenatal membranous glomerulonephritis due to anti-neutral endopeptidase antibodies. N Engl J Med 2002; 346(26):2053–60.

67. Debiec H, Nauta J, Coulet F, et al. Role of truncating mutations in MME gene in fetomaternal alloimmunisation and antenatal glomerulopathies. Lancet 2004; 364(9441):1252–9.

68. Lee LA. Neonatal lupus: clinical features and management. Paediatr Drugs 2004;6(2):71–8.

69. Lam C, Imundo L, Hirsch D, et al. Glomerulonephritis in a neonate with atypical congenital lupus and toxoplasmosis. Pediatr Nephrol 1999;13(9):850–3.

70. Westenend PJ. Congenital nephrotic syndrome in neonatal lupus syndrome. J Pediatr 1995;126(5 Pt 1):851.

71. Massengill SF, Richard GA, Donnelly WH. Infantile systemic lupus erythematosus with onset simulating congenital nephrotic syndrome. J Pediatr 1994;124(1): 27–31.

Renal Teratogens

Thomas M. Morgan, MD[a], Deborah P. Jones, MD, MS[b],
William O. Cooper, MD, MPH[c],*

KEYWORDS

- Kidney development • Teratogens • Pregnancy • Drug safety

KEY POINTS

- As the average age of childbearing increases, so does fetal exposure to potentially nephroteratogenic drugs.
- Renin-angiotensin system inhibitors should be avoided in pregnancy, and fetal exposure in the second half of pregnancy can cause a distinctive fetopathy, characterized by renal tubular dysplasia, oligohydramnios, hypertension, and hypocalvaria.
- Nonsteroidal antiinflammatory drugs taken late in pregnancy may cause oligohydramnios and should be avoided unless potential benefits (eg, for tocolysis) outweigh risks.
- Women of childbearing potential and their physicians should communicate clearly and frequently about the potential fetal risks of medications, and steps to avert or mitigate harm should be taken if clinically indicated.
- There is an urgent need for further research on fetal effects of maternally administered drugs, and study design, whenever possible, should include assessment of short-term and long-term renal harms.

INTRODUCTION

The average age of women at first childbirth has increased dramatically over the past several decades, having reached 30 years of age (the highest worldwide) in the United Kingdom and Germany and 25 years of age in the United States.[1] With the trend toward increased maternal age, as well as the declining state of preconception health

Potential conflicts of interest: T.M. Morgan served as an expert witness in litigation involving Janssen Pharmaceuticals and on the Liver Disease Board of Arrowhead Research Group. His service did not pertain to any of the medications included in this review.
Disclosures: none.
[a] Division of Medical Genetics, Department of Pediatrics, Vanderbilt University School of Medicine, 2200 Children's Way, 6120 Doctor's Office Tower, Nashville, TN 37232, USA; [b] Division of Pediatric Nephrology, Department of Pediatrics, Vanderbilt University School of Medicine, 2200 Children's Way, 10110 Doctor's Office Tower, Nashville, TN 37232, USA; [c] Division of General Pediatrics, Department of Pediatrics, Vanderbilt University School of Medicine, 1313 21st Avenue South, Suite 313, Nashville, TN 37232, USA
* Corresponding author.
E-mail address: william.cooper@vanderbilt.edu

Clin Perinatol 41 (2014) 619–632
http://dx.doi.org/10.1016/j.clp.2014.05.010
perinatology.theclinics.com

among women of childbearing age, there is an increasing prevalence of maternal chronic medical conditions, such as diabetes and hypertension, requiring prescription medication, which may result in fetal drug exposure.[2] In addition, as the evidence of the developmental origins of adult chronic diseases such as hypertension accumulates, fetal renal drug safety is likely to have long-term public health significance.[3]

Existing knowledge about the effects of maternal drug exposure on fetal kidneys is limited and derives mostly from case reports and observational studies. Thus, for most medication exposures, causality of adverse fetal consequences must be indirectly inferred according to the epidemiologic principles articulated by Doll and Hill.[4,5] Using the term teratogen broadly to include any substance that has the potential, under certain exposure conditions, to have a clinically significant harmful effect on fetal formation or organ function allows one to consider both congenital malformations of the kidney and impacts on renal function as potential outcomes of exposure. To understand fully whether or not a particular drug is a teratogen, the effects of disruptions in renal development and the functional sequelae of reduced nephron number and renal function resulting from in utero exposures should be considered.

Teratogens, per the US Food and Drug Administration (FDA) recommended use of the term,[6] have the "capacity under certain exposure conditions to produce abnormal development in an embryo or fetus." Most clinicians are familiar with the FDA fetal and infant risk classification of drugs used by pregnant or lactating women according to the A, B, C, D, or X system, explained as follows: class A, adequate and well-controlled (AWC) studies failing to show risk; B, animal reproduction studies show no risk, but AWC studies are lacking; C, adverse fetal effect in animal studies, with no AWC human studies available; D, positive evidence of human fetal risk, but benefits may justify use in appropriately compelling clinical scenarios; and X, positive evidence of risk that outweighs any possible benefit.[7] However, the FDA has proposed to eliminate the foregoing classification scheme and substitute a more detailed narrative description with 3 key elements: risk summary, clinical considerations, and data,[7] with the final rule to be implemented in 2014.[8]

In this article, the existing literature on suspected human nephroteratogenic drugs is summarized and critically appraised and brief clinical considerations are presented with risk/benefit/alternative analysis for each drug class during the relevant period of pregnancy, citing currently preferred drugs or treatment strategies that are believed to minimize the potential for maternal-fetal harm. We begin, to place in developmental context the potential for nephroteratogenicity, with an illustrative case (**Box 1**). The case described in **Box 1** shows several questions that arise when an individual with preexisting hypertension who is taking an angiotensin-converting enzyme (ACE) inhibitor or angiotensin receptor blocker (ARB) becomes pregnant. What is the risk of exposure to potentially teratogenic medication and to maternal hypertension to her baby? Which medications should be used to control blood pressure? Should the pregnancy be terminated because of conception while on valsartan? How should the infant be assessed for ARB exposure-related effect? What are the long-term effects of fetal exposure to medications that have the potential to alter kidney development?

OVERVIEW OF NEPHROGENESIS

It is useful to consider the major stages of nephrogenesis, because the timing of fetal exposure is likely to affect the observed phenotype. As shown in **Fig. 1**, kidney development in the human embryo begins before the end of the fifth week of gestation (ie, third embryonic week). Normal development is initiated with formation of the ureteric

---

Box 1
Case 1

A 16-year-old woman had been followed in the pediatric nephrology clinic since the age of 9 years for hypertension secondary to renal scarring (right upper pole scar) and vesicoureteral reflux, which had resolved. She was treated with valsartan 160 mg daily and amlodipine 5 mg daily. Past medical history was remarkable for imperforate anus, s/p repair as an infant, linear growth delay, delayed puberty, and recurrent urinary tract infections. The family history was negative for end-stage renal disease or known kidney disease. Her electrolytes were normal and serum creatinine level was 0.7 mg/dL. Her urine protein excretion was abnormal, with a baseline urine protein/creatinine ratio of 0.5 (normal <0.2). Her follow-up to clinic was sporadic, because she missed about 50% of scheduled appointments. Her mother called to report that she was pregnant and requested advice on continuation of her antihypertensive medications. She was advised to discontinue valsartan and was scheduled to see a high-risk obstetrician for care during her pregnancy. She was seen during the 24th week of gestation by a high-risk obstetrician/gynecologist, who recommended starting labetalol 200 mg by mouth twice daily, and continued the amlodipine. She did not return for the next assessment until she was in labor at 34 weeks. Fetal ultrasonography showed a normal volume of amniotic fluid and no fetal anomalies. A female infant with birth weight 2100 g was delivered by spontaneous vaginal delivery and taken to the neonatal intensive care unit for observation.

---

bud, which arises from the Wolffian duct; the surrounding metanephric mesenchyme induces ureteric bud development by elaboration of multiple factors.[9,10] Ureteric bud induction, growth, and branching are necessary for normal kidney development to proceed. Through a series of orchestrated chemical signaling events, branching morphogenesis results in the formation of approximately 15 generations of branches. The first 6 to 10 form the pelvis and calyces and the final 6 to 9 form the collecting ducts. The process of branching morphogenesis is complete by 20 to 22 weeks.[11] Thereafter, nephrons are induced in clusters around the terminal collecting duct branches, because they maintain the ability to induce surrounding mesenchyme.[9,11] The mesenchyme forms the glomeruli, proximal tubules, the loops of Henle, and the distal convoluted tubules. Differentiation into distinct epithelial subtypes proceeds in parallel with canalization and results in formation of the renal vesicle. The renal vesicle becomes connected with the adjacent ureteric bud ampulla to form the renal tubular lumen.[11] Nephron formation is typically completed by 36 weeks' gestation.

Disruption of the sequence of events described earlier results in a variety of renal phenotypes (congenital renal diseases); some are structural disorders and others are identified by their histopathologic features. In general, failure of ureteric bud outgrowth results in complete lack of kidney formation, a condition known as renal agenesis. Decreased ureteric bud branching may result in renal dysplasia or renal hypoplasia.

The most severe type of renal dysplasia includes the multicystic dysplastic kidney (large cysts replace normal parenchyma) and renal cystic dysplasia; both have reduced normal tissue because of incomplete differentiation and primitive, nonrenal tissues such as neural, cartilaginous, and muscular. Dysplastic kidneys are characterized by incomplete branching of the ureteric buds and undifferentiated mesenchyme and generally show reduced function. Cystic dysplasia refers to a form of dysplasia in which cysts and primitive tubules are scattered among otherwise normal nephrons; these kidneys usually have some function.

Renal hypoplasia refers to kidneys that contain mature nephrons in reduced number. In general, renal mass and dimensions are less than normal.[11] It is possible to have renal hypoplasia and normal renal appearance on ultrasonography, given the ability to compensate for reduced nephron number with hypertrophy of the remaining nephrons.[12]

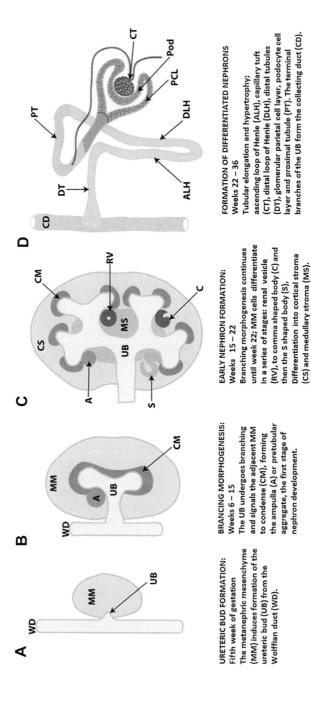

A

URETERIC BUD FORMATION:
Fifth week of gestation
The metanephric mesenchyme (MM) induces formation of the ureteric bud (UB) from the Wolffian duct (WD).

B

BRANCING MORPHOGENESIS:
Weeks 6 – 15
The UB undergoes branching and signals the adjacent MM to condense (CM), forming the ampulla (A) or pretubular aggregate, the first stage of nephron development.

C

EARLY NEPHRON FORMATION:
Weeks 15 – 22
Branching morphogenesis continues until week 22; MM cells differentiate in a series of stages: renal vesicle (RV), to comma shaped body (C) and then the S shaped body (S). Differentiation into cortical stroma (CS) and medullary stroma (MS).

D

FORMATION OF DIFFERENTIATED NEPHRONS
Weeks 22 – 36
Tubular elongation and hypertrophy; ascending loop of Henle (ALH), capillary tuft (CT), distal loop of Henle (DLH), distal tubules (DT), glomerular parietal cell layer, podocyte cell layer and proximal tubule (PT). The terminal branches of the UB form the collecting duct (CD).

Fig. 1. Overview of renal development. (*From* Cain JE, Di Giovanni V, Smeeton J, et al. Genetics of renal hypoplasia: insights into the mechanisms controlling nephron endowment. Pediatr Res 2010;68(2):92. Macmillan Publishers LTD; with permission.)

Ectopic ureteric bud outgrowth results in duplex or obstructed collecting systems or vesicoureteral reflux; however, renal dysplasia may also be observed. Renal dysplasia is often observed in the setting of obstruction and poor urinary flow. Because abnormalities of the ureters and bladder often occur in parallel with defects in parenchymal differentiation, indicating an intimate relationship between nephronal and urinary tract development, the term congenital anomalies of the kidney and urinary tract is used to refer to the variety of developmental diseases seen in children.[12]

Detection of the effect of renal teratogens on the developing kidney depends on the expected phenotype. Diagnostic imaging readily shows certain phenotypes (eg, aplasia, obstruction, hypoplasia, and cystic dysplasia), whereas others may be identified only by histopathology, which is not generally clinically available. Some developmental anomalies may be ascertained early in life, whereas others, such as reduced nephron number, may not be clinically consequential until adulthood.

THE RENIN-ANGIOTENSIN SYSTEM DURING DEVELOPMENT

In addition to direct effects on nephrogenesis and kidney function, some medications may affect the complex renin-angiotensin system (RAS), resulting in various consequences. Limited data are available for the human fetus; the mouse has most often been used as an alternative model system. In these mouse models, angiotensinogen messenger RNA is localized to the proximal tubule by the eighth week of gestation. Renin RNA expression is detected in midgestation in the mouse embryo, where it localizes to the renal arteries and in the juxtaglomerular cells.[13]

Pharmacologic inhibition with ACE inhibitors or ARBs in rodents postnatally (because nephrogenesis continues for 2 to 3 weeks) results in abnormalities in vasculature and nephrogenesis, leading to reduced nephron number and disorganization of the medulla.[13] Similarly, disruption of any one of the RAS component genes results in renal tubular dysgenesis, with reduced number and shortening of renal tubules as well as architectural disorganization.

KNOWN OR SUSPECTED NEPHROTERATOGENIC DRUG CLASSES
ACE Inhibitors and ARBs

ACE inhibitors block the conversion of angiotensin I to angiotensin II, whereas ARBs antagonize the type I receptor of angiotensin II (**Table 1**). Both classes are widely used antihypertensive agents, either as monotherapy or in combination with thiazide diuretics, and they readily cross the placenta. ACE inhibitors are first-line agents for the management of hypertension in diabetics, and the frequency of use in pregnancy increased 4-fold from the late 1980s to 2003, despite the 1992 FDA black box warning against intrapartum ACE inhibitor use, reaching 6 exposures per thousand pregnancies.[14]

Data on the effects of ACE inhibitors and ARBs on the RAS system and the developing kidney in animal models suggest that RAS is involved in ureteric bud branching morphogenesis; inhibition of the normal RAS pathway is associated with decreased nephron number along with a variety of malformations (ureteropelvic junction obstruction, megaureter, aplasia, and hypoplasia) in a subset of exposed animals.[13,15] Later exposure exerts hemodynamic effects on tubular differentiation, leading to tubular dysgenesis as well as reduced renal perfusion, reduced glomerular filtration rate, and fetal hypotension (ACE fetopathy).[13,16]

In humans, the so-called ACE inhibitor fetopathy[17,18] may be caused by exposure to either ACE inhibitors or ARBs in approximately the second half of pregnancy. It is characterized by fetal renal tubular dysplasia, oliguria or anuria, oligohydramnios with

Table 1 Renal teratogens		
Drug or Drug Class	**Relevant Timing of Exposure**	**Teratogenic Outcome**
ACE inhibitors and ARBs	Second half of pregnancy	ACE inhibitor fetopathy (renal tubular dysplasia, oligohydramnios, resistant hypertension, hypocalvaria
Nonsteroidal antiinflammatory drugs	After 30 wk gestation	Oligohydramnios, premature fetal ductus arteriosus closure
Tacrolimus	Indeterminate (likely late)	Mild, transient oliguria
Trastuzumab	Second/third trimester of pregnancy	Oligohydramnios or anhydramnios
Mycophenolate mofetil	First trimester	EMFO: ear, mouth, finger, and other (including renal) organ malformations
Thalidomide	First trimester	Thalidomide embryopathy: limb reduction defects, gastrointestinal, cardiac, otic, cranial nerve, and renal malformations

potential for pulmonary hypoplasia and Potter sequence, intrauterine growth retardation, and treatment-resistant fetal and postnatal hypotension with hypocalvaria (underdeveloped mesenchyme-derived, directly ossified, membrane skull bones but normal cartilage-derived skull base, with enlarged fontanelle and wide cranial sutures). The mechanism of hypocalvaria is unknown, but skull bone growth proceeds postnatally, and it is considered a potentially reversible feature in survivors of ACE inhibitor fetopathy.[18] Exposure during the first trimester does not produce distinctive ACE inhibitor fetopathy, but is associated with a 2-fold increased rate of major congenital malformations in newborns[19,20]; alternatives to ACE inhibitors should be considered in women who may become pregnant while taking an antihypertensive drug.

Safer alternatives to RAS blockers for chronic hypertension management in pregnancy, according to evidence-based guidelines, include labetalol (preferred first-line option), nifedipine, and methydopa, but other antihypertensive agents may also be considered, including other β-blockers (except atenolol, which is associated with intrauterine growth restriction), calcium channel blockers, diuretics, and hydralazine (note risk of neonatal thrombocytopenia), according to American College of Obstetrics and Gynecology (ACOG) guidelines.[20] RAS blockers are contraindicated throughout pregnancy.[21]

Nonsteroidal Antiinflammatory Drugs (Selective/Nonselective)

Nonsteroidal antiinflammatory drugs (NSAIDs) are taken in pregnancy for acute pain or chronic conditions such as rheumatologic disorders. NSAIDs are effective tocolytic agents, but cross the placenta and inhibit fetal prostaglandin and thromboxane production, leading to increased risks, which differ in early and late pregnancy. Early exposure has been reported to increase spontaneous abortion rate[22] and possibly cause congenital malformations, but a recent large Israeli retrospective cohort study[23] showed no increase in renal or other malformations among infants whose mothers were exposed to NSAIDs in pregnancy, and no increase in stillbirths. When NSAIDs are used late in pregnancy, premature fetal ductus arteriosus closure may occur, and NSAIDs rapidly reduce fetal urine production, causing oligohydramnios; NSAIDs have a therapeutic use in polyhydramnios.[24] NSAID-induced renal effects can in rare instances be severe, particularly after 32 weeks' gestation, with potential for neonatal renal failure, but the magnitude of risk in various clinical scenarios remains unclear and may vary with the dose, duration, timing of therapy, and maternal indication for use. NSAIDs should generally be avoided in pregnancy unless maternal benefits substantially outweigh fetal risks.

Indomethacin, an NSAID used for tocolysis, has been associated with a 2% to 20% incidence of fetal/neonatal renal impairment.[25] Although the optimal treatment of preterm labor has not been established, some guidelines support short-term use of indomethacin ($\leq$48 hours) as first-line tocolytic treatment to delay parturition long enough for maternally administered corticosteroids to promote fetal lung maturity.[26] Information about the risks and benefits of tocolysis with indomethacin should be shared with pregnant women to facilitate their understanding of whether to proceed with this treatment option.

Corticosteroids

Corticosteroids (prednisone, methylprednisolone) may be prescribed early in pregnancy and in some cases throughout pregnancy for acute conditions such as maternal asthma, or for immunosuppression in transplant recipients or patients with other chronic immunologic or rheumatologic disorders. Another indication for administration of glucocorticoids to women in preterm labor is to hasten the process of fetal lung maturation (eg, betamethasone, dexamethasone). Existing analyses of glucocorticoids on fetal renal function in such complicated clinical settings are highly confounded by maternal comorbidity and polypharmacy. Although animal studies have raised concerns about the potential for excessive corticosteroid exposure to impair nephrogenesis,[27] there are few data in humans from which to draw conclusions regarding fetal kidney safety.[28]

Intrauterine growth retardation is strongly suspected to be a consequence of prolonged exposure to maternally administered glucocorticoids, but specific influences on fetal renal development, maturation, and postnatal function have not been studied extensively. Postnatal increased glomerular filtration rate and sodium reabsorption have been observed during the first 2 weeks of life after prenatal exposure to glucocorticoids for fetal lung maturity, and such effects may to some extent be salutary in the preterm infant, with lesser need for vasopressors or treatment of hyperkalemia.[25] A meta-analysis of clinical trials of antenatal steroids for fetal lung maturity showed extensive trial design gaps in secondary safety end points, including renal safety,[29] and long-term renal effects are almost entirely unknown, although 1 study[30] suggested a possible association with hypertension in adolescence.

Cancer Chemotherapeutics

Given the fundamental cellular pathways targeted by antineoplastics, these agents are suspect with respect to fetal renal and general teratogenesis, but data necessarily are derived only from case reports or case series, because of the infrequency of use of particular agents, and even when substantial data are available, analysis is complicated by polypharmacy and widespread variation in dosing, timing of fetal exposure, and severity and type of maternal disease. Thus, without observation of a recurrent, distinctive, teratogenic pattern, most renal safety concerns remain inconclusive. There is no example, to our knowledge, of a particular rare renal anomaly that predictably occurs in relation to maternal exposure to an antineoplastic drug.

A recent meta-analysis of trastuzumab, a HER2-receptor antagonist used for breast cancer treatment, found that oligohydramnios/anhydramnios during pregnancy incidence was 61%, the most frequent adverse event in relation to trastuzumab exposure, with risk confined to fetuses exposed in second and third trimester, perhaps via an epidermal growth factor receptor–blocking mechanism.[31] Its FDA pregnancy category is D, partly because of the oligohydramnios/anhydramnios risk, and the investigators of the meta-analysis concluded (in keeping with National Comprehensive Cancer Network guidelines) that trastuzumab should not be used during pregnancy, but that clinicians may reasonably recommend pregnancy continuation in the event of inadvertent in utero exposure.

Immunosuppressives

The topic of pregnancy in renal transplant recipients has recently been reviewed.[32] The risks of azathioprine, cyclosporine, and tacrolimus were characterized as surprisingly low by the study, based on the expanding observational literature documenting pregnancy outcomes in the increasing number of long-term survivors of renal transplantation. Experience with rapamycin inhibitors sirolimus and everolimus is too limited to draw any conclusions about safety during pregnancy, and there are no renal-specific data pertaining to the fetus or newborn.

Cyclosporine nephrotoxicity has been established in rabbits,[33] and adults exposed to cyclosporine sustain dose-related acute kidney injury,[34] but nephroteratology data in humans are inconclusive, although small studies have shown no obvious fetal renal effects. In animal models, exposure to cyclosporine in early gestation is associated with as much as a 50% reduction in nephron number, indicating interruption of branching morphogenesis.[35]

Limited data on postnatal renal function after prolonged in utero exposure to cyclosporine in pregnancies to female recipients of organ transplants have detected no renal impairment,[36] including no significant impairment of renal function using sensitive (inulin and para-aminohippuric acid) clearance measures in 12 children aged 1 to 7 years.[37] Cyclosporine is not established as a nephroteratogen.

Mycophenolate mofetil, by contrast, is classified as an established teratogen, with an FDA black box warning against use in the first trimester because of the increased risks of spontaneous abortion as well as craniofacial, digital, and other congenital anomalies attributable to this drug.[38] Renal malformations are infrequently reported, and the EMFO tetrad succinctly characterizes the risk of multiple congenital anomalies as follows: ear (microtia and auditory canal atresia); mouth (cleft lip and palate); fingers (brachydactyly fifth fingers and hypoplastic toenails); organs (ocular and other different visceral malformations [cardiac, renal, diaphragmatic and central nervous system]).

Existing evidence suggests that tacrolimus may have a mild, transient, functional, adverse renal effect. Oliguria and hyperkalemia have been observed in exposed neonates. Transplacental passage of tacrolimus is inefficient, with median ratio of cord plasma to maternal plasma concentration of 0.36,[39] and partial placental protection has been proposed to explain the lack of serious renal impairment in neonates exposed in utero. The mechanism by which tacrolimus may cause transient neonatal renal impairment is unknown, but the incidence of such impairment has been estimated (8 of 54 infants) at approximately 15%.[40]

Aminoglycosides/Other Antibiotics

The potential dose-dependent nephrotoxicity of aminoglycoside antibiotics (eg, gentamicin, tobramycin), because of accumulation and progressive damage in renal proximal tubular cells, has been extensively documented to occur in adults and children.[41,42] Because aminoglycoside antibiotics generally have limited use in pregnant women for maternal conditions, including pyelonephritis, and pelvic inflammatory disease or abscess, less is known about their potential effects on fetal kidney development and function, despite ample experimental data in animals.[40] Fetal exposure to gentamicin during early gestation perturbs branching morphogenesis and results in reduced nephron number and abnormal proximal tubular differentiation.[25,43,44]

Because of its proven efficacy in serious gram-negative infections, gentamicin is one of the more frequently prescribed aminoglycosides. Single-dose gentamicin for chorioamnionitis has no apparent adverse effects on neonatal renal function, with peak fetal gentamicin concentration averaging one-third of maternal concentration.[45,46] Despite nephrotoxicity shown by animal studies,[47] there are no documented human cases of clinically significant fetal nephrotoxicity in relation to maternally administered gentamicin. There has been a single case report of renal hypoplasia, cysts, and hydronephrosis after in utero exposure to gentamicin,[46] and another of renal cystic dysplasia after gentamicin and corticosteroids were prescribed to the mother,[48] but no human structural nephroteratogenic effect has been detected in observational studies.[49]

Aminoglycosides as a class are designated category D by the FDA, but this classification is apparently based on sporadic reports of potential fetal ototoxicity in mothers who had taken streptomycin. A recent ACOG Committee opinion concluded, with respect to aminoglycosides and other antibiotics prescribed during pregnancy, that "Pregnant women should not be denied appropriate treatment for infections because untreated infections can commonly lead to serious maternal and fetal complications." Clinical judgment, taking into account risks, benefits, and alternative antibiotic options, is required in the context of shared decision making with the pregnant patient with an infection potentially requiring aminoglycoside therapy.

Renal Effects of Selected General Teratogens

Although renal development or function may not be the primary target of classic teratogens, renal adverse effects may variably be observed after in utero exposure. Early first-trimester exposure to thalidomide causes a recognizable embryopathy, the best-known feature of which is limb reduction defects. However, renal agenesis may also occur, along with gastrointestinal, cardiac, otic, and cranial nerve abnormalities.[50] Other renal malformations have been observed in thalidomide embryopathy including ectopic kidney, horseshoe kidney, and hydronephrosis. Isotretinoin embryopathy presents mainly with craniofacial, cardiac, thymic, and central nervous system malformations, but dysplastic multicystic kidneys have also been observed in a case report.[51] The natural retinoid vitamin A is not nephroteratogenic in high doses in humans, but may cause cranial-neural crest–derived malformations[52]; deficiency of vitamin A has been reported in association with renal hypoplasia.

Teratogenic methotrexate exposure presents classically with intrauterine growth restriction as well as cardiac, craniofacial, and skeletal anomalies, but renal malformations such as unilateral renal agenesis or horseshoe kidney have also been reported in the context of misdiagnosed ectopic pregnancy treated with methotrexate.[53] Cocaine[54] and alcohol[55] have been reported as risk factors for renal hypoplasia,[10] but confounding involving maternal nutritional status and other substance use is likely and causation has not been established.

SUMMARY/DISCUSSION

As more and more women with chronic health conditions conceive and carry pregnancies to viability, there is greater need to make informed decisions about the risks and benefits of various treatments, including potential renal teratogens. Clinicians and patients need information about the risks and benefits of all of the medications discussed in this article to make informed decisions about a variety of critical issues related to the health of the mother and her developing fetus. As shown here, the available information is limited. For example, most of the currently marketed medications used to treat chronic health conditions in women of childbearing age have almost no data on pregnancy-related risks because of ethical challenges of conducting randomized controlled trials in pregnant women and the fact that pregnancy occurring during a clinical trial typically results in cessation of the medication exposure. Furthermore, for many conditions, discontinuing treatments during pregnancy or not treating a condition at all during pregnancy may pose specific risks. Providing answers to questions about the safest medications will improve the overall quality of care for pregnant women with chronic health conditions, because they are able to better balance the risks and benefits of medication treatment with respect to their fetus. Minimizing exposures with known fetal harm will also result in less need for subsequent care for the infant after birth, further improving the efficiency and quality of care.

Studies specifically focusing on renal effects of medications, related to timing, dose, and duration, would be helpful to inform decision making. Clinical data describing risks of treated versus untreated conditions at various stages of pregnancy would also be of benefit. Furthermore, data on short-term neonatal outcomes and long-term child health outcomes related to infants with in utero exposures to renal teratogens would help to inform providers and patients. Study design is particularly challenging for detection of potential long-term impact of in utero exposure to various pharmaceutical classes. In addition, renal function is not routinely assayed in children who appear clinically well. One possible epidemiologic data resource is electronic medical records, but only if it becomes feasible to link children to maternal records for retrospective studies, but many decades may elapse until late adulthood when diminished renal reserve may become clinically evident.

RECOMMENDATIONS

Ideally, considerations of risks and benefits would occur before a woman becomes pregnant and would involve the patient and her family, as well as providers. Discussions should address the risks and benefits to the mother of becoming pregnant, the potential changes in the disease course that may occur as a result of pregnancy, risks of treating versus not treating, and strategies to optimize the mother's health in the preconception period to increase the likelihood of a successful outcome.

For women taking a medication with known effects on the developing kidney who discover that they are pregnant, similar discussions should address risks of continued exposure for the mother and her developing fetus versus discontinuing the exposure. Given that 52% of pregnancies in the United States are unplanned,[56] this is a likely scenario and necessitates careful communication between health care providers managing the mother's health and providers managing the pregnancy.

For children's health providers, information from the mother and her providers about potentially harmful exposures should be shared prenatally to allow for appropriate delivery in a facility equipped to address the potential health care needs of the infant. Infants with exposures who also have evidence of impaired renal function (ie, oligohydramnios) should be monitored closely for urine output, blood pressure dysregulation, and electrolyte abnormalities. For infants with prenatal exposures to medications known to be associated with a high risk of structural defects, ultrasonography should be performed in the first week of life. Typically, it is ideal to wait a minimum of 48 hours (if possible) to perform renal ultrasonography to ensure that hydronephrosis is not missed as a result of low urinary flow in the first 24 to 48 hours of life. This strategy would not apply to infants in whom antenatal ultrasonography showed significant kidney malformations, in which case the ultrasonography could be performed on the first day of life.[57,58]

There are several practical considerations for the clinician concerned about general drug safety in pregnancy. The first is to gather current best evidence. Reprotox or a similar, continuously updated database (eg, TERIS, REPRORISK, or Shepard's Catalog of Teratogenic Agents) should be consulted when prescribing for women of childbearing potential when pregnancy is known, planned, or likely to occur, for discussion of risks, benefits, and potential alternatives. Clinicians should routinely perform contraceptive counseling when prescribing or renewing potentially teratogenic medications, and contraceptive use status has been proposed as a vital sign, meaning information that should be collected at each clinical encounter that involves prescribing or medication review.[59] With half of conceptions being unintended, and 6% occurring while the woman is already taking a potentially teratogenic drug (FDA class D or X), there is a compelling need for improved communication with women (including teens) of childbearing potential who take medications without contraception.[60]

ACKNOWLEDGMENTS

The authors acknowledge the assistance of Casey H. Braddy, who helped with article preparation and submission.

REFERENCES

1. OECD Family Database. OECD. 2012. Available at: http://www.oecd.org/social/family/database. Accessed December 4, 2013.
2. Johnson K, Posner SF, Biermann J, et al. Recommendations to improve preconception health and health care–United States. A report of the CDC/ATSDR Preconception Care Work Group and the Select Panel on Preconception Care. MMWR Recomm Rep 2006;55(RR-6):1–23.
3. Boubred F, Saint-Faust M, Buffat C, et al. Developmental origins of chronic renal disease: an integrative hypothesis. International journal of nephrology 2013; 2013:346067.
4. Doll R. Proof of causality: deduction from epidemiological observation. Perspect Biol Med 2002;45(4):499–515.
5. Scialli AR. The National Birth Defects Prevention Study: how to communicate data. Semin Fetal Neonatal Med 2014;19(3):170–6.
6. Evaluating the risks of drug exposure in human pregnancies. Rockville (MD): Food and Drug Administration; 2005.
7. Feibus KB. FDA's proposed rule for pregnancy and lactation labeling: improving maternal child health through well-informed medicine use. J Med Toxicol 2008; 4(4):284–8.
8. Content and format of labeling for human prescription drug and biological products; requirements for pregnancy and lactation labeling. Rockville (MD): Food and Drug Adminstration; 2008. 0910–AF11.
9. Piscione TD, Waters AM. Structural and functional development of the kidney. In: Geary DF, Schaefer F, editors. Comprehensive Pediatric Nephrology. 1st Edition. Philadelphia: Mosby Elsevier; 2008. p. 91–110.

10. Cain JE, Di Giovanni V, Smeeton J, et al. Genetics of renal hypoplasia: insights into the mechanisms controlling nephron endowment. Pediatr Res 2010;68(2):91–8.

11. Woolf AS. A molecular and genetic view of human renal and urinary tract malformations. Kidney Int 2000;58(2):500–12.

12. Ichikawa I, Kuwayama F, Pope JC, et al. Paradigm shift from classic anatomic theories to contemporary cell biological views of CAKUT. Kidney Int 2002; 61(3):889–98.

13. Yosypiv IV. Renin-angiotensin system in ureteric bud branching morphogenesis: implications for kidney disease. Pediatr Nephrol 2014;29(4):609–20.

14. Bowen ME, Ray WA, Arbogast PG, et al. Increasing exposure to angiotensin-converting enzyme inhibitors in pregnancy. Am J Obstet Gynecol 2008; 198(3):291–5.

15. Nishimura H, Yerkes E, Hohenfellner K, et al. Role of the angiotensin type 2 receptor gene in congenital anomalies of the kidney and urinary tract, CAKUT, of mice and men. Mol Cell 1999;3(1):1–10.

16. Lasaitiene D, Chen Y, Guron G, et al. Perturbed medullary tubulogenesis in neonatal rat exposed to renin-angiotensin system inhibition. Nephrol Dial Transplant 2003;18(12):2534–41.

17. Quan A. Fetopathy associated with exposure to angiotensin converting enzyme inhibitors and angiotensin receptor antagonists. Early Hum Dev 2006;82(1):23–8.

18. Pryde PG, Sedman AB, Nugent CE, et al. Angiotensin-converting enzyme inhibitor fetopathy. Journal of the American Society of Nephrology: JASN 1993;3(9): 1575–82.

19. Cooper WO, Hernandez-Diaz S, Arbogast PG, et al. Major congenital malformations after first-trimester exposure to ACE inhibitors. N Engl J Med 2006;354(23): 2443–51.

20. Cooper WO. Clinical implications of increased congenital malformations after first trimester exposures to angiotensin-converting enzyme inhibitors. J Cardiovasc Nurs 2008;23(1):20–4.

21. American College of Obstetricians and Gynecologists. ACOG practice bulletin No. 125: chronic hypertension in pregnancy. Obstet Gynecol 2012;119(2 Pt 1): 396–407.

22. Nielsen GL, Sorensen HT, Larsen H, et al. Risk of adverse birth outcome and miscarriage in pregnant users of non-steroidal anti-inflammatory drugs: population based observational study and case-control study. BMJ 2001;322(7281): 266–70.

23. Daniel S, Matok I, Gorodischer R, et al. Major malformations following exposure to nonsteroidal antiinflammatory drugs during the first trimester of pregnancy. J Rheumatol 2012;39(11):2163–9.

24. Cabrol D, Jannet D, Pannier E. Treatment of symptomatic polyhydramnios with indomethacin. Eur J Obstet Gynecol Reprod Biol 1996;66(1):11–5.

25. Boubred F, Vendemmia M, Garcia-Meric P, et al. Effects of maternally administered drugs on the fetal and neonatal kidney. Drug Saf 2006;29(5):397–419.

26. American College of Obstetricians and Gynecologists, Committee on Practice Bulletins–Obstetrics. ACOG practice bulletin no. 127: management of preterm labor. Obstet Gynecol 2012;119(6):1308–17.

27. Paixao AD, Alexander BT. How the kidney is impacted by the perinatal maternal environment to develop hypertension. Biol Reprod 2013;89(6):144.

28. Reynolds RM. Glucocorticoid excess and the developmental origins of disease: two decades of testing the hypothesis–2012 Curt Richter Award Winner. Psychoneuroendocrinology 2013;38(1):1–11.

29. Crowley PA. Antenatal corticosteroid therapy: a meta-analysis of the randomized trials, 1972 to 1994. Am J Obstet Gynecol 1995;173(1):322–35.
30. Doyle LW, Ford GW, Davis NM, et al. Antenatal corticosteroid therapy and blood pressure at 14 years of age in preterm children. Clin Sci (Lond) 2000;98(2): 137–42.
31. Zagouri F, Sergentanis TN, Chrysikos D, et al. Trastuzumab administration during pregnancy: a systematic review and meta-analysis. Breast Cancer Res Treat 2013;137(2):349–57.
32. Hou S. Pregnancy in renal transplant recipients. Adv Chronic Kidney Dis 2013; 20(3):253–9.
33. Tendron A, Decramer S, Justrabo E, et al. Cyclosporin A administration during pregnancy induces a permanent nephron deficit in young rabbits. J Am Soc Nephrol 2003;14(12):3188–96.
34. Issa N, Kukla A, Ibrahim HN. Calcineurin inhibitor nephrotoxicity: a review and perspective of the evidence. Am J Nephrol 2013;37(6):602–12.
35. Prevot A, Martini S, Guignard JP. In utero exposure to immunosuppressive drugs. Biol Neonate 2002;81(2):73–81.
36. Giudice PL, Dubourg L, Hadj-Aissa A, et al. Renal function of children exposed to cyclosporin in utero. Nephrol Dial Transplant 2000;15(10):1575–9.
37. Cochat P, Decramer S, Robert-Gnansia E, et al. Renal outcome of children exposed to cyclosporine in utero. Transplant Proc 2004;36(Suppl 2):208S–10S.
38. Merlob P, Stahl B, Klinger G. Tetrada of the possible mycophenolate mofetil embryopathy: a review. Reprod Toxicol 2009;28(1):105–8.
39. Jain A, Venkataramanan R, Fung JJ, et al. Pregnancy after liver transplantation under tacrolimus. Transplantation 1997;64(4):559–65.
40. Kainz A, Harabacz I, Cowlrick IS, et al. Review of the course and outcome of 100 pregnancies in 84 women treated with tacrolimus. Transplantation 2000;70(12): 1718–21.
41. Quiros Y, Vicente-Vicente L, Morales AI, et al. An integrative overview on the mechanisms underlying the renal tubular cytotoxicity of gentamicin. Toxicol Sci 2011;119(2):245–56.
42. Lopez-Novoa JM, Quiros Y, Vicente L, et al. New insights into the mechanism of aminoglycoside nephrotoxicity: an integrative point of view. Kidney Int 2011; 79(1):33–45.
43. Gilbert T, Gaonach S, Moreau E, et al. Defect of nephrogenesis induced by gentamicin in rat metanephric organ culture. Lab Invest 1994;70(5):656–66.
44. Mantovani A, Macri C, Stazi AV, et al. Tobramycin-induced changes in renal histology of fetal and newborn Sprague-Dawley rats. Teratog Carcinog Mutagen 1992;12(1):19–30.
45. Ward K, Theiler RN. Once-daily dosing of gentamicin in obstetrics and gynecology. Clin Obstet Gynecol 2008;51(3):498–506.
46. Locksmith GJ, Chin A, Vu T, et al. High compared with standard gentamicin dosing for chorioamnionitis: a comparison of maternal and fetal serum drug levels. Obstet Gynecol 2005;105(3):473–9.
47. Suzuki M. Children's toxicology from bench to bed-drug-induced renal injury (4): effects of nephrotoxic compounds on fetal and developing kidney. J Toxicol Sci 2009;34(Suppl 2):SP267–71.
48. Hulton SA, Kaplan BS. Renal dysplasia associated with in utero exposure to gentamicin and corticosteroids. Am J Med Genet 1995;58(1):91–3.
49. Czeizel AE, Rockenbauer M, Olsen J, et al. A teratological study of aminoglycoside antibiotic treatment during pregnancy. Scand J Infect Dis 2000;32(3):309–13.

50. Vianna FS, Schuler-Faccini L, Leite JC, et al. Recognition of the phenotype of thalidomide embryopathy in countries endemic for leprosy: new cases and review of the main dysmorphological findings. Clin Dysmorphol 2013;22(2):59–63.
51. Rizzo R, Lammer EJ, Parano E, et al. Limb reduction defects in humans associated with prenatal isotretinoin exposure. Teratology 1991;44(6):599–604.
52. Rothman KJ, Moore LL, Singer MR, et al. Teratogenicity of high vitamin A intake. N Engl J Med 1995;333(21):1369–73.
53. Nurmohamed L, Moretti ME, Schechter T, et al. Outcome following high-dose methotrexate in pregnancies misdiagnosed as ectopic. Am J ObstetGynecol 2011;205(6):533.e1–3.
54. Battin M, Albersheim S, Newman D. Congenital genitourinary tract abnormalities following cocaine exposure in utero. Am J Perinatol 1995;12(6):425–8.
55. Taylor CL, Jones KL, Jones MC, et al. Incidence of renal anomalies in children prenatally exposed to ethanol. Pediatrics 1994;94(2 Pt 1):209–12.
56. Secura G. Long-acting reversible contraception: a practical solution to reduce unintended pregnancy. Minerva Ginecol 2013;65(3):271–7.
57. Nguyen HT, Herndon CD, Cooper C, et al. The Society for Fetal Urology consensus statement on the evaluation and management of antenatal hydronephrosis. J Pediatr Urol 2010;6(3):212–31.
58. Aksu N, Yavascan O, Kangin M, et al. Postnatal management of infants with antenatally detected hydronephrosis. Pediatr Nephrol 2005;20(9):1253–9.
59. Schwarz EB, Parisi SM, Williams SL, et al. Promoting safe prescribing in primary care with a contraceptive vital sign: a cluster-randomized controlled trial. Ann Fam Med 2012;10(6):516–22.
60. Andrade SE, Raebel MA, Morse AN, et al. Use of prescription medications with a potential for fetal harm among pregnant women. Pharmacoepidemiol Drug Saf 2006;15(8):546–54.

Diagnosis and Management of Urinary Tract Infection and Vesicoureteral Reflux in the Neonate

CrossMark

Rossana Baracco, MD, Tej K. Mattoo, MD, DCH, FRCP*

KEYWORDS

- Neonates • Urinary tract infection • UTI • Vesicoureteral reflux • VUR • Diagnosis
- Investigations

KEY POINTS

- Urinary tract infection (UTI) is the most common bacterial infection in febrile newborns.
- Male newborns, in particular if uncircumcised, are at increased risk of UTI.
- Clinical presentation of UTI in the newborn is nonspecific, and jaundice may be the only clinical manifestation.
- Newborns with UTI have a high incidence of congenital anomalies of the kidneys and urinary tract.
- Prophylaxis with antibiotics is recommended in newborns with vesicoureteral reflux.

EPIDEMIOLOGY AND RISK FACTORS

Urinary tract infection (UTI) is the most common bacterial infection in febrile new-borns.[1,2] The exact prevalence is difficult to determine, but studies that included infants younger than 2 months reported a prevalence of 4.6% to 7.5%.[3–5] Additionally, most of these studies were performed in febrile infants, which could potentially underestimate the true prevalence of UTI in newborns because a large proportion of newborns do not present with fever. A recent study that prospectively evaluated asymptomatic jaundiced infants found that 7.5% of them had a UTI, which is consistent with the findings of the previous studies.[6]

In premature and low-birth-weight (LBW) infants, the prevalence of UTI can be as high as 20%.[7] This high rate may be secondary to hospital-acquired infections and

Disclosures: The authors have no financial interests or conflicts of interest to disclose.
Division of Pediatric Nephrology, Children's Hospital of Michigan, Wayne State University, 3901 Beaubien Boulevard, Detroit, MI 48201, USA
* Corresponding author.
E-mail address: tmattoo@med.wayne.edu

this population's increased susceptibility. Premature and LBW infants often require prolonged hospitalizations in neonatal intensive care units and multiple interventions that place them at risk for infection. Mechanical ventilation, parenteral nutrition, intravascular catheters, and associated infectious pathologies have been identified as risk factors for UTI in neonates.[8]

A strong male predominance is seen in infants younger than 3 months with UTI, mainly because of a higher likelihood of UTI in uncircumcised patients. Absence of circumcision is a well-known risk factor for UTI in male young infants, and increases the risk of UTI by 10-fold.[9] Uncircumcised infants have a UTI prevalence of 20.1% compared with 7.5% in female infants and 2.4% in circumcised infants.[10] Other risk factors for UTI in newborns are prematurity, white race,[11] and renal and urinary tract malformations. Although breast-feeding has been found to protect infants from respiratory and gastrointestinal infections, a recent study showed that it does not protect against UTI in the first 3 months of life.[12]

VESICOURETERAL REFLUX

Vesicoureteral reflux (VUR) is associated with increased risk of UTI and renal scarring. The grading of VUR, which was standardized in 1982[13] by using the radiographic voiding cystourethrogram (VCUG), divides VUR into 5 grades, with grade 5 being the most severe (**Fig. 1**). Vesicoureteral reflux is the most common congenital urinary tract abnormality in children, including neonates. In a study exclusively involving 45 male neonates with UTI, 43.0% had VUR.[14] In another study of 95 patients younger than 4 months and hospitalized with UTI, VUR was diagnosed in 31.7% of patients.[15]

In a study that evaluated the gender distribution of VUR, the incidence of VUR was equal at 20% among male and female neonates with UTI, even though the incidence of UTI was 6 times more common in boys. The same study also reported that the VUR was diagnosed at a 4-fold higher rate in neonates with *Klebsiella*-induced UTI compared with those with *Escherichia Coli*–induced UTI.[16] The incidence of VUR

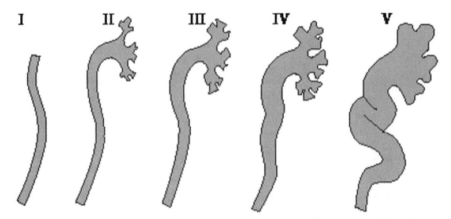

Fig. 1. International reflux study grading scheme. Grade 1, reflux into nondilated ureter. Grade 2, reflux into the renal pelvis and calyces without dilatation. Grade 3, mild/moderate dilatation of ureter and pelvicalyceal system. Grade 4, dilation of the renal pelvis and calyces with moderate ureteral tortuosity, blunting of fornices. Grade 5, gross dilatation of the ureter, pelvis, and calyces; ureteral tortuosity; loss of papillary impressions. (*Adapted from* Lebowitz RL, Olbing H, Parkkulainen KV, et al. International system of radiographic grading of vesicoureteric reflux. Pediatr Radiol 1985;15(2):106; with permission.)

seems to be lower in preterm neonates than in full-term neonates with UTI. In a study of 118 hospitalized preterm infants younger than 2 months, a major abnormality was found on at least one imaging study for 4% (5 of 118) of infants and on 4% of renal ultrasounds and 2% of VCUG examinations.[17]

In most neonates, VUR is diagnosed after an episode of UTI (primary VUR), although in many it is diagnosed during follow-up for antenatally diagnosed congenital anomalies of the kidney and urinary tract (CAKUT), such as multicystic dysplastic kidney, renal agenesis, or ureteral ectopia. Approximately 10% of patients, mostly boys, with antenatally diagnosed hydronephrosis (antenatal VUR) are found to have VUR during routine postnatal follow-up.[18] Vesicoureteral reflux can also occur secondary to bladder outlet obstruction or neurogenic bladder (secondary VUR).

VUR AND RENAL SCARRING

Vesicoureteral reflux increases the risk of UTI and renal scarring, which is called *reflux nephropathy*. The presence of reflux nephropathy puts affected patients at higher risk of developing hypertension, proteinuria, and progression of renal disease later in life. Renal scarring that occurs because of acute pyelonephritis is called *acquired reflux nephropathy*, as opposed to the renal scarring that may be present from birth, even before the occurrence of UTI, which is called *congenital reflux nephropathy*.[19] The current gold standard for diagnosing renal scarring is a technetium-99m-labeled dimercaptosuccinic acid (DMSA) renal scan, which should be performed a few months after acute infection, only if clinically indicated. Routine DMSA renal scans have no role in the acute management of UTI in neonates.

CAUSATIVE ORGANISMS FOR UTI

Although traditionally the source of infection in neonatal UTI has been thought to be hematogenous, the microbiology of the infections makes ascending infection from the urethra the most likely source. Vesicoureteral reflux predisposes to pyelonephritis. The most common bacterial pathogen identified in neonatal UTI is *E coli* (80%–88% of cases),[9,20,21] followed by *Enterobacter* spp and *Klebsiella pneumonia*. Other less common pathogens include *Pseudomonas aeruginosa, Enterococcus* spp, group B streptococcus, *Staphylococcus aureus, Citrobacter freundii, Serratia marcescens*, and *K oxytoca*. The less common bacterial pathogens are more frequent in neonates who acquire a UTI in the hospital. Fungal UTI is predominantly found in nosocomial UTI and is mainly caused by *Candida* spp.[22]

CLINICAL PRESENTATION

The symptoms of UTI in a newborn infant are generally nonspecific and similar to those seen in the clinical presentation of neonatal sepsis.[22] Young infants with high fever ($\geq$39°C) are more likely to have a UTI.[9] However, newborns with a UTI do not always present with fever. In fact, as many as half of the neonates with a UTI may have only low-grade fever or none at all.[7]

Other associated symptoms of UTI in neonates include poor feeding, failure to thrive, vomiting, diarrhea, prolonged jaundice, lethargy, and irritability. Jaundice in the absence of any other symptoms or indications has been identified as a presenting sign of UTI in neonates.[6]

Newborns with UTI are at a higher risk for bacteremia than older infants. Bachur and Caputo[23] found that bacteremia associated with UTI in infants is inversely related to age. The rate of bacteremia in neonates with UTI varies in different studies. Ginsburg and colleagues[24] found positive blood culture results in 31% of neonates with UTI. Other studies have reported lower rates of 4%[21] to 6%.[4] This discrepancy is likely because of the differences in study populations, including age group; hospital setup; and institutional protocols in infants with fever. Neonates with hospital-acquired UTI have a higher risk of bacteremia than neonates who present with a UTI from home (community-acquired). Lopez Sastre and colleagues[22] found that 24.2% of neonates who acquired a UTI in the hospital had positive blood culture results, compared with 10.8% of neonates with a community-acquired UTI (P<.05). The clinical presentation of infants who have UTI with bacteremia is not any different from those without bacteremia.[25]

Infants with bacteremia secondary to a UTI, especially if the pathogen is not the typical E coli, have a higher frequency of anatomic abnormalities of the urinary tract, including grade 3 to 5 VUR and obstruction.[25] The study analysis included infants and older children in addition to neonates. A small percentage of neonates with UTI also have meningitis.[23] Neonates who are investigated for a UTI should undergo a lumbar puncture as part of the sepsis workup.

DIAGNOSIS OF UTI
Urinalysis and Culture

A urine specimen in neonates should be obtained through suprapubic aspiration or catheterization of the bladder. The collection of urine with the use of adhesive bags in the perineal area has a high risk of contamination and has no role in the diagnosis of UTI.[26]

The diagnosis of a UTI in older children is typically based on the presence of pyuria on urinalysis and bacteriuria on urine culture. Because urine culture results take approximately 48 hours to obtain, empiric treatment is usually started when a UTI is suspected based on positive urinalysis results. However, the sensitivity of urinalysis in neonates and young infants with a UTI is low (**Table 1**); as many as half of neonates with a UTI have been reported to have negative urinalysis results.[4,6] Because of the low yield of the standard urinalysis, some studies have used an enhanced urinalysis to predict UTI in infants, which is obtained using a hemocytometer cell count and Gram staining on uncentrifuged urine. Results are reported as the number of white blood cells (WBC) per microliter; a cutoff of 10/μL or more is used to define pyuria.[11,27] The sensitivity and negative predictive value of the enhanced urinalysis are higher than those of the standard urinalysis (see **Table 1**).[1,28,29] Therefore, infants with no pyuria or bacteriuria, determined using enhanced urinalysis, have a very low likelihood of UTI. Although this method is thought to be more accurate than the standard urinalysis,[1,29] it is not widely used.

Table 1
Sensitivity, specificity, and positive and negative predictive values of laboratory tests in neonates and young infants with urinary tract infection

	Standard UA (%)	Enhanced UA (%)	Gram Stain (%)	C-RP >20%	ESR >30%
Sensitivity	54–82	82.0–96.0	64–85	59	73
Specificity	92–98	94.0	63–99	90	78
PPV	45		11		
NPV	97	99.7	99		

Abbreviations: C-RP, C-reactive protein; ESR, erythrocyte sedimentation rate; NPV, negative predictive value; PPV, positive predictive value; UA, urinalysis.
Data from Refs.[1,2,28,29,31]

The gold standard for diagnosing UTI is a positive urine culture for a single organism. A positive culture is defined as growth of 10,000 or more colony-forming units (CFU) per milliliter if the urine is obtained using suprapubic aspiration, or 100,000 CFU/mL or more if it is obtained through catheterization.[2,11] Although some studies suggest that urine cultures obtained with catheterization of the bladder that grow 10,000 to 50,000 CFU/mL may represent asymptomatic bacteriuria,[27] other studies have shown that as many as 20% of infants younger than 12 months with symptomatic UTI show low bacterial counts ($<10^5$ CFU/mL).[30] It is better to err on the side of caution with neonates, because they are at higher risk for bacteremia. Santoro and colleagues[11] recently proposed criteria to diagnose UTI in neonates, which include 10 WBC/μL or more determined through enhanced urinalysis, and a urine culture with 10,000 CFU/mL or more of a single organism obtained with a catheter sample or suprapubic aspiration.

Inflammatory Markers

C-reactive protein (CRP) and erythrocyte sedimentation rate (ESR) are frequently obtained to predict the likelihood of bacterial infection in infants. Lin and colleagues[31] studied the sensitivity and specificity of these markers for UTI in infants younger than 8 weeks, and found low sensitivity for both, suggesting that these markers are poor predictors of UTI in febrile young infants (see **Table 1**). Specificity was higher, and when CRP greater than 20 was combined with pyuria on enhanced urinalysis, the specificity increased to 98%. Similarly, the specificity of ESR greater than 30 increased to 97% when combined with pyuria on enhanced urinalysis. Procalcitonin is another marker that has been studied and found to be both sensitive and specific for acute pyelonephritis. However, most of these studies have been performed in older infants and children[32,33]; studies in neonates with UTI are lacking.

RENAL IMAGING AFTER UTI IN NEONATE

Because of a high risk of underlying CAKUT anomalies, renal imaging is important in the management of neonates with UTI.

Renal Ultrasound

All neonates with first febrile UTI should have a renal ultrasound examination because of a high incidence of CAKUT anomalies, the diagnosis of which may have a bearing on the management of the patient, both short-term and long-term. Hydronephrosis is the most frequent abnormal finding and has been found in 25% of babies younger than 60 days,[21] and 45% of neonates[6] with UTI. The importance of performing routine renal ultrasound examination after first febrile UTI in neonates can also be extrapolated from American Academy of Pediatrics (AAP)[34] and the Italian Society of Pediatric Nephrology (ISPN)[35] guidelines for children older than 2 months.

The AAP[34] and ISPN[35] guidelines recommend routine renal ultrasound in infants with first febrile UTI. National Institute for Health and Care Excellence (NICE) guidelines[36] from Great Britain also recommend routine renal ultrasound examination in children younger than 6 months. According to the AAP recommendations, the timing for renal ultrasound depends on the clinical situation and can be performed during the first 2 days of treatment, unless substantial clinical improvement is seen, in which case it can be performed later. According to the NICE and ISPN guidelines, a renal ultrasound can be performed 4 to 8 weeks after UTI unless it is atypical or does not respond promptly to antibiotic therapy within 48 hours, in which case it should be performed during acute infection. Further details on these guidelines are provided in **Table 2**.

Voiding Cystourethrogram

Voiding cystourethrogram is the gold standard for diagnosing VUR in any age group. In a study in neonates, 80% of those with significantly abnormal ultrasonographic findings were found to have VUR on VCUG.[16] A contrast VCUG is preferred over a nuclear VCUG because it allows grading of VUR, defines bladder anatomy, and identifies obstructive uropathy, such as posterior urethral valves.

Recently, the importance of diagnosing VUR, low-grade in particular, has come under scrutiny because of the emerging evidence about VUR management. As a result, none of the recent guidelines recommend routine VCUG in infants with first febrile UTI. All recommend VCUG if renal ultrasound is abnormal, the UTI is atypical, or the patient has other risk factors. The current practice in the authors' institution is to routinely perform a VCUG in newborns with a UTI, because of a poor correlation between severity of VUR and hydronephrosis as diagnosed using renal ultrasound examination.

Renal Scan

Technetium-99m-labeled dimercaptosuccinic acid helps diagnose acute pyelonephritis and renal scarring, and is not necessary for acute management of UTI. Depending on the clinical course, it may be performed selectively 4 to 6 months later to assess the presence and severity of renal scarring. On the contrary, a diuretic renal scan, such as diethylenetriaminepentaacetic acid renal scan with Lasix, may be necessary in babies to rule out upper urinary tract obstruction, if suspected on renal ultrasound examination. Diethylenetriaminepentaacetic acid scan also provides a differential renal function, which along with renal clearance may have a bearing on acute management of the patient.

TREATMENT
Treatment of UTI

Empirical parenteral antibiotic treatment of neonatal sepsis is routinely started in febrile neonates and neonates who exhibit nonspecific signs of infection. Ampicillin and gentamicin cover most bacteria that cause sepsis in the early neonatal period; an alternate regimen is ampicillin and cefotaxime. Once UTI is diagnosed and the urine

Table 2					
Recommendations on renal imaging after first febrile UTI in infants younger than 6 months					
			Renal/Bladder Imaging		
Source	Year of Publication	Age Group Covered	Routine US	Routine VCUG	Indications for VCUG
Sweden[48]	1999	All children	Yes	Yes	—
NICE[36]	2007	All children	Yes	No	Consider if renal US is abnormal. UTI recurrence or atypical UTI
AAP[34]	2011	2–24 mo	Yes	No	Abnormal renal US, atypical or complex clinical circumstances
ISPN[35]	2012	2 mo–3 y	Yes	No	Abnormal renal US or presence of risk factors

Abbreviations: AAP, American Academy of Pediatrics; ISPN, Italian Society of Pediatric Nephrology; NICE, National Institute for Health and Care Excellence; US, ultrasound; UTI, urinary tract infection; VCUG, voiding cystourethrogram.

culture and susceptibilities are available, antibiotic therapy is tailored according to these results. In addition to the importance of prompt initiation of parenteral antibiotics because of the high risk for bacteremia and sepsis in the newborn period, another important goal of early treatment is the prevention of renal scars. The risk of renal scars after a first UTI in infants younger than 1 year is 43%.[37] Renal scarring can lead to future risk for hypertension and chronic kidney disease.

No data are available in neonates with UTI to guide duration of parenteral antibiotics. Infants with bacteremia are usually treated with parenteral antibiotics for 10 to 14 days. Management of infants with UTI without bacteremia varies, with most centers completing treatment with parenteral antibiotics. The use of oral antibiotics to treat UTI in neonates has not been studied. After initial treatment with parenteral antibiotics, and if blood culture results are negative, completion of treatment with oral antibiotics in a newborn who is doing well clinically may be considered.

For infants younger than 2 months who present to the emergency department with fever or strong suspicion for infection and are found to have a UTI, the clinical course is generally benign, with resolution of fever within 48 hours after the first dose of parenteral antibiotics in 96% of patients.[21] A repeat culture is unnecessary if the patient shows clinical improvement.[21]

Management of VUR

The natural course of VUR diagnosed after UTI depends on multiple factors, most importantly the severity of the VUR. Depending on the duration of follow-up, VUR diagnosed after a UTI undergoes spontaneous resolution in 25% to 80% of cases. Schwab and colleagues[38] reported that grades 1 through 3 VUR diagnosed after UTI resolved at a rate of 13.0% per year for the first 5 years of follow-up, and 3.5% per year during subsequent years, and grades 4 and 5 VUR resolved at a rate of 5.0% per year. In a study involving black children, the mean duration for spontaneous resolution was 14.6 months, which was significantly shorter than the 21.4 months in white children.[39] In neonates with VUR diagnosed after abnormal prenatal renal ultrasound (prenatal VUR), 67% of severe VUR and 78% of mild or moderate VUR resolved by the age of 2 years.[40]

The 3 management options in older children with VUR are long-term antimicrobial prophylaxis, surgical correction, or surveillance only. The first 2 have been practiced for many decades, whereas surveillance only is a recent development prompted by some prospective, randomized studies[41–44] and the NICE,[36] AAP,[34] and ISPN[35] practice guidelines. However, none of these prospective studies generated data exclusively for the neonatal patient population, and none of the published guidelines specifically addressed the neonatal age group.

Antimicrobial prophylaxis

Of the options mentioned previously, antimicrobial prophylaxis is most practiced in neonates with VUR and UTI, partly because most of these neonates with normal renal ultrasound findings are unlikely to undergo VCUG in the neonatal period, and hence remain on prophylaxis until the procedure is performed a few weeks later. Even if a VCUG is performed sooner and VUR diagnosed, it is unlikely that any surgical intervention will be recommended, unless VUR is secondary to posterior urethral valves. Furthermore, studies in children have revealed that medical management of VUR is as effective as surgical treatment, and that these treatment modalities show no significant difference in outcome.[45–47]

Unlike in older children, ampicillin or amoxicillin are the commonly used antibiotics for UTI prophylaxis in neonates with VUR. Trimethoprim-sulfamethoxazole should be avoided because of the immaturity of the newborn liver and kidneys, which causes slower metabolism and excretion of this antibiotic. The prophylactic dose of antimicrobials is one-fourth to one-half of the therapeutic dose for acute infection, and the dosage for commonly used antimicrobials is as follows:

Cephalexin: 10 mg/kg as a single daily dose
Ampicillin: 20 mg/kg as a single daily dose
Amoxicillin: 10 mg/kg, as a single daily dose.

FOLLOW-UP

Appropriate monitoring for possible recurrence of UTI is important to prevent long-term morbidity, particularly in infants diagnosed with VUR or any other CAKUT abnormality. Early detection and prompt treatment of UTI, management with antimicrobial prophylaxis if clinically indicated, and appropriate follow-up with renal imaging are advisable.

REFERENCES

1. Herr S, Wald E, Pitetti R, et al. Enhanced urinalysis improves identification of febrile infants ages 60 days and younger at low risk for serious bacterial illness. Pediatrics 2001;108:866–71.
2. Dayan P, Bennett J, Best R, et al. Test characteristics of the urine gram stain in infants ≤60 days of age with fever. Pediatr Emerg Care 2002;18:12–4.
3. Hoberman A, Chao H, Keller D, et al. Prevalence of urinary tract infection in febrile infants. J Pediatr 1993;123:17–23.
4. Crain E, Gershel J. Urinary tract infections in febrile infants younger than 8 weeks of age. Pediatrics 1990;86:363–7.
5. Bachur R, Harper M. Reliability of the urinalysis for predicting urinary tract infections in young febrile children. Arch Pediatr Adolesc Med 2001;155(1):60–5.
6. Garcia F, Nager A. Jaundice as an early diagnostic sign of urinary tract infection in infants. Pediatrics 2002;109:846–51.
7. Cataldi L, Zaffanello M, Gnarra M, et al. Urinary tract infection in the newborn and the infants: state of the art. J Matern Fetal Neonatal Med 2010;23:90–3.
8. Cicero Falcao M, Rodrigues Leone C, D'Andrea R, et al. Urinary tract infection in full-term newborn infants: risk factor analysis. Rev Hosp Clin Fac Med Sao Paulo 2000;55:9–16.
9. Zorc J, Levine D, Platt S, et al. Clinical and demographic factors associated with urinary tract infection in young febrile infants. Pediatrics 2005;116:644–8.
10. Shaikh N, Morone N, Bost J, et al. Prevalence of urinary tract infection in childhood: a meta-analysis. Pediatr Infect Dis J 2008;27:302–8.
11. Santoro J, Carroll V, Steele R. Diagnosis and management of urinary tract infections in neonates and young infants. Clin Pediatr 2012;52:111–4.
12. Katikaneni R, Ponnapakkam T, Ponnapakkam A, et al. Breastfeeding does not protect against urinary tract infection in the first 3 months of life, but vitamin D supplementation increases the risk by 67%. Clin Pediatr 2009;48:750–5.
13. Duckett JW, Bellinger MF. A plea for standardized grading of vesicoureteral reflux. Eur Urol 1982;8:74–7.
14. Goldman M, Lahat E, Strauss S, et al. Imaging after urinary tract infection in male neonates. Pediatrics 2000;105:1232–5.
15. Wang SF, Huang FY, Chiu NC, et al. Urinary tract infection in infants less than 2 months of age. Zhonghua Min Guo Xiao Er Ke Yi Xue Hui Za Zhi 1994;35:294–300.

16. Cleper R, Krause I, Eisenstein B, et al. Prevalence of vesicoureteral reflux in neonatal urinary tract infection. Clin Pediatr 2004;43:619–25.

17. Nowell L, Moran C, Smith PB, et al. Prevalence of renal anomalies after urinary tract infections in hospitalized infants less than 2 months of age. J Perinatol 2010;30:281–5.

18. Ismaili K, Hall M, Piepsz A, et al. Primary vesicoureteral reflux detected in neonates with a history of fetal renal pelvis dilatation: a prospective clinical and imaging study. J Pediatr 2006;148:222–7.

19. Mattoo TK. Vesicoureteral reflux and reflux nephropathy. Adv Chronic Kidney Dis 2011;18:348–54.

20. Ismaili K, Lolin K, Damry N, et al. Febrile urinary tract infections in 0- to 3-month old infants: a prospective follow-up study. J Pediatr 2011;158:91–4.

21. Dayan P, Hanson E, Bennett J, et al. Clinical course of urinary tract infections in infants younger than 60 days of age. Pediatr Emerg Care 2004;20:85–8.

22. Lopez Sastre J, Ramos Aparicio A, Coto Cotallo G, et al. Urinary tract infection in the newborn: clinical and radio imaging studies. Pediatr Nephrol 2007;22: 1735–41.

23. Bachur R, Caputo G. Bacteremia and meningitis among infants with urinary tract infections. Pediatr Emerg Care 1995;11:280–4.

24. Ginsburg CM, McCracken GH Jr. Urinary tract infections in young infants. Pediatrics 1982;69(4):409–12.

25. Honkinen O, Jahnukainen T, Mertsola J, et al. Bacteremic urinary tract infection in children. Pediatr Infect Dis J 2000;19:630–4.

26. Saadeh S, Mattoo T. Managing urinary tract infections. Pediatr Nephrol 2011;26: 1967–76.

27. Hoberman A, Wald E, Reynolds E, et al. Pyuria and bacteriuria in urine specimens obtained by catheter from young children with fever. J Pediatr 1994;124:513–9.

28. Lin D, Huang F, Chiu N, et al. Comparison of hemocytometer leukocyte counts and standard urinalyses for predicting urinary tract infections in febrile infants. Pediatr Infect Dis J 2000;19:223–7.

29. Hoberman A, Wald E, Penchansky L, et al. Enhanced urinalysis as a screening test for urinary tract infection. Pediatrics 1993;91:1196–9.

30. Hansson S, Brandstrom P, Jodal U, et al. Low bacterial counts in infants with urinary tract infection. J Pediatr 1998;132:180–2.

31. Lin D, Huang S, Lin C, et al. Urinary tract infection in febrile infants younger than eight weeks of age. Pediatrics 2000;105:E20.

32. Pecile P, Romanello C. Procalcitonin and pyelonephritis in children. Curr Opin Infect Dis 2007;20:83–7.

33. Smolkin V, Koren A, Raz R, et al. Procalcitonin as a marker of acute pyelonephritis. Pediatr Nephrol 2002;17:409–12.

34. Roberts KB. Urinary tract infection: clinical practice guideline for the diagnosis and management of the initial UTI in febrile infants and children 2 to 24 months. Pediatrics 2011;128:595–610.

35. Ammenti A, Cataldi L, Chimenz R, et al. Febrile urinary tract infections in young children: recommendations for the diagnosis, treatment and follow-up. Acta Paediatr 2012;101:451–7.

36. National Institute for Health and Care Excellence. Urinary tract infection (UTI) in children. London: NICE; 2001. Available at: http://guidance.nice.org.uk/CG054. Accessed February 10, 2014.

37. Benador D, Benador N, Slosman D, et al. Are younger children at highest risk of renal sequelae after pyelonephritis? Lancet 1997;349:17–9.

38. Schwab CW Jr, Wu HY, Selman H, et al. Spontaneous resolution of vesicoureteral reflux: a 15-year perspective. J Urol 2002;168:2594–9.

39. Skoog SJ, Belman AB. Primary vesicoureteral reflux in the black child. Pediatrics 1991;87:538–43.

40. Steele BT, Robitaille P, DeMaria J, et al. Follow-up evaluation of prenatally recognized vesicoureteric reflux. J Pediatr 1989;115:95–6.

41. Garin EH, Olavarria F, Garcia Nieto V, et al. Clinical significance of primary vesicoureteral reflux and urinary antibiotic prophylaxis after acute pyelonephritis: a multicenter, randomized, controlled study. Pediatrics 2006;117:626–32.

42. Pennesi M, Travan L, Peratoner L, et al, North East Italy Prophylaxis in VUR study group. Is antibiotic prophylaxis in children with vesicoureteral reflux effective in preventing pyelonephritis and renal scars? A randomized, controlled trial. Pediatrics 2008;121:e1489–94.

43. Montini G, Rigon L, Zucchetta P, et al. Prophylaxis after first febrile urinary tract infection in children? A multicenter, randomized, controlled, noninferiority trial. Pediatrics 2008;122:1064–71.

44. Craig JC, Simpson JM, Williams GJ, et al. Antibiotic prophylaxis and recurrent urinary tract infection in children. N Engl J Med 2009;361:1748–59.

45. Prospective trial of operative versus non-operative treatment of severe vesicoureteric reflux in children: five years' observation. Birmingham Reflux Study Group. Br Med J (Clin Res Ed) 1987;295:237–41.

46. Piepsz A, Tamminen-Mobius T, Reiners C, et al. Five-year study of medical or surgical treatment in children with severe vesico-ureteral reflux dimercaptosuccinic acid findings. International Reflux Study Group in Europe. Eur J Pediatr 1998;157:753–8.

47. Brandstrom P, Esbjorner E, Herthelius M, et al. The Swedish reflux trial in children: III. Urinary tract infection pattern. J Urol 2010;184:286–91.

48. Jodal U, Lindberg U. Guidelines for management of children with urinary tract infection and vesico-ureteric reflux. Recommendations from a Swedish state-of-the-art conference. Swedish Medical Research Council. Acta Paediatr Suppl 1999;88:87–9.

Lower Urinary Tract Obstruction in the Fetus and Neonate

Douglass B. Clayton, MD*, John W. Brock III, MD

KEYWORDS

- Urethral obstruction • Prenatal diagnosis • Prune-belly syndrome
- Prenatal ultrasonography • Posterior urethral valves • Fetal intervention

KEY POINTS

- Congenital lower urinary tract obstruction in the fetus and neonate is rare but is increasingly identified in the era of prenatal sonography and can result in substantial perinatal mortality with lifelong morbidity.
- Posterior urethral valves, urethral atresia, and prune-belly syndrome are the frequently reported causes of lower urinary tract obstruction, with posterior urethral valves seen most often.
- The management of these diseases in the newborn period requires appropriate urinary tract decompression, subspecialty support, and definitive diagnosis with endoscopy and radiography.
- Despite numerous human series and the recent publication of a randomized trial, the survival benefit in lower urinary tract obstruction afforded by fetal intervention with vesicoamniotic shunt placement remains unclear.

INTRODUCTION

Routine prenatal sonography has made prenatal anomaly detection a reality. Congenital anomalies affect up to 2% of all pregnancies,[1,2] and ultrasound technology has high sensitivity for urologic anomalies, particularly diagnoses involving obstruction. Urologic diagnoses account for 20% of all prenatally identified congenital anomalies.[3] Fetal hydronephrosis is one of the most commonly detected findings, but alone it does not necessarily portend a persistent postnatal obstruction.[1,2,4] Prenatal care providers must rely on additional findings to increase the degree of suspicion for urinary tract obstruction.

Funding Sources: None.

Conflict of Interest: None.

Division of Pediatric Urologic Surgery, Department of Urologic Surgery, Monroe Carrel Jr. Children's Hospital, 2200 Children's Way, 4102 DOT, Nashville, TN 37232, USA

* Corresponding author.

E-mail address: douglass.b.clayton@vanderbilt.edu

Several genitourinary anomalies with a high propensity for morbidity and mortality are causes of lower urinary tract obstruction (LUTO).[5] **Box 1** lists the causes of LUTO that are discussed in this article. The article focuses on:

- Review of the current literature regarding LUTO in the fetus and newborn
- Clinical aspects of each diagnosis and management strategies
- Prenatal sonographic appearance suggesting LUTO
- Fetal intervention for LUTO

EPIDEMIOLOGY AND INTRODUCTION OF LUTO

Congenital LUTO is a rare phenomenon primarily affecting the male fetus.[6] Epidemiologic data suggest that the birth prevalence of LUTO is stable. In a large population-based study from the United Kingdom, the birth prevalence of postnatally confirmed LUTO was 3.34 per 10,000 live births, with no significant change in birth prevalence occurring between 1995 and 2007.[7] **Table 1** shows the birth prevalence of LUTO diagnoses. A United States report using the kids inpatient database also found no significant changes in the prevalence of prune-belly syndrome (PBS) or posterior urethral valves (PUV) between 1997 and 2009.[8]

PUV

The most common cause of LUTO is PUV, with a birth prevalence of 1 to 2 per 10,000 live male births.[8,9] The male urethra consists of the posterior urethra, which comprises the prostatic and membranous sections, and the anterior urethra, which is distal to the membranous urethra and traverses the entire penis.[10] A posterior urethral valve is an obstructing membrane or mucosal fold within the posterior urethra leading to complete or partial bladder outlet obstruction.[11] Hugh Hampton Young[12] originally described 3 types of PUV in the early 1900s. Type I valves are most common and appear as leaflets that extend in an inferior and anterior direction originating posteriorly from the verumontanum. Type II valves are not obstructive and represent mucosal folds extending superiorly from the verumontanum to the bladder neck. Type III valves

---

Box 1
Congenital LUTO diagnoses

1. Most common
   a. Posterior urethral valves
   b. Urethral atresia
   c. Prune-belly syndrome
2. Less common
   a. Anterior urethral valves/anterior urethral diverticulum
   b. Congenital megalourethra
   c. Obstructing ureterocele
3. Rare mimics
   a. Isolated megacystis
   b. MMIHS
   c. Megacystis-megaureter association

Table 1
Birth prevalence of congenital LUTO in 284 pregnancies with LUTO

Diagnosis	%	Prevalence per 10,000 Live Births
PUV	63	2.10
UA	9.9	0.33
Urethral Stenosis	7.0	0.23
PBS	2.5	0.08
Unspecified	17.6	0.59

Abbreviations: PBS, prune-belly syndrome; PUV, posterior urethral valves; UA, urethral atresia.
  Data from Malin G, Tonks AM, Morris RK, et al. Congenital lower urinary tract obstruction: a population-based epidemiological study. BJOG 2012;119(12):1455–64.

appear as an annular ring or membrane in the posterior urethra.[10,13] The classification of PUV has no bearing on the diagnosis, management, or outcome of the child.[10] Irrespective of valve type, progressive prenatal obstruction can result in variable effects, including megacystis, bladder wall fibrosis, unilateral or bilateral hydronephrosis, renal dysplasia, vesicoureteral reflux, oligohydramnios, and pulmonary insufficiency.

Urethral Atresia

Urethral atresia (UA) has a prevalence of 0.3 per 10,000 live births.[7] UA has been defined as complete infravesical obstruction caused by a membrane that obliterates the lumen at the distalmost aspect of the prostatic urethra.[14] Most reported cases have been in male fetuses and it may occur in isolation or with other anomalies. Accurate birth prevalence is difficult to ascertain given the near-universal mortality of UA without some means of fetal bladder decompression either by prenatal intervention or spontaneous egress via a patent urachus or a vesicocutaneous fistula.[14–16] A less common and potentially less severe variant form of UA is urethral stenosis in which narrowing of the urethra is present without complete obliteration of the urethral lumen.[17,18]

PBS

PBS is a disease of male newborns characterized by intra-abdominal cryptorchidism, upper urinary tract dilatation with megacystis, and a redundant anterior abdominal wall with muscular deficiency.[19] Features of PBS can be present in female newborns but without gonadal abnormalities. PBS affects between 1 in 29,000 and 1 in 40,000 fetuses (prevalence of 0.4 per 10,000 live births).[8,19,20] Two key theories exist to explain the constellation of findings in children with PBS. One theory supports developmental arrest of the lateral plate mesoderm during the 6th to 10th weeks of gestation leading to a malformation of the muscular component of the abdominal wall and the urinary tract. Another prominent theory posits that an infravesical obstruction is present during critical phases of development causing bladder distension, upper urinary tract dilatation, and muscular atrophy, and resulting in the prototypical findings of PBS.[21–23]

LUTO in the fetus with PBS is variable given that some boys maintain normal amniotic fluid volumes despite megacystis and upper tract dilatation, do not show anatomic obstructive lesions postnatally, and are able to void spontaneously. When postnatally confirmed LUTO is coexistent with PBS, the obstruction may be caused by prostatic hypoplasia, causing a functional rather than an anatomic obstruction that impairs emptying during voiding, sometimes referred to as a type IV urethral valve.[19] Overt UA and urethral stenosis have also been reported in association with PBS.[24,25] Additional sequelae of PBS include renal dysplasia, pulmonary hypoplasia, gastrointestinal anomalies, cardiac anomalies, and lower limb deformities.[23]

Anterior Urethral Obstruction

Anterior urethral valves (AUV) and their associated variant anterior urethral diverticulum (AUD) are rare forms of anterior urethral obstruction causing LUTO. The name denotes an obstruction that may occur at any point between the meatus and the membranous urethra, with slightly less than half located in the bulbar urethra and approximately one-third each being in either the penile urethra or at the penoscrotal junction.[26] AUV/AUD is reported to be 30 times less common than PUV,[26,27] and occurs from a mucosal fold arising from the floor of the urethra to coapt with the roof, thus creating an antegrade obstruction with variable degrees of diverticulum formation.[28,29] In the era of prenatal sonography, as many as 45% are diagnosed prenatally.[26] Fetal presentation might include bilateral hydronephrosis, megacystis, and possibly a perineal cyst. Neonatal presentation may include the findings discussed earlier and penile swelling or megalourethra.[26,30]

Congenital megalourethra (CM) is a rare anterior urethral disorder in boys, characterized by variable deficiency of penile tissue causing dilatation of the anterior urethra. CM occurs in 2 variants, scaphoid and fusiform, with both involving absence of penile tissue. Scaphoid CM variants have deficient corpus spongiosum only and fusiform variants are deficient in corpus cavernosum and corpus spongiosum tissue.[31,32] Fusiform CM is more often lethal compared with the scaphoid variant.[33] Each form can be associated with lower and upper urinary tract dilatation, and prenatal diagnosis has been reported.[32] Impaired egress of urine in CM is caused by functional obstruction. Prenatal appearance suggesting CM includes urinary tract dilatation along with penile ballooning, phallic distension, or a perineal cyst.[32,34,35]

Obstructing Ureterocele

A ureterocele is a cystic dilatation of the distal ureter that leads to ballooning of the ureter into the bladder.[36] Ureteroceles most commonly occur in an ectopic location within the bladder and are usually associated with the upper pole of a duplicated collecting system.[37] Although obstruction of the upper pole segment is common, ureteroceles do not often cause LUTO. However, several reports now exist in the literature describing this rare cause of fetal LUTO. When LUTO does occur, the ureterocele has either prolapsed into the bladder neck creating a ball-valve effect or a cecoureterocele variant is present in which the ureterocele tracks distally into the proximal urethra creating a windsock-type obstruction.[37] Obstructing ureteroceles may be amenable to fetal intervention and there are several reports of prenatal puncture using a variety of techniques.[36,38,39] More commonly, ureteroceles are punctured postnatally using endoscopic techniques.

Mimics of LUTO

Several rare entities mimicking LUTO should be considered if megacystis is present but other corroborating signs of obstruction are absent:

- Megacystis-microcolon-intestinal hypoperistalsis syndrome (MMIHS)
- Isolated congenital megacystis
- Megacystis-megaureter association[40]

True anatomic obstruction is not usually present in any of these entities. MMIHS is predominately a female disease (3:1 preponderance) characterized by dilated small bowel, microcolon, and megacystis with or without hydronephrosis.[41] Female gender along with high digestive enzymes on amniocentesis and increased calcium levels on vesicocentesis suggest MMIHS.[42] MMIHS is often lethal but not as a result of LUTO because the megacystis is nonobstructive. Isolated congenital megacystis has been reported and is theorized to be a milder variant of MMIHS or a variant form of visceral myopathy.[43,44] Megacystis-megaureter association is characterized by a massive thin-walled bladder with upper urinary tract dilatation and is the result of large-volume urinary reflux that repetitively cycles urine back and forth between the bladder and upper tracts. This type of yo-yo reflux causes progressive bladder and ureteral distension. The association has been shown on prenatal ultrasonography and is characterized by a thin bladder, hydroureteronephrosis, and normal amniotic fluid volumes.[45]

Voluntary Termination of Pregnancy

The combined effects of epidemiologic rarity, potential for fetal demise, and voluntary termination of pregnancy create challenges for studying LUTO. Previous data suggested that increasing prenatal ultrasonography use does not correlate with increasing pregnancy terminations.[46] By contrast, one French report of 165,000 pregnancies over a 7-year period found significantly higher rates of voluntary termination over time that paralleled increases in prenatal sonogram use. Voluntary terminations with multiple anomalies remained stable but terminations increased significantly in pregnancies with isolated anomalies. For single-system anomalies, voluntary termination of pregnancy occurred in 22% with spina bifida, 20% with genitourinary anomalies, and 55% with suspected LUTO.[47] A review over a 20-year period in the United States found voluntary termination in 46% of PUV cases, and 31% of PBS cases.[48] Similar epidemiologic trials show early termination rates of 20% in isolated LUTO cases and 41% in LUTO associated with multiple anomalies.[7]

ANTENATAL SUSPICION OF LUTO

Suspicion of LUTO is prompted during routine second-trimester fetal anomaly sonograms, and often requires rapid escalation in care during this critical window of time. Distinguishing between the different causes of fetal LUTO is challenging given the overlap in sonographic characteristics. No single finding is most predictive of LUTO; multiple findings typically guide decision making. The constellation of findings most consistent with fetal LUTO includes male gender, bilateral hydronephrosis, enlargement of the fetal bladder (megacystis), a dilated posterior urethra (a keyhole sign), and oligohydramnios.[49]

Timing

Timing is the most important overarching theme in fetal diagnosis of LUTO, with earlier findings being more worrisome for both fetal survival and renal function. Beyond 16 weeks of gestation, fetal urine becomes the foremost constituent of amniotic fluid. Simultaneous with this process, fetal nephrogenesis is occurring and renal mass is undergoing rapid, exponential growth between weeks 16 and 35. It is during this critical developmental window that LUTO is often identified and subsequent decisions must be made about intervention.

Amniotic Fluid Volume

A reduction in amniotic fluid index or frank anhydramnios is a poor prognostic sign when LUTO is suspected. The natural history of LUTO is predicated on the status of the amniotic fluid, and untreated second-trimester oligohydramnios results in fetal demise in up to 80% of cases.[15] In a prospective analysis of 145 fetuses with hydronephrosis, a multivariable logistic regression model identified second-trimester oligohydramnios as a significant and independent predictor of diagnosing PUV.[6] A retrospective review of 65 boys with PUV reported oligohydramnios and sonographic detection at a gestational age less than 24 weeks as significant predictors of poor postnatal renal function.[50] Moreover, in a meta-analysis including 10 studies and 215 pregnancies affected by LUTO, oligohydramnios was a significant predictor of poor postnatal renal function in children.[51]

Renal Appearance

The appearance of the kidneys, specifically the cortex and the collecting system, provide some insight into the severity of LUTO and possibly even postnatal renal function. Hydronephrosis associated with LUTO may be unilateral or bilateral and may also include dilatation of the ureters. Unilateral hydronephrosis does not eliminate the possibility of LUTO and should still raise suspicion. However, in one study, isolated unilateral hydronephrosis with no other findings was significantly associated with the absence of LUTO.[6] Objective methods have been reported to quantify fetal hydronephrosis. Measurement of the anterior-posterior diameter of the renal pelvis in a transverse plane are often used with diameters greater than 4 mm in the second trimester or greater than 7 mm in the third trimester considered abnormal in the pediatric urology literature.[52,53] More severe hydronephrosis increases the risk for postnatal urologic abnormality to be present.[54]

Evaluating the appearance of the fetal renal parenchyma may help with predicting the presence of LUTO and renal dysplasia. Important characteristics that are worrisome include increased renal echogenicity and the presence of cystic parenchymal changes.[55,56] Arguments for and against the predictive capacity of fetal renal cortical appearance have been made.[6,50,56,57] However, in a published meta-analysis of LUTO series, abnormal renal cortical appearance showed the best accuracy in predicting poor postnatal renal function with an area under the curve of 0.78. The investigators of the meta-analysis admitted that the inherent heterogeneity of the reviewed studies limited the precision of the predictive capacity.[51]

Bladder Appearance

Sonographic enlargement of the fetal bladder is termed megacystis and is reported to be present in less than 1% of pregnancies by late first trimester.[58] Few objective definitions of megacystis are present in the literature. In a prospective study evaluating more than 24,000 pregnancies between 10 and 14 weeks, a longitudinal bladder diameter of greater than 7 mm and a ratio of longitudinal bladder diameter to crown-rump length of greater than 10% defined megacystis.[58] Between weeks 10 and 14 of gestation, longitudinal bladder measurements exceeding 15 mm suggest a fetal LUTO, whereas measurements between 7 and 15 mm are more often associated with chromosomal or congenital anomalies.[59] In the second trimester, megacystis is characterized as an enlarged bladder failing to empty during 45 minutes of sonographic observation.[60] Third-trimester definitions are nonexistent. A recent French report examined 84 cases of fetal megacystis using these definitions, and **Table 2** shows the outcomes of megacystis by trimester, highlighting the importance of timing.[61]

A sonographic keyhole sign indicates dilatation of the male posterior urethra and is sometimes considered diagnostic of PUV.[62] **Fig. 1** shows the prenatal appearance of a keyhole sign in 2 male fetuses. However, a positive keyhole sign does not guarantee a postnatal diagnosis of PUV.[63] In one series, prenatal sonograms were found to be

Table 2
Outcome by trimester of fetal megacystis

Trimester (n = 84 Total)	Live Births (%)	Chromosomal/Congenital Anomalies (%)	LUTO (%)	Normal Bladder (%)
First (n = 8)	0 (0)	17 (68)	8 (32)	0 (0)
Second (n = 31)	11 (35)	11 (35)	16 (51)	1 (3)
Third (n = 28)	25 (89)	4 (14)	14 (50)	4 (14)

Data from Bornes M, Spaggiari E, Schmitz T, et al. Outcome and etiologies of fetal megacystis according to the gestational age at diagnosis. Prenat Diagn 2013;33:1162–6.

94% sensitive but only 43% specific for a diagnosis of PUV. A keyhole sign was present in 51% of patients with PUV and in 34% without PUV, and was not a significant predictor of postnatal diagnosis of PUV.[63]

Urinary Extravasation

Urinary extravasation may be present on sonography, supporting a diagnosis of LUTO. The most commonly reported anatomic sites include urinary ascites, perinephric urinoma, and urinothorax.[64,65] PUV is the most common entity associated with extravasation, and causes include bladder rupture, urinary transudate, and forniceal rupture. Up to 15% of boys with PUV show urinary extravasation on prenatal sonograms.[64,66] It has been postulated that urinomas may protect renal function by acting as a pop-off valve for the high-pressure urinary tract.[66]

NEONATAL DIAGNOSIS AND MANAGEMENT
Standard Work-up

The neonatal management of the entities causing LUTO should be standard irrespective of the ultimate diagnosis and include the following:

- Availability of neonatology and intensive care unit support
- Pediatric subspecialty consultation including nephrology and urology
- Prophylactic antibiotics using penicillins or first-generation cephalosporins

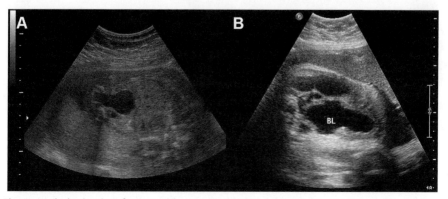

Fig. 1. Keyhole sign in 2 fetuses with presumed LUTO. (*A*) Male fetus at 28 weeks' gestation eventually diagnosed with PUV. (*B*) Male fetus at 34 weeks' gestation diagnosed postnatally with PBS. BL, bladder.

- Thorough physical examination with attention to abdominal wall and external genitalia
- Adequate bladder drainage
- Radiographic work-up with renal-bladder ultrasonography and voiding cystourethrogram

Most term neonates should be able to accept an 8-French catheter per urethra. Smaller 5-French feeding tubes may be used in premature infants but should be exchanged for 8-French tubes as soon as feasible to allow for optimal drainage. In some patients, a suprapubic cystotomy or cutaneous vesicostomy may be necessary to achieve adequate drainage. Circumcision should be offered in the newborn period to reduce the risk of urinary tract infection. Retrospective data have shown up to 83% reduction in urinary tract infection following circumcision in boys with PUV.[67,68] At present, a randomized clinical trial is being conducted to study the effect of routine neonatal circumcision with antibiotic prophylaxis versus antibiotic prophylaxis alone on the relative risk of febrile urinary tract infection in boys with PUV.[69]

PUV

The critical diagnostic test in PUV is the voiding cystourethrogram (VCUG), which confirms the presence of the obstructing valve, shows the contour and appearance of the bladder, and shows any vesicoureteral reflux (**Fig. 2**). Neonates with PUV need definitive valve ablation in the operating room before discharge from the hospital.

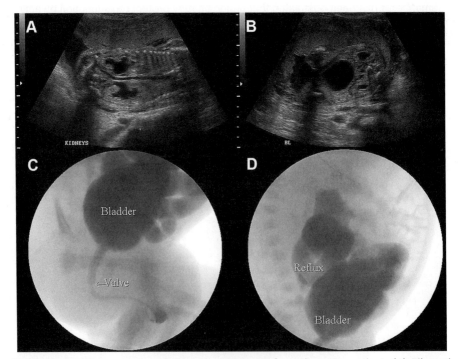

Fig. 2. Postnatal appearance of PUV. All images are from the same patient. (*A*) Bilateral hydronephrosis on fetal ultrasonography. (*B*) Dilated fetal bladder on ultrasonography. (*C*) The presence of the obstructing valve is noted during the voiding phase of the VCUG study performed on day of life 2. (*D*) High-grade vesicoureteral reflux into the left collecting system.

In some cases, prematurity may prevent endoscopic treatment because of the size of the urethra, and a cutaneous vesicostomy may be necessary. A variety of instruments and surgical energies are available to ablate valve leaflets endoscopically, including cold-knife incision, electrosurgical ablation, hook fulguration, and holmium:YAG laser incision.[70]

UA

In the fetus with UA who survives either by spontaneous egress of urine or by fetal intervention, cutaneous vesicostomy has been the procedure of choice to establish adequate drainage of the urinary tract early in the neonatal period.[14] Additional procedures are necessary in most patients and include endoscopic puncture of the obstructing membrane, endoscopic urethral dilatation, formal open urethroplasty, and in some cases a continent urinary diversion.[14]

PBS

A spectrum of disease severity exists in PBS with extremely severe variants (type 1) having little chance for neonatal survival and milder variants having fewer sequelae (type 3). Boys with intermediate severity (type 2) require the most attention because of improved chance of survival, but with greater morbidity, including renal dysplasia, upper tract dilatation, and abdominal wall redundancy. Many boys with type 2 and 3 PBS can void spontaneously at birth, but placement of an indwelling urinary catheter may help in identifying baseline renal function. VCUG and renal ultrasonography are important in establishing the anatomy of the urinary tract. **Fig. 3** shows the ectatic, dilated appearance of the urinary tract in 2 different boys with PBS. Because of massive upper tract dilatation, some boys may require intermittent catheterization to ensure good drainage.

LONG-TERM OUTCOME OF LUTO

The long-term outcome of LUTO in neonatal survivors is primarily related to future renal function; however, other important lifelong considerations include bladder and lung function, as well as neurocognitive development. In both PUV and PBS, the initial

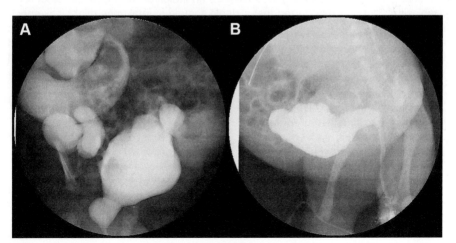

Fig. 3. VCUG appearance of PBS. (*A*) Massive vesicoureteral reflux with upper tract dilatation, a large bladder, and a dilated posterior urethra. (*B*) A large irregular bladder with posterior urethral dilatation and an abnormal angle of the urethra on the voiding phase.

creatinine nadir after bladder drainage most strongly predicts future renal function with values less than 0.8 mg/dL in PUV and less than 0.7 mg/dL in PBS being considered good prognostic signs for future renal function. As many as 30% of boys with PUV and 20% with PBS develop end stage renal disease later in adolescence or early adulthood.[71–73] In boys with PUV, renal failure is considered to be multifactorial, resulting from progressive bladder dysfunction, renal hyperfiltration injury, vesicoureteral reflux, renal dysplasia, and recurrent urinary tract infections.[74] Infertility can be an issue in PBS caused by hypoplasia of the prostate. Prevention of urinary tract infection, which is secondary to massive upper tract dilatation and reflux, is important to help preserve nephron mass in all boys with LUTO. Depending on the severity of the phenotype, boys with PBS require surgical intervention that may include:

- Bilateral orchiopexy for intra-abdominal testicles (required in all boys)
- Reduction cystoplasty (in isolated cases)
- Abdominal wall reconstruction (commonly delayed until adolescence)

ANTENATAL INTERVENTION

Fetal intervention for LUTO was pioneered at the University of California at San Francisco in the 1980s using a fetal lamb model.[75–78] Numerous single-institution reports in human fetuses have subsequently been published, as has been highlighted in several meta-analyses and systematic reviews.[79,80] Interventional approaches for fetal LUTO that have been reported include fetal vesicostomy, repetitive vesicocentesis, vesicoamniotic shunt (VAS), fetal cystoscopy with or without ablation of the obstructing lesion, and fetal ureterostomy.[49,81] The most commonly reported single technique today is percutaneous placement of a VAS.[80]

Preservation of Renal Function

After showing technically feasibility, attention was primarily directed to patient selection on the grounds of renal preservation. Fetal urine is hypotonic to serum and becomes increasingly hypotonic as gestation progresses.[82] Thus, sampling of fetal urine via vesicocentesis was introduced as a method for quantifying fetal renal tubular function, and increased tonicity was used as an indicator for the presence of renal dysplasia.[83,84] It was recognized that a single sample of fetal urine might lack specificity and thus repetitive vesicocentesis was introduced.[85,86] Fetuses could then be stratified into good and poor prognosis groups for expected renal function based on the hypotonicity of the urine.[85] Absolute cutoffs for urinary analysis (increased values suggest a poor prognosis) used in multiple studies[87,88] include:

- Sodium less than 100 mmol/L
- Chloride less than 90 mmol/L
- Calcium less than 8 mg/dL
- Osmolality less than 200 mmol/L
- Total protein less than 20 mg/dL
- β2-Microglobulin less than 6 mg/L

Debate has existed over the accuracy of fetal urine analysis with respect to future renal function.[89,90] A systematic review published in 2007 examining 23 articles and 572 pregnancies found no single urinary analyte to be clinically significant in its accuracy for predicting poor renal function. However, studies using pooled analysis and cutoffs of greater than the 95th percentile for gestational age (cutoffs that have not been routinely used in most studies), showed that calcium and sodium had the best accuracy for predicting postnatal renal function. The review also identified multiple critical problems in the available literature, including poorly reported methodologies as well as variable thresholds and reference standards.[91]

Renal Function in LUTO Survivors

Despite these criticisms, fetal urine analysis remains a part of the evaluation in many centers. In series with long-term follow-up after fetal intervention, the rate of renal insufficiency among survivors ranges from 50% to 66%.[49,83,87,88,92] Even the presence of good prognosis electrolytes on serial vesicocentesis does not guarantee optimal renal outcomes after intervention.[88] The current limitations of early LUTO combined with the rapid growth of the kidney during early gestation make salvage of renal function with fetal intervention an elusive target.

Pulmonary Survival

The primary goal of fetal intervention currently is to improve survival by supporting pulmonary development. Published rates of survival after VAS vary widely, ranging from 40% to 91%.[83,87,88,93] In general, fetuses with PUV and PBS have higher survival rates after VAS than do those with UA.[87] In the 1986 report from the International Fetal Surgery Registry, survival after VAS placement without fetal electrolyte analysis was 48% in nonterminated fetuses, and by postnatal diagnosis, survival was 76% for PUV, 100% for PBS, and 20% for UA.[94] By contrast, in a highly refined population of singleton male gestations with primarily good or borderline prognosis published 20 years later, VAS placement achieved 91% survival at 1 year of age.[88] However, the survival benefit of intervention remains unproved. In a 2010 meta-analysis of 12 intervention studies, fetal survival with LUTO was significantly improved after VAS placement (odds ratio, 3.86) compared with no treatment. The observed benefit was driven largely by the inclusion of 2 studies reporting intervention in fetuses with poor prognosis electrolytes.[83,87] Once the investigators of the meta-analysis excluded voluntary pregnancy termination and intrauterine death, VAS placement showed a survival benefit only in the fetuses with poor prognosis.[80]

Percutaneous Shunting for LUTO Trial

With the inherent heterogeneity of LUTO intervention series, a randomized trial of intervention for fetal LUTO was needed. The Percutaneous Shunting for LUTO (PLUTO) trial represents the only randomized trial of fetal intervention in urology. Performed in the United Kingdom and Ireland, the study compared fetal VAS placement with conservative management.[95] The results of the PLUTO trial were recently published. Eligibility criteria for enrollment and randomization included:

- Singleton male gestation without chromosomal or other structural anomaly
- Sonography showing LUTO (enlarged bladder, dilated proximal urethra, hydronephrosis, and cystic renal parenchyma)
- Clinician uncertainty regarding the benefit of shunt placement

The primary outcome measure was survival at 28 days, and the study was powered to detect improvement in survival from 39% to 61%, which correlated with a relative risk of 1.55 with VAS placement. At 80% power, sample size calculations required 75 pregnancies per arm. A nonrandomized registry component was included as an alternative to randomization. In the end, the trial did not meet recruitment goals and was underpowered to analyze the intended outcomes. Key findings of the trial include:

- Thirty-one women randomized; 16 to VAS placement and 15 to conservative management

- Forty-five women enrolled in the registry component
- Sixty-eight women voluntary terminated pregnancy
- Twelve live births occurred in each group
- Twenty-eight-day survival was 50% (8 of 16) after VAS and 26% (4 of 15) in the conservative group

All neonatal deaths were caused by pulmonary hypoplasia. At 2 years of age, 7 patients in the VAS group and 3 in the conservative group were alive. Even though survival was higher in the VAS group (50%) versus conservative management (26%), the differences were not statistically significant by intention-to-treat analysis. Of the 10 children alive at 2 years of age, only 2 had normal renal function (defined as serum creatinine <50 μmol/L), both of whom had received a VAS.

SUMMARY

LUTO is a rare congenital anomaly and PUV is the most common cause. The critical consideration after fetal detection of LUTO is determining the likelihood for survival and the potential for morbidity, both of which are closely associated with the timing of diagnosis and the status of the amniotic fluid. For neonatal survivors with LUTO, postnatal pulmonary and renal function is the major concern initially. For fetuses surviving to term, aggressive treatment is needed to address the anatomic cause of obstruction, improve and protect bladder function, and preserve functional nephron mass. The characteristics of the ideal candidate for antenatal intervention remain elusive. Despite the completion of a randomized trial, the benefit of prenatal intervention with VAS placement remains unclear.

REFERENCES

1. Clementi M, Stoll C. The Euroscan study. Ultrasound Obstet Gynecol 2001; 18(4):297–300.
2. Grandjean H, Larroque D, Levi S. The performance of routine ultrasonographic screening of pregnancies in the Eurofetus Study. Am J Obstet Gynecol 1999; 181(2):446–54.
3. Grandjean H, Larroque D, Levi S. Sensitivity of routine ultrasound screening of pregnancies in the Eurofetus database. The Eurofetus Team. Ann N Y Acad Sci 1998;847:118–24.
4. Stefos T, Plachouras N, Sotiriadis A, et al. Routine obstetrical ultrasound at 18-22 weeks: our experience on 7,236 fetuses. J Matern Fetal Med 1999;8(2):64–9.
5. Clayton DB, Brock JW 3rd. In utero intervention for urologic diseases. Nat Rev Urol 2012;9(4):207–17.
6. Oliveira EA, Diniz JS, Cabral AC, et al. Prognostic factors in fetal hydronephrosis: a multivariate analysis. Pediatr Nephrol 1999;13(9):859–64.
7. Malin G, Tonks AM, Morris RK, et al. Congenital lower urinary tract obstruction: a population-based epidemiological study. BJOG 2012;119(12):1455–64.
8. Lloyd JC, Wiener JS, Gargollo PC, et al. Contemporary epidemiological trends in complex congenital genitourinary anomalies. J Urol 2013;190(Suppl 4): 1590–5.
9. Hodges SJ, Patel B, McLorie G, et al. Posterior urethral valves. ScientificWorldJournal 2009;9:1119–26.
10. Kajbafzadeh A. Congenital urethral anomalies in boys. Part I: posterior urethral valves. Urol J 2005;2(2):59–78.

11. Krishnan A, de Souza A, Konijeti R, et al. The anatomy and embryology of posterior urethral valves. J Urol 2006;175(4):1214–20.
12. Young HH, Frontz WA, Baldwin JC. Congenital obstruction of the posterior urethra. J Urol, 3: 289–365, 1919. J Urol 2002;167(1):265–7 [discussion: 268].
13. Zderic SA, Canning DA. Posterior urethral valves. London: Informa; 2007.
14. Gonzalez R, De Filippo R, Jednak R, et al. Urethral atresia: long-term outcome in 6 children who survived the neonatal period. J Urol 2001;165(6 Pt 2):2241–4.
15. Reuss A, Wladimiroff JW, Stewart PA, et al. Non-invasive management of fetal obstructive uropathy. Lancet 1988;2(8617):949–51.
16. Stalberg K, Gonzalez R. Urethral atresia and anhydramnios at 18 weeks of gestation can result in normal development. J Pediatr Urol 2012;8(3):e33–5.
17. Ruano R, Yoshizaki CT, Giron AM, et al. Fetal cystoscopic placement of transurethral stent in a fetus with urethral stenosis. Ultrasound Obstet Gynecol 2013. [Epub ahead of print].
18. Robyr R, Benachi A, Daikha-Dahmane F, et al. Correlation between ultrasound and anatomical findings in fetuses with lower urinary tract obstruction in the first half of pregnancy. Ultrasound Obstet Gynecol 2005;25(5):478–82.
19. Caldamone A, Woodard J. Prune belly syndrome. In: Wein AJ, editor. Campbell Walsh urology. vol. 4. Philadelphia: Elsevier; 2012. p. 3310–24.
20. Routh JC, Huang L, Retik AB, et al. Contemporary epidemiology and characterization of newborn males with prune belly syndrome. Urology 2010;76(1):44–8.
21. Granberg CF, Harrison SM, Dajusta D, et al. Genetic basis of prune belly syndrome: screening for HNF1beta gene. J Urol 2012;187(1):272–8.
22. Herman TE, Siegel MJ. Prune belly syndrome. J Perinatol 2009;29(1):69–71.
23. Hudson RG, Skoog SJ. Prune belly syndrome. London: Informa; 2007.
24. Reinberg Y, Chelimsky G, Gonzalez R. Urethral atresia and the prune belly syndrome. Report of 6 cases. Br J Urol 1993;72(1):112–4.
25. Kuga T, Esato K, Sase M, et al. Prune belly syndrome with penile and urethral agenesis: report of a case. J Pediatr Surg 1998;33(12):1825–8.
26. Cruz-Diaz O, Salomon A, Rosenberg E, et al. Anterior urethral valves: not such a benign condition. Front Pediatr 2013;1:35.
27. Jehannin B. Congenital obstructive valves and diverticula of the anterior urethra. Chir Pediatr 1990;31(3):173–80 [in French].
28. Kibar Y, Coban H, Irkilata HC, et al. Anterior urethral valves: an uncommon cause of obstructive uropathy in children. J Pediatr Urol 2007;3(5):350–3.
29. Firlit RS, Firlit CF, King LR. Obstructing anterior urethral valves in children. J Urol 1978;119(6):819–21.
30. Confer SD, Galati V, Frimberger D, et al. Megacystis with an anterior urethral valve: case report and review of literature. J Pediatr Urol 2010;6(5):459–62.
31. Sepulveda W, Elorza C, Gutierrez J, et al. Congenital megalourethra: outcome after prenatal diagnosis in a series of 4 cases. J Ultrasound Med 2005;24(9): 1303–8.
32. Promsonthi P, Viseshsindh W. Case report and review: prenatal diagnosis of congenital megalourethra. Fetal Diagn Ther 2010;28(2):123–8.
33. Jones EA, Freedman AL, Ehrlich RM. Megalourethra and urethral diverticula. Urol Clin North Am 2002;29(2):341–8, vi.
34. Amsalem H, Fitzgerald B, Keating S, et al. Congenital megalourethra: prenatal diagnosis and postnatal/autopsy findings in 10 cases. Ultrasound Obstet Gynecol 2011;37(6):678–83.
35. Yamamoto R, Ishii K, Ukita S, et al. Fetoscopic diagnosis of congenital megalourethra at early second trimester. Fetal Diagn Ther 2013;34(1):63–5.

36. Ashmead GG, Mercer B, Herbst M, et al. Fetal bladder outlet obstruction due to ureterocele: in utero "colander" therapy. J Ultrasound Med 2004;23(4): 565–8.

37. Austin PF, Cain MP, Casale AJ, et al. Prenatal bladder outlet obstruction secondary to ureterocele. Urology 1998;52(6):1132–5.

38. Soothill PW, Bartha JL, Tizard J. Ultrasound-guided laser treatment for fetal bladder outlet obstruction resulting from ureterocele. Am J Obstet Gynecol 2003;188(4):1107–8.

39. Quintero RA, Homsy Y, Bornick PW, et al. In-utero treatment of fetal bladder-outlet obstruction by a ureterocele. Lancet 2001;357(9272):1947–8.

40. Osborne NG, Bonilla-Musoles F, Machado LE, et al. Fetal megacystis: differential diagnosis. J Ultrasound Med 2011;30(6):833–41.

41. Machado L, Matias A, Rodrigues M, et al. Fetal megacystis as a prenatal challenge: megacystis-microcolon-intestinal hypoperistalsis syndrome in a male fetus. Ultrasound Obstet Gynecol 2013;41(3):345–7.

42. Muller F, Dreux S, Vaast P, et al. Prenatal diagnosis of megacystis-microcolon-intestinal hypoperistalsis syndrome: contribution of amniotic fluid digestive enzyme assay and fetal urinalysis. Prenat Diagn 2005;25(3):203–9.

43. Johnson EK, Nelson CP. Spontaneous resolution of isolated congenital megacystis: the incredible shrinking bladder. J Pediatr Urol 2013;9(1):e46–50.

44. Shimizu M, Nishio S, Ueno K, et al. Isolated congenital megacystis without intestinal obstruction: a mild variant of chronic intestinal pseudoobstruction syndrome? J Pediatr Surg 2011;46(11):e29–32.

45. Mandell J, Lebowitz RL, Peters CA, et al. Prenatal diagnosis of the megacystis-megaureter association. J Urol 1992;148(5):1487–9.

46. Hsieh MH, Lai J, Saigal CS. Trends in prenatal sonography use and subsequent urologic diagnoses and abortions in the United States. J Pediatr Urol 2009;5(6): 490–4.

47. Julian-Reynier C, Philip N, Scheiner C, et al. Impact of prenatal diagnosis by ultrasound on the prevalence of congenital anomalies at birth in southern France. J Epidemiol Community Health 1994;48(3):290–6.

48. Cromie WJ, Lee K, Houde K, et al. Implications of prenatal ultrasound screening in the incidence of major genitourinary malformations. J Urol 2001;165(5): 1677–80.

49. Holmes N, Harrison MR, Baskin LS. Fetal surgery for posterior urethral valves: long-term postnatal outcomes. Pediatrics 2001;108(1):1–7.

50. Sarhan O, Zaccaria I, Macher MA, et al. Long-term outcome of prenatally detected posterior urethral valves: single center study of 65 cases managed by primary valve ablation. J Urol 2008;179(1):307–12 [discussion: 312–3].

51. Morris RK, Malin GL, Khan KS, et al. Antenatal ultrasound to predict postnatal renal function in congenital lower urinary tract obstruction: systematic review of test accuracy. BJOG 2009;116(10):1290–9.

52. Coplen DE, Austin PF, Yan Y, et al. The magnitude of fetal renal pelvic dilatation can identify obstructive postnatal hydronephrosis, and direct postnatal evaluation and management. J Urol 2006;176(2):724–7 [discussion: 727].

53. Nguyen HT, Herndon CD, Cooper C, et al. The Society for Fetal Urology consensus statement on the evaluation and management of antenatal hydronephrosis. J Pediatr Urol 2010;6(3):212–31.

54. Lee RS, Cendron M, Kinnamon DD, et al. Antenatal hydronephrosis as a predictor of postnatal outcome: a meta-analysis. Pediatrics 2006;118(2): 586–93.

55. Anumba DO, Scott JE, Plant ND, et al. Diagnosis and outcome of fetal lower urinary tract obstruction in the northern region of England. Prenat Diagn 2005; 25(1):7–13.
56. Hutton KA, Thomas DF, Davies BW. Prenatally detected posterior urethral valves: qualitative assessment of second trimester scans and prediction of outcome. J Urol 1997;158(3 Pt 2):1022–5.
57. Kaefer M, Peters CA, Retik AB, et al. Increased renal echogenicity: a sonographic sign for differentiating between obstructive and nonobstructive etiologies of in utero bladder distension. J Urol 1997;158(3 Pt 2):1026–9.
58. Sebire NJ, Von Kaisenberg C, Rubio C, et al. Fetal megacystis at 10-14 weeks of gestation. Ultrasound Obstet Gynecol 1996;8:387–90.
59. Liao AW, Sebire NJ, Geerts L, et al. Megacystis at 10-14 weeks of gestation: chromosomal defects and outcome according to bladder length. Ultrasound Obstet Gynecol 2003;21(4):338–41.
60. Montemarano H, Bulas DI, Rushton HG, et al. Bladder distention and pyelectasis in the male fetus: causes, comparisons, and contrasts. J Ultrasound Med 1998;17(12):743–9.
61. Bornes M, Spaggiari E, Schmitz T, et al. Outcome and etiologies of fetal megacystis according to the gestational age at diagnosis. Prenat Diagn 2013;33(12): 1162–6.
62. Mahony BS, Callen PW, Filly RA. Fetal urethral obstruction: US evaluation. Radiology 1985;157(1):221–4.
63. Bernardes LS, Aksnes G, Saada J, et al. Keyhole sign: how specific is it for the diagnosis of posterior urethral valves? Ultrasound Obstet Gynecol 2009;34(4): 419–23.
64. Heikkila J, Taskinen S, Rintala R. Urinomas associated with posterior urethral valves. J Urol 2008;180(4):1476–8.
65. Yitta S, Saadai P, Filly RA. The fetal urinoma revisited. J Ultrasound Med 2014; 33(1):161–6.
66. Wells JM, Mukerji S, Chandran H, et al. Urinomas protect renal function in posterior urethral valves–a population based study. J Pediatr Surg 2010;45(2): 407–10.
67. Bader M, McCarthy L. What is the efficacy of circumcision in boys with complex urinary tract abnormalities? Pediatr Nephrol 2013;28(12):2267–72.
68. Mukherjee S, Joshi A, Carroll D, et al. What is the effect of circumcision on risk of urinary tract infection in boys with posterior urethral valves? J Pediatr Surg 2009; 44(2):417–21.
69. Réunion CHUdl. Circumcision and urinary tracting infections in boys with posterior urethral valves. Bethesda (MD): National Library of Medicine (US); 2000. In: ClinicalTrials.gov [Internet]. Available at: http://clinicaltrials.gov/ct2/show/record/NCT01537601. Accessed February 1, 2014.
70. Mandal S, Goel A, Kumar M, et al. Use of holmium:YAG laser in posterior urethral valves: another method of fulguration. J Pediatr Urol 2013;9(6 Pt B):1093–7.
71. Smith GH, Canning DA, Schulman SL, et al. The long-term outcome of posterior urethral valves treated with primary valve ablation and observation. J Urol 1996; 155(5):1730–4.
72. Ylinen E, Ala-Houhala M, Wikstrom S. Prognostic factors of posterior urethral valves and the role of antenatal detection. Pediatr Nephrol 2004;19(8): 874–9.
73. Heikkila J, Holmberg C, Kyllonen L, et al. Long-term risk of end stage renal disease in patients with posterior urethral valves. J Urol 2011;186(6):2392–6.

74. Lopez Pereira P, Martinez Urrutia MJ, Espinosa L, et al. Long-term consequences of posterior urethral valves. J Pediatr Urol 2013;9(5):590–6.

75. Harrison MR, Nakayama DK, Noall R, et al. Correction of congenital hydronephrosis in utero II. Decompression reverses the effects of obstruction on the fetal lung and urinary tract. J Pediatr Surg 1982;17(6):965–74.

76. Glick PL, Harrison MR, Adzick NS, et al. Correction of congenital hydronephrosis in utero IV: in utero decompression prevents renal dysplasia. J Pediatr Surg 1984;19(6):649–57.

77. Glick PL, Harrison MR, Halks-Miller M, et al. Correction of congenital hydrocephalus in utero II: Efficacy of in utero shunting. J Pediatr Surg 1984;19(6):870–81.

78. Glick PL, Harrison MR, Noall RA, et al. Correction of congenital hydronephrosis in utero III. Early mid-trimester ureteral obstruction produces renal dysplasia. J Pediatr Surg 1983;18(6):681–7.

79. Clark TJ, Martin WL, Divakaran TG, et al. Prenatal bladder drainage in the management of fetal lower urinary tract obstruction: a systematic review and meta-analysis. Obstet Gynecol 2003;102(2):367–82.

80. Morris RK, Malin GL, Khan KS, et al. Systematic review of the effectiveness of antenatal intervention for the treatment of congenital lower urinary tract obstruction. BJOG 2010;117(4):382–90.

81. Quintero RA, Hume R, Smith C, et al. Percutaneous fetal cystoscopy and endoscopic fulguration of posterior urethral valves. Am J Obstet Gynecol 1995;172(1 Pt 1):206–9.

82. Nicolini U, Spelzini F. Invasive assessment of fetal renal abnormalities: urinalysis, fetal blood sampling and biopsy. Prenat Diagn 2001;21(11):964–9.

83. Crombleholme TM, Harrison MR, Golbus MS, et al. Fetal intervention in obstructive uropathy: prognostic indicators and efficacy of intervention. Am J Obstet Gynecol 1990;162(5):1239–44.

84. Nicolaides KH, Cheng HH, Snijders RJ, et al. Fetal urine biochemistry in the assessment of obstructive uropathy. Am J Obstet Gynecol 1992;166(3):932–7.

85. Johnson MP, Corsi P, Bradfield W, et al. Sequential urinalysis improves evaluation of fetal renal function in obstructive uropathy. Am J Obstet Gynecol 1995;173(1):59–65.

86. Evans MI, Sacks AJ, Johnson MP, et al. Sequential invasive assessment of fetal renal function and the intrauterine treatment of fetal obstructive uropathies. Obstet Gynecol 1991;77(4):545–50.

87. Freedman AL, Bukowski TP, Smith CA, et al. Fetal therapy for obstructive uropathy: diagnosis specific outcomes [corrected]. J Urol 1996;156(2 Pt 2):720–4.

88. Biard JM, Johnson MP, Carr MC, et al. Long-term outcomes in children treated by prenatal vesicoamniotic shunting for lower urinary tract obstruction. Obstet Gynecol 2005;106(3):503–8.

89. Wilkins IA, Chitkara U, Lynch L, et al. The nonpredictive value of fetal urinary electrolytes: preliminary report of outcomes and correlations with pathologic diagnosis. Am J Obstet Gynecol 1987;157(3):694–8.

90. Elder JS, O'Grady JP, Ashmead G, et al. Evaluation of fetal renal function: unreliability of fetal urinary electrolytes. J Urol 1990;144(2 Pt 2):574–8 [discussion: 593–4].

91. Morris RK, Quinlan-Jones E, Kilby MD, et al. Systematic review of accuracy of fetal urine analysis to predict poor postnatal renal function in cases of congenital urinary tract obstruction. Prenat Diagn 2007;27(10):900–11.

92. Salam MA. Posterior urethral valve: outcome of antenatal intervention. Int J Urol 2006;13(10):1317–22.

93. McLorie G, Farhat W, Khoury A, et al. Outcome analysis of vesicoamniotic shunting in a comprehensive population. J Urol 2001;166(3):1036–40.
94. Manning FA, Harrison MR, Rodeck C. Catheter shunts for fetal hydronephrosis and hydrocephalus. Report of the International Fetal Surgery Registry. N Engl J Med 1986;315(5):336–40.
95. Morris RK, Malin GL, Quinlan-Jones E, et al. Percutaneous vesicoamniotic shunting versus conservative management for fetal lower urinary tract obstruction (PLUTO): a randomised trial. Lancet 2013;382:1496–506.

Hydronephrosis

Prenatal and Postnatal Evaluation and Management

Dennis B. Liu, MD[a],*, William R. Armstrong III, MD[b],
Max Maizels, MD[a]

KEYWORDS

- Hydronephrosis • Radiology • Antenatal diagnosis • Vesicoureteral reflux
- Obstructive uropathy • Urinary tract infections

KEY POINTS

- An anterior-posterior diameter (APD) of greater than or equal to 4 mm at less than 33 weeks gestation and 7 mm at greater than 33 weeks gestation most commonly define antenatal hydronephrosis.
- The likelihood of significant postnatal urologic pathologic abnormality correlates with the grade of APD and the gestational age at the time of measurement.
- Prenatal management is predominately expectant. Fetal intervention is rarely needed and remains controversial.
- Ureteropelvic junction obstruction and vesicoureteral reflux are the 2 most common post-natal diagnoses.
- The renal and bladder ultrasound is the mainstay of the postnatal evaluation and helps guide further testing with voiding cystourethrography and diuretic renography.

INTRODUCTION

The widespread use of routine second-trimester ultrasounds has increased the detection of congenital anomalies. One of the most frequently detected abnormalities is the dilation of the fetal renal collecting system, affecting 1% to 4.5% of all pregnancies.[1–4] This finding, however, is of uncertain clinical significance as this may be due to a wide spectrum of causes, ranging from insignificant transient physiologic development to

Disclosure: Co-founder and co-Executive Director of CEVL for Healthcare, Inc.
[a] Ann and Robert H. Lurie Children's Hospital of Chicago, Department of Urology, Northwestern University Feinberg School of Medicine, 225 East Chicago Avenue, Box 24, Chicago, IL 60611, USA; [b] Department of Urology, University of Illinois Chicago College of Medicine, 820 South Wood Street, M/C 955, Chicago, IL 60612, USA
* Corresponding author.
E-mail address: dbliu@luriechildrens.org

significant uropathies, such as urinary obstruction to vesicoureteral reflux (VUR) with the potential for renal compromise. Detection of urologic anomalies prenatally permits interventions that avoid complications (eg, pyelonephritis, flank or abdominal pain, renal calculi, hypertension, and renal failure); however, upwards of 64% to 94% of affected patients will ultimately not have significant urologic pathologic abnormality.[3–7] The clinical challenge, therefore, exists to differentiate those cases with significant pathologic abnormalities, which would benefit from early detection from those who would not, thereby reducing the performance of prenatal and postnatal testing to those who really benefit.

This review summarizes the current literature on the topic of prenatal diagnosis and postnatal assessment and management. The review highlights controversies that stem from a lack of consensus on the definition of antenatal hydronephrosis (ANH) and of evidence-based data to guide both prenatal and postnatal management.

PRENATAL DIAGNOSIS AND MANAGEMENT
Defining ANH

Terms such as "pyelectasis" and hydronephrosis are often used interchangeably and thus have become associated with implied pathologic abnormality, whereby these findings may instead reflect normal physiology. Therefore, the prefered term is SERP (sonographically evident renal pelvis) instead of pyelectasis to connote a neutral position.[8] The term hydronephrosis is reserved for dilation of the renal pelvis and calices.

Anterior-Posterior Diameter

The measurement of the anterior-posterior diameter (APD) of the renal pelvis in a transverse plane is currently the most widely accepted parameter to define SERP (**Fig. 1**).[9] Although there is a lack of uniformity in cutoff values for significant APD, the most commonly accepted values are those described initially by Corteville and colleagues.[10] In their study, an APD greater than or equal to 4 mm before 33 weeks gestation or 7 mm after 33 weeks gestation allowed for identification of 100% of fetuses that ultimately had impaired renal function or require surgery.

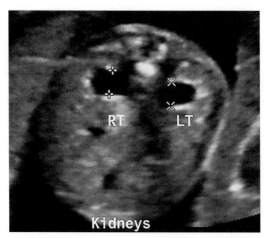

Fig. 1. Prenatal diagnosis of SERP. 20-week prenatal ultrasound depicting a transverse image of the fetal kidneys. APD measurements of the renal pelvis are 6.2 mm on the right (*RT*) and 6.1 mm on the left (*LT*). Postnatal ultrasound revealed SFU grade 1 on the right and SFU grade 2 on the left.

The difficulty in establishing cutoff values of APD lies in the balance between achieving high sensitivity while limiting false positives. If the value is too high, patients who will ultimately have significant urologic pathologic abnormality may be missed. However, if the value is lowered, the potential exists to overdiagnose and lead to over-testing. Corteville's APD cutoffs have been criticized on both accounts. It has previously been found that 35% of patients with APD less than these values still required extensive postnatal urologic care, suggesting that the current cutoff values are too high.[11] On the other hand, Bassanese and colleagues[12] identified higher cutoff APDs of 6 mm at 20 weeks of gestation and 10 mm at 30 weeks for isolated pyelectasis and APD of 10 mm at 20 weeks and 12 mm at 30 weeks for hydronephrosis and reported that these values achieved 100% sensitivity for detecting significant urologic abnormalities with specificities of 84%, 92%, 86%, and 67%, respectively. Similarly, Siemens and colleagues[13] suggested that postnatal follow-up was unnecessary for APDs of less than 6 mm at less than 20 weeks, less than 8 mm at 20 to 30 weeks, and 10 mm at greater than 30 weeks of gestation.

Differential Diagnosis

Up to 64% to 94% of fetuses, identified as having prenatal hydronephrosis, will ultimately have no identifiable postnatal urologic abnormality.[2,4-7] These patients are considered to have idiopathic ANH by Sidhu and colleagues.[6] The most common urologic pathologic diagnoses with their characteristic ultrasound findings and suggested postnatal evaluations are found in **Table 1**.[14,15]

Prognosis

Determining the prognosis of the fetus after discovery of SERP remains a critical but challenging component of prenatal counseling. To assist in predicting postnatal outcome, several ultrasonic features have been associated with an increased risk of urologic abnormalities. These abnormalities include the grade or severity of ANH, renal parenchymal abnormalities, low amniotic fluid levels, and the presence of additional features. The following link demonstrates a method of prenatal counseling on the significance of SERP: http://www.cevlforhealthcare.org/cevl/cevl_ver_2/MENUS/PrenatalConsultationProtocol/PCPU_for_pediatricians/story.html.

Grading and severity of ANH

The extent of APD dilatation is the key prognosticator for postnatal urologic diagnoses (see **Fig. 1**). Although there is no universally accepted grading system, 91% of maternal-fetal medicine (MFM) specialists and 45% of pediatric urologists use APD for grading.[9] One such classification system and the frequency of urologic pathologies are shown in **Table 2**. As expected, higher grades of APD were associated with higher rates of postnatal urologic pathologies with the notable exception of VUR.[7] Although most studies on APD use diagnosis as the outcome measure, Kim and colleagues[16] showed that the severity of APD also accurately predicted the loss of renal function of the involved kidney. In a study of 229 infants, the probability of a split differential function of less than 35% in infants with median APD of 11 mm at 20 to 24 weeks gestational age and 22 mm at 28 to 32 weeks was 28% and 30%, respectively.[6]

Although originally described for grading postnatal hydronephrosis, an adaptation of the Society for Fetal Urology (SFU) grading system is the second most commonly used grading system among pediatric urologists.[9,14,17] As with APD classification systems, higher SFU grades of hydronephrosis were associated with higher rates of postnatal persistence, as shown in **Fig. 5**.[6,18]

Table 1
Diagnosis-specific findings on prenatal ultrasound and recommended postnatal confirmatory tests

Diagnosis	US Findings	VCUG	DRS
UPJ obstruction	Hydronephrosis	Yes	Yes
VUR	Dilated (FSBL > GA + 2)[14] Increased APD after voiding[15]	Yes	Optional if concern for UPJ obstruction
PUV	Dilated (FSBL > GA + 2) Megacystis (FSBL > GA + 12)[14] Thick-walled bladder Dilated posterior urethra ("keyhole" sign) Bilateral hydronephrosis	Yes	No
Prune belly syndrome	Megacystis (FSBL > GA + 12)[14] Bilateral hydroureteronephrosis Distended bladder Irregular abdominal circumference	Yes	Optional to rule out obstruction and/or assess renal dysplasia (DMSA)
Megaureter	Ureteral dilatation/hydroureter	Yes	Yes
Megacystis/megaureter VUR syndrome	Ureteral dilatation/hydroureter Megacystis (FSBL > GA + 12)[14]	Yes	Optional if concern for obstruction
Duplicated collecting system	Segmental hydronephrosis	Yes	Yes
Ureterocele	Thin-walled cystic structure in the bladder	Yes	Yes
Ectopic ureter	Hydroureter without ureterocele in a duplex system	Yes	Yes
MCDK	Multiple cysts of varying sizes Absent normal parenchyma Contralateral compensatory hypertrophy	Optional	Optional

Abbreviations: ARPCKD, autosomal-recessive polycystic kidney disease; DMSA, dimercaptosuccinic acid; FSBL, fetal sagittal bladder length.

Table 2
Classification system for ANH and risk of postnatal uropathy

	APD		Risk of Uropathology[a]
Grade	2nd Trimester	3rd Trimester	Percent (95% CI)
Mild	4 to <7 mm	7 to <9 mm	11.9 (4.5–28.0)
Moderate	7 to 10 mm	9 to 15 mm	45.1 (25.3–66.6)
Severe	>10 mm	>15 mm	88.3 (53.7–98.0)

Abbreviation: CI, confidence interval.

[a] *Data from* Lee RS, Cendron M, Kinnamon DD, et al. Antenatal hydronephrosis as a predictor of postnatal outcome: a meta-analysis. Pediatrics 2006;118:586–96.

Adapted from Nguyen HT, Herndon CD, Cooper C, et al. The Society for Fetal Urology Consensus Statement on the evaluation and management of antenatal hydronephrosis. J Pediatr Urol 2010;6:215; with permission.

Although the absolute measure of APD can be used to prognosticate postnatal outcomes, the relationship of the APD to gestational age should also be considered. Hothi and colleagues[4] showed that the risk of postnatal renal dilation increased with each 1-mm increase in APD, but decreased 16% to 18% per week of pregnancy for any given fetal APD. Thus, an APD of 5 mm at 20 weeks would be associated with a higher risk of postnatal pathologic abnormality than a fetus with the same APD diagnosed at 34 weeks. This finding is reflective of the normal growth of the renal pelvis during development and is useful in providing prenatal counseling (**Fig. 2**).[19]

Renal parenychmal assessment
Another important sonographic predictor of postnatal urologic pathologic abnormality is the prenatal appearance of the renal parenchyma. The lack of a reniform shape, presence of renal cysts, and increased echogenicity of the renal parenchyma are all findings suggestive of significant renal pathologic abnormality and impaired renal function.[20–22] The "eggshell sign," a thin hyperechogenic crescent over a dilated calyx, may indicate elevated intrarenal pressures and is more commonly associated with obstructive uropathies.[23] Differentiation of severe hydronephrosis from cystic renal diseases, such as multicystic dysplastic kidneys (MCDK), can be challenging. MCDK lack a reniform shape and have a disorganized cystic architecture. Hydronephrosis, on the other hand, retains its reniform shape and demonstrates organization around a central anechoic structure with communication between the dilated renal pelvis and calyces.

Amniotic fluid level
One of the most important determinants of fetal renal health and survival is the amniotic fluid volume. Amniotic fluid is principally maintained by fetal urine production beginning the 16th week of development, and it reaches a constant volume by around the 28th week.[17] It is best measured by determining the amniotic fluid index (AFI). This AFI is determined by ultrasonic measurement of the deepest pocket of fluid in 4 quadrants. Normative AFI ranges between 5 and 20 cm.[24,25] Oligohydramnios, defined by an AFI of less than 5, is particularly concerning for bladder outlet obstruction.[26]

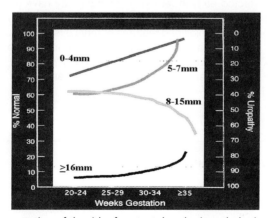

Fig. 2. Visual representation of the risk of postnatal urologic pathologic abnormality based on APD relative to gestational age. Note that for each measurement, the risk varies and decreases with increased gestational age. (*From* Wickstrom E, Maizels M, Sabbagha RE, et al. Isolated fetal pyelectasis: assessment of risk for postnatal uropathy and Down syndrome. Ultrasound Obstet Gynecol 1996;8:238; with permission.)

Because of its importance in fetal lung development, especially during the second trimester, oligohydramnios is an important predictor of adverse postnatal outcomes, such as neonatal death and chronic renal failure in patients with obstructive uropathies on multivariant analysis.[27,28]

Additional features

In addition to the presence of SERP, the presence of other additional features helps predict the presence of postnatal uropathy. These additional features include calyceal involvement, dilated ureters, elongated renal length, enlarged fetal bladder, progression of SERP, and ureteral duplication.[12,14,29–32] The presence of these abnormal findings has been associated with a 12.9 times increased risk of requiring extensive postnatal urologic care when present on a second-trimester ultrasound as opposed to fetuses with normal additional features.[8] Definitions of these specific features are shown in **Box 1**.

Visualization of in utero bladder cycling and its relationship to renal pelvic dilatation are further important prognosticators of postnatal urologic pathologies. The normal fetal bladder cycles every 30 to 45 minutes in utero.[32,33] Failure of the bladder to empty after 45 minutes or the presence of a distended bladder has been associated with posterior urethral valves (PUV) and prune belly syndrome.[32] Similarly, Herndon and colleagues[15] reported an increased incidence in postnatal VUR in fetuses with increased renal pelvic diameter at bladder emptying.

Prenatal Management

Prenatal management options for fetuses with hydronephrosis include elective termination, early delivery, expectant management, and fetal intervention. Considerations in determining optimal management include gestational age at diagnosis, the severity and laterality of the condition, suspected diagnosis, presence of unfavorable features of renal development, amniotic fluid volume, associated chromosomal or other structural anomalies, and fetal lung development. **Fig. 3** shows an algorithm for the prenatal management of hydronephrosis.

Elective termination

Hydronephrosis detected early in fetal development may have a significant impact on fetal lung and kidney development. First-trimester fetuses with bilateral disease associated with oligohydramnios and features of renal dysplasia, such as renal cysts and hyperechoic parenchyma, have poor prognoses, and elective termination may be considered. Chromosomal abnormalities and other systemic abnormalities of the fetus may also portend a poor prognosis and may warrant similar considerations.

Box 1
Additional features on second-trimester ultrasound

Progression	>4 mm per month
Fetal sagittal bladder length (FSBL)	
Dilated	>GA + 2 mm
Megacystis	>GA + 12 mm
Elongated renal length	>GA + 5 mm
Hydronephrosis	>4 mm APD + calyceal dilation

Abbreviations: APD, Anterior-posterior diameter; GA, gestational age.

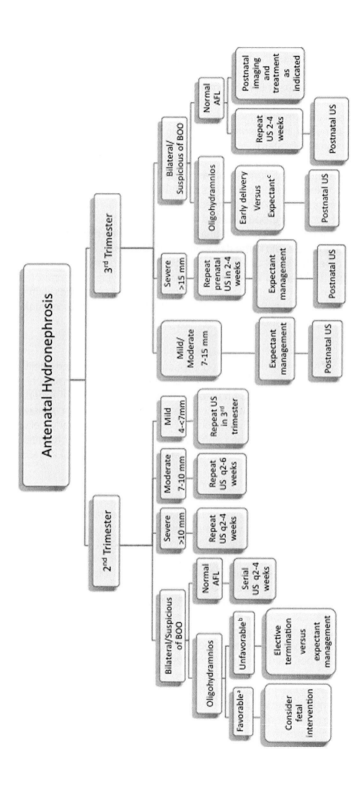

Fig. 3. Prenatal management of ANH. AFL, amniotic fluid level; BOO, bladder outlet obstruction; US, ultrasound.

[a] favorable urine parameters AND no chromosomal/structural abnormalities
[b] unfavorable urine parameters OR chromosomal/structural abnormalities
[c] Dependent on expectant fetal lung maturity.

Expectant management

As up to 88% of prenatal hydronephrosis will resolve during the duration of the pregnancy, there has been an increasing trend toward expectant management.[34] With the rare exception, all fetuses with unilateral ANH and most with bilateral ANH may be managed expectantly. However, it is recommended that repeat prenatal imaging be performed. The optimal timing of the repeat ultrasound depends on the gestational age of initial diagnosis and the severity of the condition. In most cases of unilateral SERP in the second-trimester, it is reasonable to obtain a repeat ultrasound in the third trimester. Severe unilateral, bilateral, solitary kidneys and cases in which bladder outlet obstruction is suspected require more frequent ultrasounds, with most MFMs specialists recommending repeat prenatal ultrasounds in 4 to 6 weeks with a smaller group recommending follow-up in 2 to 4 weeks.[9,17] Late third-trimester diagnoses or persistence of hydronephrosis in the third trimester merit postnatal follow-up because of the increased risk of postnatal uropathies and the need for surgical intervention.[17,35]

In determining which fetuses are safe to manage expectantly, the presence of oligohydramnios plays an important role in the decision-making process. Herndon and colleagues[36] surveyed members of the SFU in their management decisions in 7 hypothetical scenarios. In all cases with normal amniotic fluid levels, expectant management was the treatment of choice for most respondents. Only scenarios with low amniotic fluid levels garnered consideration of intervention with either vesicoamniotic shunt or early delivery dependent on fetal lung maturation.

Early delivery

Although most cases of ANH may be managed expectantly to full term, early delivery may be considered in fetuses with oligohydramnios with documented lung maturation. Typically this can be expected by the 34th week of pregnancy. Non-North American pediatric urologists favor this approach more readily than their North American colleagues.[36] However, to date, there has been no clear evidence that early delivery offers long-term benefits.[37] In fact, on the contrary, emerging data appear to indicate that early term neonates (gestational age <39 weeks) have a small but real increased risk of neonatal morbidity.[37,38]

Fetal intervention

Prenatal intervention for ANH continues to be rarely used and remains controversial. Indication for fetal intervention has largely been isolated to mid-second-trimester fetuses with suspected bladder outlet obstruction in the setting of oligohydramnios and preserved renal function. Assessment of renal function can be made based on an analysis of urine electrolytes obtained from sequential fetal bladder taps within 48 hours of an initial bladder tap.[39] This sequence is thought to be a more accurate reflection on current tubular function because it reflects the urine most recently produced by the kidney rather than urine that has been retained in the obstructed bladder.[39] Favorable urine parameters include urinary sodium less than 100 mg/dl, calcium less than 8 mg/dl, osmolarity less than 200 mOsm/L, β-2 microglobulin less than 4 mg/L, and total protein less than 40 mg/dl.[40] It is thought that on sequential bladder taps, a decrease in urine values would be reflective of good tubular function, whereas an increase in parameters would indicate renal dysplasia and thus be a poor candidate for intervention.[39] The most commonly performed fetal intervention is the vesicoamniotic shunt. The ability to correct oligohydramnios secondary to a urinary obstructive process by diverting urine into the amniotic space should offer benefits in fetal renal and lung development and ultimately improve fetal health. However, to date, there have been insufficient data to demonstrate the benefits of fetal intervention. Although some studies have shown modest benefits in pulmonary outcomes,[41,42] long-term improvement in renal function has yet to be established.[43,44] Complications such as shunt migration, urinary ascites, bladder fistula, and bowel herniation have been reported as high as 48% and fetal mortalities have been reported up to 43%.[44,45] Most recently, a multicenter, prospective Percutaneous shunting for Lower Urinary Tract Obstruction (PLUTO) randomized trial was completed in Europe. Results from this trial showed that, although survival was higher in fetuses undergoing fetal intervention with vesicoamniotic shunting, the benefit of intervention remains inconclusive, as only 2 of 31 fetuses (both shunted) survived with normal renal function at 2 years. Thus, survival of these fetuses with normal renal function is very low regardless of whether fetal intervention was performed or not.[46] Due to the high complication rate and as-yet unproven medical benefit, fetal intervention should only be considered in a select patient population and after extensive counseling of the parents.

POSTNATAL EVALUATION AND MANAGEMENT

The postnatal management of ANH has been a topic of significant debate. Inherent to the difficulty in establishing a unified approach is the continuous evolution of management strategies for the urologic sequelae of ANH, ureteropelvic junction (UPJ) obstruction, and VUR. Furthermore, as upwards of 88% of mild cases of AHN will not result in uropathies, the challenge exists to provide appropriate and indicated postnatal evaluation while weighing the invasiveness, radiation, and cost of testing against the benefits of urinary tract infection (UTI) prevention and resultant renal preservation.[34] There are several imaging modalities commonly used in the postnatal evaluation of ANH. These imaging modalities include renal and bladder ultrasound (RBUS), voiding cystourethrography (VCUG), and diuretic renal scintigraphy (DRS). Determination of which ANH patients would benefit from surgical intervention and which may be best served with continued surveillance remains the ultimate goal of any imaging strategy. Our current imaging algorithm is shown in **Fig. 4**.

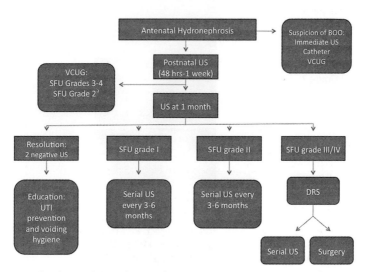

Fig. 4. Postnatal radiographic evaluation for ANH. [a] Patients at high risk of risk (eg, females, uncircumcised males), or have ureteral dilatation. BOO, bladder outlet obstruction; US, ultrasound.

Evaluation

Renal and bladder ultrasound

The postnatal evaluation of the neonate with a history of ANH begins with the RBUS. Careful evaluation of the renal parenchyma, the degree of postnatal hydronephrosis, presence of ureteral dilation, and assessment of the urinary bladder should be undertaken. Although the predictive value of RBUS for obstruction and VUR is poor, findings on serial imaging may help in the decision-making process of long-term management of these conditions. Diagnoses such as MCDK and duplicated collecting systems associated with ectopic ureters and ureteroceles may also be more readily identified postnatally based on their characteristic RBUS findings.

Grading of hydronephrosis on RBUS Various grading systems have been used for the assessment of hydronephrosis postnatally. In an effort to standardize the interpretation of this study, the SFU introduced the SFU grading system for postnatal assessment of hydronephrosis, shown in **Fig. 5**. Grading of ureteral dilation as measured by the retrovesical ureter may also be accomplished with the SFU grading system. Ureteral dilation is graded as follows: grade 1, less than 7 mm; grade 2, between 7 and 10 mm; and Grade 3, greater than 10 mm.[47] Although this grading system has enjoyed popularity among pediatric urologists, subjective personalized grading systems continue to be used by up to 35.8% of pediatric radiologists.[9] However, to better facilitate interspecialty communication and consistency in reporting for outcome analysis, the authors strongly advocate for the universal adoption of the SFU grading system for the ultrasonic assessment of postnatal hydronephrosis.

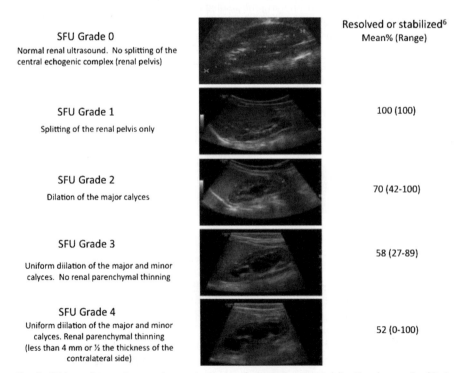

		Resolved or stabilized[6] Mean% (Range)
SFU Grade 0 Normal renal ultrasound. No splitting of the central echogenic complex (renal pelvis)		
SFU Grade 1 Splitting of the renal pelvis only		100 (100)
SFU Grade 2 Dilation of the major calyces		70 (42-100)
SFU Grade 3 Uniform diilation of the major and minor calyces. No renal parenchymal thinning		58 (27-89)
SFU Grade 4 Uniform diilation of the major and minor calyces. Renal parenchymal thinning (less than 4 mm or ½ the thickness of the contralateral side)		52 (0-100)

Fig. 5. SFU grading system and expected rate of resolution or stablization by grade. (*Data from* Sidhu G, Beyene J, Rosenblum ND. Outcome of isolated antenatal hydronephrosis: a systemic review and meta-analysis. Pediatr Nephrol 2006;21:218–24; with permission.)

Which patients need evaluation? The management of ANH that resolves on serial prenatal ultrasound is also of clinical importance. Current SFU guidelines suggest that ANH diagnosed in the second trimester that resolves on repeat ultrasound in the third trimester does not require postnatal evaluation, while any diagnosis of ANH in the third trimester requires postnatal evaluation, even if resolution occurs on serial prenatal ultrasound.[17] Likewise, postnatal imaging for ANH that resolves on the first postnatal ultrasound is also recommended. Approximately 25% of fetuses with prenatal hydronephrosis demonstrate resolution on the first postnatal ultrasound.[48] The likelihood of significant urologic pathologic abnormality has been reported to be low in these patients.[49] However, Aksu and colleagues[50] reported that 45% of neonates with a normal RBUS on first RBUS performed after 48 hours of life demonstrated a significant uropathy on subsequent evaluations. Because of this risk, it is commonly recommended that a follow-up ultrasound at 1 month of age is necessary to confirm resolution. Following this protocol, the negative predictive value of normal RBUS reaches 97% to 99%, with all failures presenting with UTIs.[49,51,52] **Table 2** summarizes the current recommendations from the SFU for subsequent imaging and evaluation based on initial postnatal ultrasound results.[17]

Optimal timing of RBUS Although Docimo and Silver[53] previously reported the safety of obtaining an initial postnatal ultrasound within the first 48 hours of life, most reports recommend deferring the initial RBUS until after the first 48 hours but within the first week of life.[17,49–52,54,55] This delay is recommended to overcome the potentially confounding effects of transient physiologic oliguria in the newborn that could conceivably mask the presence of or underestimate the degree of residual hydronephrosis. Exceptions to this practice include antenatal findings concerning for obstructive renal failure, such as the presence of ANH in a solitary kidney, bilateral ANH, or other findings suggestive of a bladder outlet or urethral obstruction. These clinical scenarios warrant immediate postnatal ultrasonography.

VCUG

The VCUG is another useful imaging modality for the postnatal evaluation of ANH. A VCUG is absolutely necessary as an urgent postnatal study for neonates suspicious of a bladder outlet obstruction, most commonly PUV. In addition, VCUG may be helpful in the evaluation for VUR, megaureters, ureteroceles, MCDK, and renal duplication anomalies. Although the recommended use of VCUG for severe hydronephrosis (SFU grades 3 to 4) is well established, the need for VCUG with its inherent invasiveness, radiation exposure, and risk of procedural UTI in the workup of patients with mild to moderate hydronephrosis (SFU 2 or less) remains controversial.

VUR is the second most common urologic diagnosis in patients with residual ANH, reported to be present in 7% to 35% of patients with residual ANH and up to 25% of neonates with resolved hydronephrosis.[15,56] As it is commonly recognized that APD is a poor predictor of the overall incidence of VUR,[7,56–59] many continue to advocate for the inclusion of VCUG as a necessary imaging study for all patients with hydronephrosis found on postnatal ultrasounds.[54,58–61] However, it remains unproven whether there is a clear benefit to its diagnosis and treatment. It is now clear that VUR in the setting of ANH differs from VUR diagnosed after a febrile UTI. Neonatal VUR tends to be more prevalent in male neonates, be of higher grade, have higher rates of renal parenchymal injury, yet also higher rates of spontaneous resolution as compared with VUR found following a febrile UTI.[15,56,62] In light of these attributes, some have questioned the clinical significance of neonatal VUR and, as such, have incorporated a more selective approach to the use of VCUG. APD of less than 7 mm,[49,55] SFU grade of 2 or less,[54,63] APD less than 10 mm + lack of calyceal involvement,[51,57] APD less than 10 mm on both fetal and postnatal RBUS,[59] and 2 successive normal postnatal ultrasounds[49,51] have all been used as potential criteria for the safe omission of VCUG in postnatal management.

However, the presence of VUR in the setting of ANH does appear to have clinical significance with an increase risk of UTI. In an analysis by Coelho and colleagues,[64] 44% of patients with VUR had a febrile UTI within the first 2 years with female gender as an independent risk factor on multivariant analysis. Patients with UPJ obstruction and megaureter were also at higher risk of UTI with a reported rate of 24%. Likewise, Estrada and colleagues[65] reported febrile UTIs in 4.4% of patients with SFU grade 2 hydronephrosis who had VCUGs deferred, representing a 9-fold increase from patients screened with VCUG and treated with prophylactic antibiotics.[65] The main goal of the evaluation and treatment of VUR remains the prevention of UTIs and the risk of renal parenchymal damage. Therefore, VCUG should continue to be considered for patients with ANH at higher risk of UTI, such as girls, uncircumcised boys, and neonates suspected of obstruction.

Although most algorithms continue to recommend routine VCUG for cases of suspected UPJ obstruction, Kim and colleagues recently reported that, although the incidence of VUR with UPJ obstruction was 11%, VUR was either low grade, which resolved spontaneously, or high grade, in which ureteral dilatation was readily identified on RBUS. Therefore, they recommended obtaining VCUGs in children suspected of UPJ obstruction only in those with dilated distal ureters on RBUS.[66]

Diuretic renal scintigraphy

DRS is the most commonly used modality to evaluate patients with ANH for obstruction. When indicated, DRS is typically deferred until at least 6 weeks of life to allow maturation of the kidneys and provide more accurate studies. Technetium-99m-mercaptoacetyltriglycine (Tc-MAG3) is currently the agent of choice. It is bound primarily to plasma proteins and cleared by tubular secretion. The 2 most important pieces of information that the DRS provides a urologist for the determination of significant obstruction are the spilt differential function (%df), measured by relative uptake in the radionucleotide, and the drainage curve calculated by the percent washout of tracer over time. As the interpretation of DRS is highly susceptible to technical variations, the authors strongly advocate for the use of a standardized technique that will provide consistency in interpretation. An established protocol for a "well-tempered" renogram has been established and should be adopted.[67]

Which patients with ANH need DRS? DRS should be considered in patients at increased risk for obstruction. The SFU currently recommends DRS for the following patients: moderate unilateral ANH with persistent postnatal hydronephrosis with no VUR, severe ANH regardless of postnatal ultrasound result with no VUR, moderate or severe postnatal hydronephrosis, any hydronephrosis with bladder or urethral abnormalities, any hydronephrosis with a dilated ureter, and any hydronephrosis associated with decreased amniotic fluid, without VUR.[17]

Magnetic resonance urogram

The final imaging modality used in ANH evaluation is the magnetic resonance urogram (MRU). Its pharmaceuticals are gadolinium-diethylenetriamine pentaacetic acid and furosemide. MRU provides both T1-weighted and T2-weighted images and is used to measure both GFR and renal transit time. It provides better anatomic detail than both RBUS and DRS modalities and has been suggested to be a better predictor of UPJ obstruction.[68,69] A pelvic index ratio, defined as the measurement of the distance from the lowest calyx to the UPJ (D) divided by the total length of the calyceal system (L) on MRU, of greater than 0.3 was demonstrated by Kaneyama and colleagues[70] as a predictor of a need for surgery, whereas a ratio of less than 0.1 correlates with success with observation. However, because MRU is the newest modality, it is expensive and not readily available at many centers. In addition, MRU typically requires sedation in children to obtain optimal results.[60] For these reasons MRU is not widely used, and MAG3 remains the most common imaging modality to evaluate renal function and degree of obstruction.

Evaluation of Obstruction

UPJ obstruction represents the most common uropathologic diagnosis for ANH. Other potential obstructive processes include megaureters and ureteroceles. Although there is a clear correlation of the severity of ANH with an increased risk of obstruction, the natural history of ANH with persistent postnatal hydronephrosis remains variable, and the utility of early surgical correction is debatable. To date, there is no clear imaging study that is diagnostic of obstruction. Information obtained from RBUS, DRS, and MRU may be suggestive of obstruction but has not been proven to be definitive. The difficulty in diagnosing obstruction is in large part due to recent changes in management of UPJ obstruction and the lack of agreement on who requires surgery.

Traditionally, management of UPJ obstruction was surgical. However, beginning in the 1990s, natural history studies due to a shift toward observational management have demonstrated the potential of UPJ obstruction to spontaneously resolve over time.[71,72] In a prospective randomized trial of surgery versus observation for patients with unilateral hydronephrosis (APD >15 mm) and a %df of greater than 40%, Dhillon[71] reported that 33% of infants remained stable on follow-up and 47% resolved or improved to mild dilatation. Similarly, a study by Ulman and colleagues[72] followed 104 infants with SFU grades 3 or 4 hydronephrosis conservatively and found that only 22% eventually required pyeloplasty, whereas 69% of patients resolved to an SFU grade 1 or 0.

Although DRS remains the most used modality to evaluate obstruction, the diagnostic accuracy of DRS for obstruction has been reported to be highly variable. Takla and colleagues[73] reported that the drainage curve on the initial DRS was predictive of resolution with 86% of patients with nonobstructive, 62% with indeterminate, and only 18% with obstructive curves ultimately resolving. On the other hand, Hafaz and colleagues[74] found that neither the drainage curve nor %df on initial DRS was ineffective in predicting resolution, reporting sensitivities of 63% and 56% and specificities of 59% and 66%, respectively. Because of these inaccuracies, the SFU guidelines recommend DRS more to establish baseline renal function to accompany ultrasonic follow-up in appropriate patients and less as a stand-alone predictor of obstruction.[17]

Although the extent of hydronephrosis seen on initial postnatal RBUS has also been found to be a poor predictor for the need for surgical correction,[73,74] other findings may still be useful in determining the need for pyeloplasty. Progression of hydronephrosis on 2 consecutive RBUS has been shown to be an early predictor of obstruction,[74] while an SFU grade of 3 correlated with preserved renal function (>40 %df) and thus less likely to require surgery.[75]

Which Patients Require Surgery for Obstruction

Given the variable natural history of obstruction and hydronephrosis, inconsistencies regarding indications for surgery currently persist. Most observational protocols recommend surgery if patients show a DRS revealing an obstructive washout curve and %df less than 40%, decreased %df of greater than 10% on serial DRS, and progression of hydronephrosis on serial RBUS. In cases of bilateral hydronephrosis with obstruction, the kidney with lesser differential function is typically repaired first in an attempt to preserve the remaining parenchyma. For patients followed with DRS who do not show progression on serial studies, the timing and frequency of follow-up imaging are individualized and are based on clinical experience and judgment.

Continuous Antibiotic Prophylaxis

The final area of controversy in the postnatal management of ANH involves the application of continuous antibiotic prophylaxis (CAP). Conclusive data for or against CAP are still lacking due to inconsistencies found in the literature regarding the effectiveness of prophylactic antibiotics. Proponents for CAP point to the increased risk of infection in patients with ANH. Walsh and colleagues[76] recently reported a 12 times increased risk for hospitalization for pyelonephritis in infants with ANH in their first year of life. Likewise, Song and colleagues[77] reported a UTI incidence of 36.2% in patients with severe hydronephrosis. Coelho and colleagues[64] also reported a 14% rate of UTI in all patients followed for ANH but questioned the effectiveness of prophylaxis as 74% of the patients with UTI in their study presented while on prophylaxis. Recently, Braga and colleagues[78] performed a meta-analysis examining the effectiveness of prophylactic antibiotics in preventing UTIs in children with ANH. They reported that children with high-grade ANH not receiving CAP have a significantly higher UTI risk than those receiving CAP (28.9% vs 14.6%). UTI rates in patients with low-grade ANH were similar whether or not CAP was used. Female gender and distal ureteral obstruction are also associated with a higher rate of UTI.[64,76,77] Although CAP remains controversial, it should be strongly considered in patients with ANH and at higher risk of UTI, such as patients with postnatal SFU grade 2 or higher, female patients, uncircumcised males in the first year of life, and patients with low ureteral dilation such as megaureter and ureterovesical junction obstruction.

SUMMARY

The diagnosis of ANH continues to increase as the standard of care includes performance of second-trimester prenatal ultrasound. Prenatal management of ANH continues to be expectant with fetal intervention rarely indicated. Postnatal management is often multimodal and clearly requires a systematic approach to select indicated imaging modalities, choose the most appropriate medical or surgical treatment options, and determine which patients are most appropriate for surveillance protocols. Although much has been learned about this topic recently, the lack of evidence-based guidelines continues to hamper the creation of standards of care. Adoption and utilization of common grading systems and definitions in prospective studies will greatly advance the knowledge of this complex condition and are sorely needed.

REFERENCES

1. Ismaili K, Hall M, Donner C, et al. Results of systematic screening for minor degrees of renal pelvis dilatation in an unselected population. Am J Obstet Gynecol 2003;188:242–6.
2. Coplen DE, Austin PF, Yan Y, et al. The magnitude of fetal renal pelvic dilatation can identify obstructive postnatal hydronephrosis, and direct postnatal evaluation and management. J Urol 2006;176:724–7.

3. Morin L, Cendron M, Crombleholme TM, et al. Minimal hydronephrosis in the fetus: clinical significance and implications for management. J Urol 1996;155:2047–9.
4. Hothi DK, Wade AS, Gilbert R, et al. Mild fetal renal pelvis dilatation-much ado about nothing? Clin J Am Soc Nephrol 2009;4:168–77.
5. Ahmad G, Green P. Outcome of fetal pyelectasis diagnosed antenatally. J Obstet Gynaecol 2005;25:119–22.
6. Sidhu G, Beyene J, Rosenblum ND. Outcome of isolated antenatal hydronephrosis: a systemic review and meta-analysis. Pediatr Nephrol 2006;21:218–24.
7. Lee RS, Cendron M, Kinnamon DD, et al. Antenatal hydronephrosis as a predictor of postnatal outcome: a meta-analysis. Pediatrics 2006;118:586–96.
8. Maizels MM, Wang E, Sabbagha RE, et al. Late second trimester assessment of pyelectasis (SERP) to predict pediatric urological outcome is improved by checking additional features. J Matern Fetal Neonatal Med 2006;19(5):295–303.
9. Zanetta VC, Rosman BM, Bromley B, et al. Variation in management of mild prenatal hydronephrosis among maternal-fetal medicine obstetricians, and pediatric urologists, and radiologists. J Urol 2012;188:1935–9.
10. Corteville JE, Gray DL, Crane JP. Congenital hydronephrosis: correlation of fetal ultrasonographic findings with infant outcome. Am J Obstet Gynecol 1991;165:384–8.
11. Chaviano AH, Maizels M, Yerkes EB, et al. Incidence based fetal urological counseling using the Virtual Pediatric Urology Registry: importance of insignificant fetal pyelectasis (SERP). J Urol 2007;178:1781–5.
12. Bassanese G, Travan L, D'Ottavio G, et al. Prenatal anteroposterior pelvic diameter cutoffs for postnatal referral for isolated pyelectasis and hydronephrosis: more is not always better. J Urol 2013;190:1858–63.
13. Siemens DR, Prouse KA, MacNeily AE, et al. Thresholds of renal pelvic diameter to predict insignificant postnatal pelviectasis. Tech Urol 1998;4:198–201.
14. Maizels M, Alpert SA, Houston JB, et al. Fetal bladder sagittal length: a simple monitor to assess normal and enlarged fetal bladder size, and forecast clinical outcome. J Urol 2004;172:1995–9.
15. Herndon CD, McKenna PH, Kolon TF, et al. A multicenter outcomes analysis of patients with neonatal reflux presenting with prenatal hydronephrosis. J Urol 1999;162:1203–8.
16. Kim DY, Mickelson JJ, Helfand BT, et al. Fetal pyectasis as predictor of decreased differential renal function. J Urol 2009;182:1849–53.
17. Nguyen HT, Herndon CD, Cooper C, et al. The Society for Fetal Urology consensus statement on the evaluation and management of antenatal hydronephrosis. J Pediatr Urol 2010;6:212–31.
18. Fernbach SK, Maizels M, Conway JJ. Ultrasound grading of hydronephrosis: introduction to the system used by the Society for Fetal Urology. Pediatr Radiol 1993;23:478–80.
19. Wickstrom E, Maizels M, Sabbagha RE, et al. Isolated fetal pyelectasis: assessment of risk for postnatal uropathy and Down syndrome. Ultrasound Obstet Gynecol 1996;8:236–40.
20. Estroff JA, Mandell J, Benacerraf BR. Increased renal parenchymal echogenicity in the fetus: importance and clinical outcome. Radiology 1991;181:135–9.
21. Mahony BS, Filly RA, Callen PW. Fetal renal dysplasia: sonographic evaluation. Radiology 1984;152:143–6.
22. Chi T, Feldstein VA, Nguyen HT. Increased echogenicity as a predictor of poor renal function in children with grade 3 to 4 hydronephrosis. J Urol 2006;175(5):1898–901.

23. Dewan PA, Moon D, Anderson K. Presence of the eggshell sign in obstructive uropathy. Urology 2002;59:287–9.
24. Rutherford SE, Phelan JP, Smith CV, et al. The four-quadrant assessment of amniotic fluid volume: an adjunct to antepartum fetal heart rate testing. Obstet Gynecol 1987;70:353–7.
25. Taskin S, Pabuccu EG, Kanmaz AG, et al. Perinatal outcomes of idiopathic poly-hydramnios. Interv Med Appl Sci 2013;5:21–5.
26. Zaccara A, Giorlandino C, Mobili L, et al. Amniotic fluid index and fetal bladder outlet obstruction. Do we really need more? J Urol 2005;174:1657–60.
27. Oliveira EA, Diniz JS, Cabral AC, et al. Prognostic factors in fetal hydronephro-sis: a multivariant analysis. Pediatr Nephrol 1999;13:859–64.
28. Oliveira EA, Rabelo EA, Pereira AK, et al. Prognostic factors in prenatally-detected posterior urethral valves: a multivariant analysis. Pediatr Surg Int 2002;18:662–7.
29. Broadley P, McHugo J, Morgan I, et al. The 4 year outcome following the demon-stration of bilateral renal pelvic dilatation on pre-natal renal ultrasound. Br J Ra-diol 1999;72:265–70.
30. Liu HY, Dhillon HK, Yeung CK, et al. Clinical outcome and management of pre-natally diagnosed primary megaureters. J Urol 1994;152:614–7.
31. Aviram R, Pomeranz A, Sharony R, et al. The increase of renal pelvis dilatation in the fetus and its significance. Ultrasound Obstet Gynecol 2000;16:60–2.
32. Montemarano H, Bulas DI, Rushton HG, et al. Bladder distention and pyectasis in the male fetus: causes, comparisons, and contrasts. J Ultrasound Med 1998; 17:743–9.
33. Coplen DE. Prenatal management of hydronephrosis. American Urological As-sociation Update Series 2000. Lesson 19.
34. Sairam S, Al-Habib A, Sasson S, et al. Natural history of fetal hydronephrosis diagnosed on mid-trimester ultrasound. Ultrasound Obstet Gynecol 2001;17: 191–6.
35. Wollenberg A, Neuhaus TJ, Willi UV, et al. Outcome of fetal renal pelvic dilatation diagnosed during the third trimester. Ultrasound Obstet Gynecol 2005;25: 483–8.
36. Herndon CD, Ferrer FA, Freedman A, et al. Consensus on the prenatal man-agement of antenatally detected urological abnormalities. J Urol 2000;164: 1052–6.
37. Engle WA. Morbidity and mortality in late preterm and early term newborns: a continuum. Clin Perinatol 2011;38:493–516.
38. Parikh LI, Reddy UM, Mannisto T, et al. Neonatal outcomes in early term birth. Am J Obstet Gynecol 2014. http://dx.doi.org/10.1016/j.ajog.2014.03.021.
39. Johnson MP, Corsi P, Bradfield W, et al. Sequential fetal urine aspiration in the evaluation of patients with obstructive uropathy. Am J Obstet Gynecol 1995; 173:59–65.
40. Johnson MP, Bukowski TP, Reitelman C, et al. In utero surgical treatment of fetal obstructive uropathy: a new comprehensive approach to identify appropriate candidates for vesicoamniotic shunt therapy. Am J Obstet Gynecol 1994;170: 1770.
41. Biard JM, Johnson MP, Carr MC, et al. Long-term outcomes in children treated by prenatal vesicoamniotic shunting for lower urinary tract obstruction. Obstet Gynecol 2005;106:503–8.
42. Freedman AL, Johnson MP, Smith CA, et al. Long-term outcome in children after antenatal intervention for obstructive uropathies. Lancet 1999;354:374–7.

43. McLorie G, Farhat W, Khoury A, et al. Outcome analysis of vesicoamniotic shunting in a comprehensive population. J Urol 2001;166:1036–40.
44. Holmes N, Harrison MR, Baskin LS. Fetal surgery for posterior urethral valves: long-term postnatal outcomes. Pediatrics 2001;108:e7. http://dx.doi.org/10.1542/peds.108.1.e7.
45. Freedman AL, Johnson MP, Gonzalez R. Fetal therapy for obstructive uropathy: past, present...future? Pediatr Nephrol 2000;14:167–76.
46. Morris RK, Malin GL, Quinlan-Jones E, et al. Percutaneous vesicoamniotic shunting versus conservative management for fetal lower urinary tract obstruction (PLUTO): a randomized trial. Lancet 2013;382:1496–506.
47. Maizels M, Reisman ME, Flom LS, et al. Grading nephroureteral dilatation detected in the first year of life: correlation with obstruction. J Urol 1992;148:609–14.
48. Barbosa JA, Chow JS, Benson CB, et al. Postnatal longitudinal evaluation of children diagnosed with prenatal hydronephrosis: insights in natural history and referral patterns. Prenat Diagn 2012;32:1242–9.
49. Ismaili K, Avni FE, Wissing KM, et al. Long-term clinical outcome of infants with mild and moderate fetal pyelectasis: validation of neonatal ultrasound as a screening tool to detect significant nephrouropathies. J Pediatr Urol 2004;144:759–65.
50. Aksu N, Yavascan O, Kangun M, et al. Postnatal management of infants with antenatally detected hydronephrosis. Pediatr Nephrol 2005;20:1253–9.
51. Moorthy I, Joshi N, Cook JV, et al. Antenatal hydronephrosis: negative predictive value of normal postnatal ultrasound-a 5-year study. Clin Radiol 2003;58:964–70.
52. Matui F, Shimada K, Matsumoto F, et al. Recurrence of symptomatic hydronephrosis in patients with prenatally detected hydronephrosis and spontanesou resolution. J Urol 2008;180:322–5.
53. Docimo SG, Silver RI. Ultrasonography in newborns with prenatally detected hydronephrosis: why wait? J Urol 1997;157:1387–9.
54. Riccabona M, Avni FE, Blickman JG, et al. Imaging recommendations in paediatric uroradiology: minutes of the ESPR workgroup session on urinary tract infection, fetal hydronephrosis, urinary tract ultrasonography and voiding cystourethrography, Barcelona, Spain, June 2007. Pediatr Radiol 2008;38:138–45.
55. Becker A. Postnatal evaluation of infants with an abnormal antenatal renal sonogram. Curr Opin Pediatr 2009;21:207–13.
56. Skoog SJ, Peters CA, Arant BS, et al. Pediatric Vesicoureteral reflux guidelines panel summery report: clinical practice guidelines for screening siblings of children with vesicoureteral reflux and neonate/infants with prenatal hydronephrosis. J Urol 2010;184:1145–51.
57. Coplen DE, Austin PF, Yan Y. Correlation of prenatal and postnatal ultrasound findings with the incidence of vesicoureteral reflux in children with fetal renal pelvic dilatation. J Urol 2008;180:1631–4.
58. Brophy MM, Austin PF, Yan Y, et al. Vesicoureteral reflux and clinical outcomes in infants with prenatally detected hydronephrosis. J Urol 2002;168:1716–9.
59. Diaz CS, Bouzada MC, Pereira AK, et al. Predictive factors for vesicoureteral reflux and prenatally diagnosed renal pelvic dilatation. J Urol 2009;182:2440–5.
60. Kitchens DM, Herndon CD. Antenatal hydronephrosis. Curr Urol Rep 2009;10:126–33.
61. Estrada CR. Prenatal hydronephrosis: early evaluation. Curr Opin Urol 2008;18:401–3.

62. Knudson MJ, Austin JC, McMillan ZM, et al. Predictive factors of early sponta-neous resolution in children with primary vesicoureteral reflux. J Urol 2007; 178:1684–8.

63. Yerkes EB, Adams MC, Pope JC, et al. Does every patient with prenatal hydro-nephrosis need voiding cystourethrography? J Urol 1999;162:1218–20.

64. Coelho GM, Bouzada MC, Lemos GS. Risk factors for urinary tract infection in children with prenatal renal pelvic dilatation. J Urol 2008;179:284–9.

65. Estrada CR, Peters CA, Retik AB, et al. Vesicoureteral reflux and urinary tract infection in children with a history of prenatal hydronephrosis-should voiding cystourethrography be performed in cases of postnatally persistent grade II hy-dronephrosis? J Urol 2009;181:801–7.

66. Kim YS, Do SH, Hong CH, et al. Does every patient with ureteropelvic junction obstruction need voiding cystourethrography? J Urol 2001;165:2305–7.

67. Conway JJ, Maizels M. The "well tempered" diuretic renogram: a standard method to examine the asymptomatic neonate with hydronephrosis or hydrour-eteronephrosis. A report from combined meetings of the Society for Fetal Uro-logy and members of the Pediatric Nuclear Medicine Council—The Society of Nuclear Medicine. J Nucl Med 1992;33:2047–51.

68. McMann LP, Kirsh AJ, Scherz HC, et al. Magnetic resonance urography in the evaluation of prenatally diagnosed hydronephrosis and renal dysgenesis. J Urol 2006;176:1786–92.

69. Perez-Braysfield MR, Kirsch AJ, Jones RA, et al. A prospective study comparing ultrasound, nuclear scintigraphy and dynamic contrast enhaced magnetic reso-nance imaging in the evaluation of hydronephrosis. J Urol 2003;170:1330–4.

70. Kaneyama K, Yamataka A, Someya T, et al. Magnetic resonance urographic -pa-rameters for predicting the need for pyeloplasty in infants with prenatally diag-nosed severe hydronephrosis. J Urol 2006;176:1781–5.

71. Dhillon HK. Prenatal diagnosed hydronephrosis: the Great Ormond Street expe-rience. Br J Urol 1998;81:39–44.

72. Ulman I, Jayanthi VR, Koff SA. The long-term followup of newborns with severe unilateral hydronephrosis initially treated nonoperatively. J Urol 2000;164: 1101–5.

73. Takla NV, Hamilton BD, Cartwright PC, et al. Apparent unilateral ureteropelvic junction obstruction in the newborn: expectations for resolution. J Urol 1998; 160:2175–8.

74. Hafaz AT, McLorie G, Bagli D, et al. Analysis of trends on serial ultrasounds for high grade neonatal hydronephrosis. J Urol 2002;168:1518–21.

75. Erickson BA, Maizels M, Shore RM, et al. Newborn Society of Fetal Urology grade 3 hydronephrosis is equivalent to preserved percentage differential func-tion. J Pediatr Urol 2007;3:382–6.

76. Walsh TJ, Hsieh S, Grady R, et al. Antenatal hydronephrosis and the risk of pyelonephritis hospitalization during the first year of life. Urology 2007;69:970–4.

77. Song SH, Lee SB, Park YS, et al. Is antibiotic prophylaxis necessary in infants with obstructive hydronephrosis? J Urol 2007;177:1098–101.

78. Braga LH, Mijovic H, Farrokhyar F, et al. Antibiotic prophylaxis for urinary tract infections in antenatal hydronephrosis. Pediatrics 2013;131:e251–61.

Upper Urinary Tract Anomalies and Perinatal Renal Tumors

 CrossMark

Ellen Shapiro, MD

KEYWORDS

- Renal agenesis • Ectopia and fusion anomalies • Renal hypoplasia and dysplasia
- Congenital mesoblastic nephroma • Wilms' tumor

KEY POINTS

- Unilateral renal agenesis occurs in 1100 births, is associated with Müllerian duct (MD) anomalies in 25% to 50% of females with unilateral renal agenesis, and requires life-long follow-up for hypertension and microalbuminuria.
- Renal ectopia, although usually asymptomatic, may have associated ureteropelvic or ureterovesical junction obstruction, reflux, or genital anomalies.
- Crossed renal ectopia occurs when a kidney is located on the side opposite from that in which its ureter inserts into the bladder. Ninety percent are fused, with the lower pole of the normal kidney fusing with the upper pole of the ectopic kidney, and they may have associated MD anomalies.
- Horseshoe kidneys occur in about 1 in 400 persons, are malrotated with calyces pointing posteriorly, have a variable blood supply, and are found in association with other congenital anomalies, including ureteropelvic junction obstruction and reflux.
- Congenital mesoblastic nephroma, the most common renal tumor in the first 3 months of life, can be diagnosed prenatally or may present as an abdominal mass, and is curable in most cases with only primary surgical excision.

RENAL EMBRYOLOGY

The mesonephric duct or Wolffian duct (WD) elongates caudally and fuses with the anterior cloaca. The metanephric blastema, which becomes the definitive kidney, differentiates from a region of intermediate mesoderm termed the metanephric mesenchyme. Signaling from the metanephric blastema leads to ureteral bud branching from the WD at the 28th day of gestation and reciprocal induction proceeds between the ureteral bud and metanephric blastema. Invasion of the metanephric blastema by

Disclosure: The authors have nothing to disclose.
Department of Urology, New York University School of Medicine, 150 32nd Street, 2nd Floor, New York, NY 10017, USA
E-mail address: ellen.shapiro@nyumc.org

Clin Perinatol 41 (2014) 679–694
http://dx.doi.org/10.1016/j.clp.2014.05.014
0095-5108/14/$ – see front matter © 2014 Elsevier Inc. All rights reserved.

the ureteral bud results in repetitive branching that forms the collecting duct system. In turn, the metanephros is complete with the induction of nephron differentiation in the surrounding mesenchyme.[1,2] When the nephric ridge fails to form, or there is failure of ureteral bud formation, a kidney will not develop, resulting in renal agenesis.

Specific anomalies of the Müllerian ducts (MD) are often seen in association with renal agenesis. This is explained by a 3-phase model of MD development: (1) Coelomic epithelium in the cervical region of the intermediate mesoderm, which are specified to become MD cells, (2) a WD-independent phase with these cells invaginating to become the MDs, which is complete when the MD extends caudally and contacts the WD, and (3) a WD-dependent phase involving elongation of the MDs posteriorly until they are joined at the urogenital sinus.[3–8] This final phase requires the MD epithelium at its posterior end to be in close physical contact with the WD epithelium, while the MDs are separated from the coelomic epithelium by only a basement membrane.[4] Because normal MD formation depends in part on a normal WD, abnormalities of the WDs result in an high incidence of anomalies of the MD structures including the fallopian tube, uterine horn and body, and proximal vagina.[9]

UNILATERAL RENAL AGENESIS
Incidence, Diagnosis, and Associated Anomalies

Unilateral renal agenesis (URA) occurs once in 1100 births in autopsy series.[10] URA may be an incidental finding on a sonogram performed after an abnormal physical examination of the external genitalia or female pelvis and/or after an abnormal radiographic evaluation of the female or male pelvis (**Fig. 1**). URA is detected with increasing frequency. Approximately 5% of URA may have been a dysplastic or multicystic dysplastic kidney (MCDK; incidence 1 in 4300) that involuted during gestation.[11–13] Renal aplasia is found in 1 in ~1300 births and is considered the most common cause of congenital solitary kidney. A renal unit with renal aplasia has rudimentary parenchyma and ureter (absent in 60%) owing to early regression of the ureteral bud, altered metanephric differentiation, or defects in the branching ureteral bud and/or the metanephric blastema, affecting reciprocal communication.[14]

URA is observed in X-linked and sporadic cases of Kallmann syndrome, Turner syndrome, Poland syndrome, Frazer syndrome, brachio-oto-renal syndrome, and maternal diabetes.[15–19] URA is seen in about 30% of neonates with VACTERL association (*V*ertebral, imperforate *A*nus, *C*ardiac, *T*racheo-*E*sophageal atresia, *R*enal, and *L*imb anomalies).[20] Associated anomalies of other organ systems involve primarily the cardiovascular, gastrointestinal, hematologic, neurologic, and musculoskeletal systems.[21] Because the ipsilateral gonad is derived from nearby mesenchyme and is usually present in its normal position, the metanephric blastema is not thought to be responsible for URA in most cases.[14] In addition, the adrenal gland is almost always found in its normal position owing to its dual origin from primitive mesoderm and ectodermal neural crests cells, but it may seem to be flattened ("lying down" sign) on ultrasonography.[22]

The contralateral ureter may be abnormal, with associated vesicoureteral reflux in 30% and obstruction at the ureteropelvic or ureterovesical junction in 11% and 7%, respectively.[23] Reproductive tract malformations in females are found in 25% to 50% despite URA being more common in males (1.8:1) in whom reproductive tract anomalies occur in only 10% to 15%.[24] About 40% of females with genital anomalies have URA. As noted, these anomalies involve the MD owing to its close developmental relationship with the WD. In males, an anomalous WD affects its derivatives, including the vas deferens, seminal vesicles, ampulla, ejaculatory duct, and the body and tail of

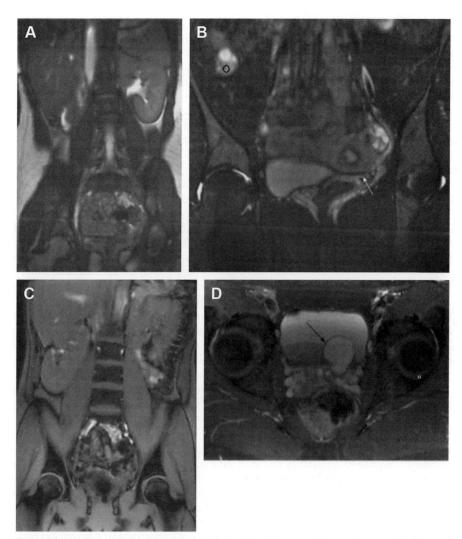

Fig. 1. Magnetic resonance imaging (MRI) showing (*A*) coronal scout image of right renal agenesis with the bowel occupying the right renal fossa. (*B*) Coronal T2 fat-saturated images show left unicornuate uterus (*arrow*), absent right cornua, and superior location of right ovary (*o*). (*C*) Coronal scout image demonstrates left renal agenesis with bowel occupying the left renal fossa and right renal malrotation. (*D*) Transverse T2 fat-saturated image of male pelvis shows left seminal vesicle cyst (*arrow*). (*From* Shapiro E, Bauer SB, Chow JS. Anomalies of the upper urinary tract. In: Wein AJ, Kavoussi LR, Novick AC, et al, editors. Campbell-Walsh urology, vol. 4. 10th edition. Philadelphia: Elsevier; 2011. p. 3123–60; with permission.)

the epididymis. A seminal vesicle cyst may form as a result of atresia of the ejaculatory duct and may be associated with URA (Zinner's syndrome).[25] The head of the epididymis is present and contains the efferent ductules; they are of mesonephric tubule origin. The fimbriated end of the fallopian tube has a similar origin, which explains their invariable presence despite anomalies of the uterus.[26] The URA-associated uterine anomalies include congenital absence of the uterus and uterus didelphys, with the most common malformations being unicornuate uterus with complete absence of the ipsilateral horn and fallopian tube and bicornuate uterus with rudimentary development of the ipsilateral horn.[27] The vagina may be absent, proximally atretic, completely duplicated, or septated.[28] A didelphys or septate uterus owing to partial or complete midline fusion of the MD may be associated with a single or duplicated cervix. Uterus didelphys commonly presents with a pelvic mass or pain in pubertal girls owing to an obstructed hemivagina and hematometrocolpos. This entity has been referred to as Herlyn-Werner-Wunderlich syndrome.[9,29] Smith and Laufer suggested the acronym OHVIRA: Obstructed Hemivagina and Ipsilateral Renal Anomaly to classify this syndrome.[30]

Another complex of malformations, which occurs in 1 in 4500 females, is the Mayer-Rokitansky-Kuster-Hauser syndrome.[31,32] All females are phenotypically 46,XX. Type I is usually characterized by MD remnants and normal fallopian tubes. Type II is characterized by asymmetrical hypoplasia of 1 or both buds with or without dysplasia of the fallopian tubes and renal anomalies in 40% to 60%, including URA primarily, ectopia of 1 or both kidneys (usually pelvic in location), and horseshoe kidney.[33] In a more severe constellation of anomalies, the MURCS association or duct aphasia (96%), Renal aplasia or ectopia (86%), and Cardiothoracic Somite dysplasia (2–4 anomalous vertebrae between C5-T1 [80%]) has been reported.[34]

Van Vuuren and investigators[35] reported that from the 20th week of gestation about 90% of solitary kidneys owing to URA or MCDK undergo compensatory hypertrophy. A retroperitoneal sonogram with color Doppler ultrasonography shows absence of renal parenchyma and ipsilateral renal vessels. A DMSA scan confirms this or may detect an ectopic (usually pelvic) or a crossed kidney.[36]

Although controversial, a voiding cystourethrogram should be considered when there is URA, because there is an incidence of contralateral reflux in 28%.[37]

Long-Term Outcomes

Brenner's "hyperfiltration" hypothesis may be extrapolated to those with solitary functioning kidney (SFK) who have reduced nephron number, especially if CAKUT or Congenital Anomalies of the Kidney and Urinary Tract affects that kidney.[38,39] This includes renal hypoplasia and/or dysplasia, segmental MCDK, ureteropelvic junction obstruction, megaureter, vesicoureteral reflux, and posterior urethral valves. Some of these anomalies may be associated with subtle defects in uteric bud branching resulting in the development of a reduced number of nephrons and subsequent renal insufficiency in late adolescence and adulthood.[40]

Sanna-Cherchi and colleagues[41] reported on long-term renal function in individuals with URA and predicted that 50% had a probability of renal failure requiring dialysis by age 30. They postulated that the number of nephrons in URA may be lower than expected, thereby increasing the risk of hypertension, albuminuria, and focal glomerulosclerosis. Westland and colleagues[42] in the KIMONO study (Kidney of MONofunctional Origin) retrospectively evaluated 116 children with congenital or primary SKF (54 with URA and 62 with MCDK) and 90 children with secondary SKF after unilateral nephrectomy for CAKUT or tumor. The solitary kidney had CAKUT in about 30%. Hypertension, albuminuria, or the use of renoprotective medication were used to define renal injury because hypertension and microalbuminuria (>30 mg/24 h) are indicators of a progressive reduction in glomerular filtration rate. These investigators found that 32% with SFK had renal injury at a mean age of 9.5 years with a decline in the glomerular filtration rate and the development of microalbuminuria as early as age 9 and 16, respectively.[42] Ipsilateral CAKUT in a SFK from any cause was associated with more renal injury than if CAKUT were not present. Although these studies are limited by selection bias, both stress the importance of identifying patients likely to develop renal insufficiency in adulthood.

Follow-up for those with SKF includes an annual blood pressure and testing for microalbuminuria (first morning specimen) when the kidney is normal and biannually when there is CAKUT.[43–45] Angiotensin-converting enzyme inhibitors may reduce progression of renal injury.[46] In addition, limiting salt and protein are recommended depending on patient age. Ultrasound examinations ensure appropriate compensatory hypertrophy and growth through childhood and adolescence.

ANOMALIES OF ASCENT
Simple Renal Ectopia

Renal ectopia refers to a kidney not located in its normal or orthotopic location in the upper retroperitoneum or "renal" fossa. The term ectopia is derived from the Greek words *ek* ("out") and *topos* ("place"). The kidney may be pelvic, iliac, abdominal, thoracic, and contralateral or crossed in location (**Fig. 2**). Renal ectopia occurs in about 1 in 900 with no gender propensity.[47]

Pelvic ectopia is observed in 1 of 2100 to 3000 autopsies.[48] A solitary ectopic kidney occurs in only 1 of 22,000 autopsies and bilateral renal ectopia is seen in 10% of those with ectopic kidneys.[49,50] The ureter enters the bladder normally, except for rare cases of ectopic kidneys with ectopic ureters.[51]

About one half of the ectopic kidneys have a hydronephrotic collecting system. Approximately one half of those with hydronephrosis have evidence of obstruction, with ureteropelvic or ureterovesical junction obstruction in 70% and 30%, respectively. Hydronephrosis may be a manifestation of vesicoureteral reflux (grade 3 or greater) in about 25%, and another 25% are hydronephrotic with malrotation alone.[52] Up to 66% of females and 20% of males with ectopic kidneys have reproductive/genital anomalies.[53] The adrenal gland is almost always in a normal position. The

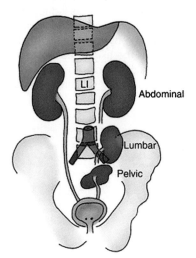

Fig. 2. Incomplete ascent of kidney. The kidney may halt at any level of its ascent from the pelvis. (*From* Shapiro E, Bauer SB, Chow JS. Anomalies of the upper urinary tract. In: Wein AJ, Kavoussi LR, Novick AC, et al, editors. Campbell-Walsh urology, vol. 4. 10th edition. Philadelphia: Elsevier; 2011; with permission.)

kidneys derive their aberrant blood supply from adjacent vessels (distal aorta, the bifurcation, the external or iliac arteries, and the inferior mesenteric artery).[54]

Most renal ectopia are asymptomatic. The lumbar and pelvic kidneys may result in a pattern of direct and referred pain that is atypical for colic and may be misdiagnosed as acute appendicitis, or as pelvic inflammatory disease in female patients. Patients may be more susceptible to stones and blunt abdominal trauma.[55]

ANOMALIES OF FORM AND FUSION
Crossed Renal Ectopia with and Without Fusion

Crossed ectopia refers to a kidney located on the side opposite from that in which its ureter inserts into the bladder. Most crossed ectopic kidneys are fused to the contralateral kidney (90%). The lower pole of the orthotopic kidney is usually joined with the upper pole of the crossed ectopic kidney. These anomalies may include crossed ectopia with fusion, crossed ectopia without fusion, solitary crossed ectopia, and bilaterally crossed ectopia.[56] The fusion anomalies have been described as (1) unilateral fused kidney with inferior ectopia, (2) sigmoid or S-shaped, (3) lump or cake, (4) L-shaped or tandem, (5) disc, shield, or doughnut, and (6) unilateral fused kidneys with superior ectopia (**Fig. 3**). The ultimate shape of the fused renal units depends on the time and extent of fusion and the degree of renal rotation. Horseshoe kidney is the most common fusion anomaly, followed by crossed renal ectopia. Fusion anomalies are found incidentally on radiographic studies evaluating other malformations or amenorrhea; most individuals are otherwise asymptomatic.[57] Skeletal and reproductive tract anomalies (including cryptorchidism or absence of the vas deferens in males and vaginal atresia or a unilateral uterine abnormality in females) are seen in 50% and 40%, respectively, in those with solitary crossed ectopic kidney.[58,59]

HORSESHOE KIDNEY
Incidence, Diagnosis, and Associated Anomalies

The horseshoe kidney is usually asymptomatic, occurs in about 1 in 400, and is the most common renal fusion anomaly. Horseshoe kidneys have 2 distinct renal masses that are low lying, oriented with a vertical or outward axis on each side of the midline and joined at the lower poles (95%) by a parenchymatous or fibrous isthmus.[60–63] The calyces point posteriorly, and the axis of each pelvis remains in the vertical or obliquely lateral plane. The isthmus of most horseshoe kidneys is located adjacent to the L3 to L4 level because the inferior mesenteric artery prevents further ascent

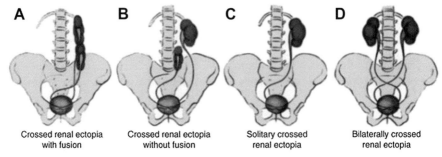

Crossed renal ectopia with fusion	Crossed renal ectopia without fusion	Solitary crossed renal ectopia	Bilaterally crossed renal ectopia

Fig. 3. (*A–D*) Four types of crossed renal ectopia. (*From* Shapiro E, Bauer SB, Chow JS. Anomalies of the upper urinary tract. In: Wein AJ, Kavoussi LR, Novick AC, et al, editors. Campbell-Walsh urology, vol. 4. 10th edition. Philadelphia: Elsevier; 2011; with permission.)

(**Fig. 4**). About one third of horseshoe kidneys have a single renal artery to the renal units, whereas the remainder have a variable blood supply from nearby vasculature.[64] In addition, about one third of horseshoe kidneys are associated with congenital anomalies, some of which may lead to early demise.[65] The most common congenital anomalies are skeletal, cardiovascular (primarily ventriculoseptal defects), central nervous system, and neural tube defects (3%), as well as anorectal malformations.[66,67] Hydronephrosis is commonly observed owing to the relationship of the ureter as it crosses over the renal pelvis and isthmus, but radionuclide scanning usually demonstrates a nonobstructed pattern.

About 50% of horseshoe kidneys have associated vesicoureteral reflux and 30% of patients develop urinary tract infections.[68] Boatman and colleagues[69] report hypospadias and undescended testes in 4% of boys and a bicornuate uterus or septate vagina in 7% of girls. Horseshoe kidney occurs in 60% of those with Turner syndrome.[70] Stone formation occurs in horseshoe kidney when there are metabolic alterations including hypercalciuria and hypocitraturia.[71]

Although renal tumors have been reported, with renal cell carcinoma being the most frequent (50%), renal cell carcinoma has no greater incidence in horseshoe kidneys than occurs in the general population.[72] Transitional cell carcinoma of the renal pelvis and Wilms' tumor (WT) each account for about 25% of the kidney cancers. WTs occur in 0.48% of horseshoe kidneys, with the incidence of WT in horseshoe kidneys being 1.76 to 7.93 times greater than that expected in the general population.[73,74] Unlike WT in a single renal unit, 37% of the tumors were inoperable at presentation and required preoperative chemotherapy. Ultimately, however, there was a 75% preservation rate of renal parenchyma in this group.[73]

RENAL HYPOPLASIA AND DYSPLASIA
Renal Hypoplasia

When normal nephrogenesis is disrupted, nephron number can be reduced or organogenesis may be disordered. The former can lead to renal hypoplasia and the latter, renal dysplasia.[75,76] Renal hypoplasia refers to a congenitally small kidney (>2 standard deviations from the mean size by age on sonography) with normal architecture and a 20% to 25% reduction in nephron number (normal nephron number ranges from 600,000 to 2 million). The kidneys seem to be hyperechogenic on sonogram. Histologically, there are hypertrophic glomeruli and tubules.

Renal hypoplasia may be unilateral or bilateral.[75] Unilateral renal hypoplasia may be associated with contralateral compensatory hypertrophy. In bilateral hypoplasia, a younger presentation is associated with greater renal impairment. During the first year of life, patients may present with anorexia, vomiting, failure to thrive, and growth retardation and usually progress to end-stage renal disease owing to focal segmental glomerulosclerosis. Renal hypoplasia may occur as an isolated finding or in association with syndromes such as renal-coloboma and brachio-oto-renal syndromes, as well as renal tubular dysgenesis.

Three forms of renal hypoplasia have been described.[75] Oligomeganephronia is the most common form, with small kidneys and decreased nephrons and calyces. Simple hypoplasia describes small kidneys with a normal number of nephrons. A unipapillary hypoplastic kidney contains a single papilla.

Renal Dysplasia

Renal dysplasia refers to abnormal renal parenchyma, histologically characterized by poor branching and maldifferentiation of nephrons with primitive tubules and

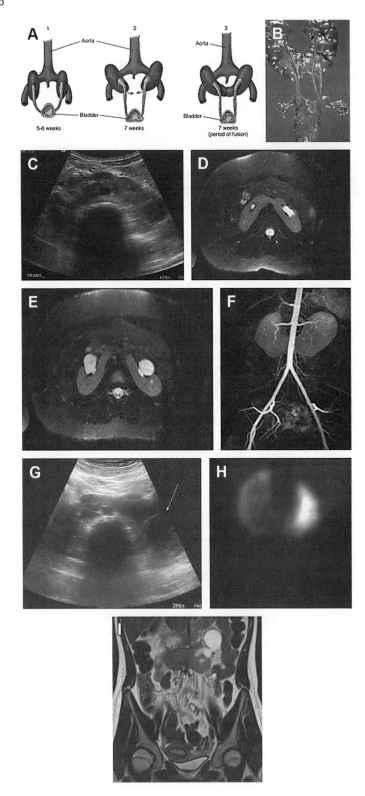

collecting ducts, interstitial fibrosis, and metaplasia of metanephric mesenchyme to cartilage and bone.[76] Renal hypodysplasia is a combination of both entities.

Renal dysplasia may be unilateral or bilateral and occurs in 0.2% to 0.4% of births.[76] Renal dysplasia may be detected prenatally or postnatally during ultrasonography of an infant with dysmorphic features. The sonogram usually shows a smaller than normal kidney with increased echogenicity, loss of corticomedullary differentiation, and cortical cysts. If renal dysplasia is bilateral, renal function will be impaired with progressive renal insufficiency. In contrast, those with unilateral renal dysplasia and a normal contralateral renal unit have a good prognosis. Renal dysplasia may be associated with ipsilateral upper tract or ureteral anomalies and bladder outlet obstruction, which may predispose to urinary tract infection. A voiding cystourethrogram should be considered as part of the initial evaluation of renal dysplasia.

NEONATAL RENAL TUMORS
Incidence, Diagnosis, and Associated Syndromes

Renal tumors in neonates are rare and account for approximately 7% of tumors in the first 30 days of life.[77] The most common neonatal renal tumor is congenital mesoblastic nephroma (CMN), which is more prevalent than WT in the first 3 months of life. Rhabdoid tumor and clear cell sarcoma of the kidney are both exceedingly rare.

Prenatal diagnosis detects only about 20% of renal tumors and about 50% present with an abdominal mass.[77,78] Polyhydramnios, fetal hydrops, hematuria, and hypertension may be present, as well as nonspecific signs, including pallor, vomiting, lethargy, abdominal distension, and failure to thrive.[77,78] Laboratory evaluation may reveal anemia, hypercalcemia, and hyperreninism. Tumor predisposing syndromes associated with WT occur in 10% and include Beckwith-Wiedemann, Denys-Drash, Perlman, Simpson-Golabi-Behmel, and WAGR syndromes (Wilms', Aniridia, Genitourinary anomalies, and mental Retardation). When an infant is found to have one of these syndromes, abdominal ultrasound is performed every 3 months until age 5 and until age 8 for those with Beckwith-Wiedemann syndrome.[79,80]

CMN

CMNs are almost always diagnosed within the first 6 months of life.[77] These tumors are usually unilateral and may be detected prenatally, but are indistinguishable from

---

Fig. 4. (A) Embryogenesis of horseshoe kidney. The lower poles of the 2 kidneys touch and fuse as they cross the iliac arteries. Ascent is stopped when the fused kidneys reach the junction of the aorta and inferior mesenteric artery. (B) Post mortem specimen showing horseshoe kidney with bilateral duplicated ureters. (C) Ultrasonography of horseshoe kidney at the level of the isthmus. (D) Magnetic resonance (MR) urogram shows axial T2 fat-saturated image at the level of the isthmus. (E) Axial T2 fat-saturated image demonstrates extrarenal pelves. (F) Angiographic sequence shows variable blood supply to the kidney. (G) Transverse sonogram of 14-year-old girl with left flank pain found to have marked left hydronephrosis in a horseshoe kidney (arrow). (H) MAG3 scan demonstrates left ureteropelvic junction obstruction. (I) Coronal T2 images of MR urogram show the isthmus (arrow) and severe left hydronephrosis occupying the left renal fossa. (From Shapiro E, Bauer SB, Chow JS. Anomalies of the upper urinary tract. In: Wein AJ, Kavoussi LR, Novick AC, et al, editors. Campbell-Walsh urology, vol. 4. 10th edition. Philadelphia: Elsevier; 2011. p. 3123–60, with permission; [A] Benjamin JA, Schullian DM. Observation on fused kidneys with horseshoe configuration: the contribution of Leonardo Botallo (1564). J Hist Med Allied Sci 1950;5:315 after Gutierrez R. The clinical management of horseshoe kidney. 1931 Am J Surg;14:657–88 and [B] Weiss MA, Mills SE. Atlas of genitourinary tract disorders. Philadelphia: JB Lippincott; 1988.)

WT.[81] Polyhydramnios may be present in up to 70% during gestation.[78] CMN is more common in boys (1.5:1) and often presents with an abdominal mass.[79] The majority of these infants have no associated anomalies.[77] Ultrasonographic findings show a solid mass with homogeneous echogenicity near the hilum and renal sinus. There is no well-defined capsule as seen in WT, and the tumor blends with the normal renal parenchyma, although it remains well demarcated from the renal tissue.[82]

Pathologically, CMN are hamartomas that originate from proliferating nephrogenic mesenchyme and infiltrate the kidney, but do not invade the renal vessels or inferior vena cava or form a pseudocapsule, which may be seen with malignant tumors and is compressed or reactive connective tissue within the renal parenchyma.[77,79] Histologically, the tumor is composed of spindle-cell bundles composed of immature renal stromal cells and is primarily low in grade. Three pathologic variants are described: Classic (rare mitoses and no necrosis), atypical or cellular (high mitotic index, hypercellularity, necrosis with invasion of adjacent structures), or mixed (classic and cellular subtypes).[77,79] CMN rarely metastasize, although the cellular variant can be more aggressive and present with distant disease to the lung, brain, liver, bone, or heart.[77–79,83] In addition to the cellular variant, older age and positive surgical margins may increase the risk of recurrence and metastasis.[80]

Treatment is radical nephrectomy with a 5-year event-free survival of 94% and overall survival of 96% for infants.[84] These rates are slightly lower for those with the cellular variant (85% and 90%, respectively).[80] There is no established role for routine chemotherapy after surgery, but adjuvant chemotherapy should be considered in patients 3 months or older with an high stage cellular variant owing to the greater risk for recurrence in this subtype.[77,79,80]

WT

WT accounts for approximately 20% of neonatal renal tumors.[77,78] The majority of WT are diagnosed postnatally and present as an abdominal mass. Because CMN and WT are indistinguishable prenatally, postnatal ultrasonography and subsequent magnetic resonance imaging may show renal vein or inferior vena cava involvement, which suggests a diagnosis of WT.[77]

Most WT (80%) are stage I or II when diagnosed.[77,79] The pathology in neonates with WT is almost invariably favorable histology.[77] The treatment for WT is radical nephrectomy.[80,85] Primary surgical resection alone is recommended in children under 2 years of age, with stage I unilateral tumors weighing less than 550 g.[85] Stage I unilateral tumors weighing less than 550 g that recur can be salvaged with chemotherapy, with the 5-year overall survival of 99% with surgery versus 98% with surgery plus chemotherapy.[85,86] Therefore, if there is a *WT1* mutation and 11p15 loss of heterozygosity, which are markers for relapse in this group, chemotherapy is now given.[85–87]

All other stage I and II favorable histology are given vincristine and dactinomycin after surgical excision.[88,89] This includes children 2 years and older or those with a tumor weighing 550 g or more. Doxorubicin is added if there is loss of heterozygosity of 1p and 16q (markers of increased rates of relapse and mortality).[88,89] When radiation is needed for local control in advanced stages, consideration is made to avoid (until age 6 months) or reduce the dose if treatment involves the hemiabdomen, whole abdomen, or lung in those younger than 1.[77] Neonatal WT has an event-free survival and overall survival of 86% and 93%, respectively.[79] Bilateral WT in this young age group are managed individually with partial nephrectomy, wedge excisions, and adjuvant chemotherapy, with the aim of nephron sparing to avoid renal failure and dialysis.[77,78,88]

Rhabdoid Tumor of the Kidney

About 11% of neonatal renal tumors are rhabdoid tumors.[77–79] Rhabdoid tumors of the kidney occur primarily in neonates and infants, with this group comprising almost 70% of all cases.[89] The tumors resemble rhabdomyosarcoma, but have no skeletal muscle markers and are associated with deletions at chromosome locus 22q11.1, which codes for a tumor suppressor gene.[90,91]

These tumors are extremely aggressive, presenting with an abdominal mass and metastases in approximately 50% in 1 series of fetal and neonatal rhabdoid tumors.[78] Hypercalcemia is common.[78] On computed tomography, curvilinear calcifications are seen around the tumor with subcapsular fluid collections.[92] Metastatic evaluation includes brain and bone imaging. Rhabdoid tumors are treated with radical nephrectomy, and adjuvant chemotherapy and radiation therapy. Younger age and metastatic disease are poor prognostic indicators, with an overall survival rate in neonates of less than 10%.[78,84]

Clear Cell Sarcoma of the Kidney

Clear cell sarcoma of the kidney is the least common neonatal neoplasm (3%), presents with an abdominal mass, and about 30% have metastatic disease at diagnosis (stage IV).[78] Although it has been referred to as the "bone metastasizing" tumor of the kidney, metastases commonly occur in the lung, liver, and lymph nodes. A metastatic evaluation should include a radionuclide bone scan.[77] Radical nephrectomy is indicated; adjuvant chemotherapy and radiation are administered for metastatic disease.[77,79] Stage I/II have very good survival (100% in this series) compared with stage IV (~50%).[78]

In summary, fetuses and neonates have reduced survival rates compared with survival rates for infants and older children. This is most likely related to prenatal and postnatal conditions, such as polyhydramnios, fetal hydrops, congestive heart failure, hypertension, and stillbirth, which prevent treatment. Chemotherapeutic doses may be limited by gestational age and the overall condition of the neonate.[78] When the clinical status of the neonate permits surgery, survival potential is similar to that of older children.[78]

Neuroblastoma

Although neuroblastoma is not a renal tumor, it deserves mention because it is the most common neonatal malignancy, accounting for greater than 20% of neonatal tumors and is, at times, in the differential diagnosis of renal tumors, especially those involving the upper pole of the kidney.[93] Recently, a case of intrarenal neuroblastoma mimicking a mesoblastic nephroma was reported on prenatal sonogram at 30 weeks. Postnatally, the infant had hypertension and cardiac failure. The tumor showed calcifications and perirenal adenopathy and pathologically was a neuroblastoma with elevated catecholamines.[94]

Neuroblastoma occurs in 1 in 7000 to 10,000 live births.[95] Neuroblastoma commonly involves the neuroectodermal sympathetic chain and the adrenal medulla.[93] The adrenal is the most common primary site in children (40%). Infants tend to have thoracic and cervical primaries with the adrenal being the primary in 25%.

Prenatally Diagnosed Adrenal Mass

Adrenal tumors may be observed incidentally at 32 weeks, but have been seen as early as 23 weeks of gestation.[93] They may range in size between 2 and 10 cm and may be solid or cystic with foci of calcifications. Adrenal hemorrhage is the most common alternative diagnosis in the differential. Adrenal hemorrhage is echogenic and does not show the vascularization of a neuroblastoma on sonography.[93,96]

When a suprarenal mass has been observed prenatally, an abdominal sonogram is performed and laboratory evaluation including urinary levels of homovanillic acid and vanillylmandelic acid are obtained. Although urinary catecholamines are elevated in greater than 90% of neuroblastomas, only 33% of perinatal neuroblastomas have elevated levels.[93] Abdominal magnetic resonance imaging may be indicated to evaluate the infant for regional or metastatic disease. These masses are often observed for the first 3 months and followed with sonograms and urinary catecholamines every 3 weeks. When regression is observed, testing may occur at increased intervals. If the tumor size enlarges by 50%, surgical resection is recommended at that time.[93]

Congenital Neuroblastomas: Special Considerations

Factors influencing prognosis include tumor stage, age at diagnosis, pathologic risk classification, cytogenetics, and molecular genetics. Neuroblastoma in infants younger than 18 months have a very good prognosis because their tumors often have favorable biological features with some spontaneously regressing, despite metastases (stage 4S).[97–99] Neuroblastomas in infants younger than 6 months who have small, localized adrenal masses or asymptomatic stage 4s ("s" refers to special) when the adrenal is the primary and the metastases are limited to the skin, liver, and/or bone marrow can be observed but followed carefully as outlined.[97–99] The exception to this good prognosis group are the neonates (<4–6 weeks of age) with Stage 4s, because liver metastases can enlarge rapidly leading to pulmonary compromise and renal failure in 30% of these cases.[97–99]

REFERENCES

1. Costantini F, Kopan R. Patterning a complex organ: branching morphogenesis and nephron segmentation in kidney development. Dev Cell 2010;18(5): 698–712.
2. Uetani N, Bouchard M. Plumbing in the embryo: developmental defects of the urinary tracts. Clin Genet 2009;75:307–17.
3. Guioli S, Ryohei S, Lovell-Badge R. The origin of the Mullerian duct in chick and mouse. Dev Biol 2007;302:389–98.
4. Orvis GD, Behringer RR. Cellular mechanisms of Müllerian duct formation in the mouse. Dev Biol 2007;306(2):493–504.
5. Kobayashi A, Kwan KM, Carroll TJ, et al. Distinct and sequential tissue-specific activities of the LIM-class homeobox gene Lim1 for tubular morphogenesis during kidney development. Development 2005;132:2809–23.
6. Masse J, Watrin T, Laurent A, et al. The developing female genital tract: from genetics to epigenetics. Int J Dev Biol 2009;53:411–24.
7. Kobayashi A, Shawlot W, Kania A, et al. Requirement of Lim1 for female reproductive tract development. Development 2004;131:539–49.
8. Carroll TJ, Park JS, Hayashi S, et al. Wnt9b plays a central role in the regulation of mesenchymal to epithelial transitions underlying organogenesis of the mammalian urogenital system. Dev Cell 2005;9:283–92.
9. Yoder IC, Pfister RC. Unilateral hematocolpos and ipsilateral renal agenesis: report of two cases and review of the literature. AJR Am J Roentgenol 1976; 127:303.
10. Doroshow LW, Abeshouse BS. Congenital unilateral solitary kidney: report of 37 cases and a review of the literature. Urol Surv 1961;11:219.

11. Sipek A, Gregor V, Horacek J, et al. Incidence of renal agenesis in the Czech Republic from 1961-1995. Ceska Gynekol 1997;62:340–3.
12. Hiraoka M, Tsukahara H, Ohshima Y, et al. Renal aplasia is the predominant cause of congenital solitary kidneys. Kidney Int 2002;61:1840–4.
13. Schreuder MF, Westland R, van Wijk JA. Unilateral multicystic dysplastic kidney: a meta-analysis of observational studies on the incidence, associated urinary tract malformations and the contralateral kidney. Nephrol Dial Transplant 2009;6:1810–8.
14. Ashley DJB, Mostofi FK. Renal agenesis and dysgenesis. J Urol 1960;83:211.
15. Quinton R, Duke VM, Robertson A, et al. Idiopathic gonadotrophin deficiency: genetic questions addressed through phenotypic characterization. Clin Endocrinol 2001;55:163–74.
16. Mace JW, Kaplan JM, Schanberger JE, et al. Poland's syndrome: report of seven cases and review of the literature. Clin Pediatr 1972;11:98.
17. Fryns JP, van Schoubroeck D, Vandenberghe K, et al. Diagnostic echographic findings in cryptophthalmos syndrome (Fraser syndrome). Prenat Diagn 1997; 17:582–4.
18. Pierides AM, Athanasiou Y, Demetriou K, et al. A family with the branchio-oto-renal syndrome: clinical and genetic correlations. Nephrol Dial Transplant 2002;17:1014–8.
19. Davis EM, Peck JD, Thompson D, et al. Maternal diabetes and renal agenesis/dysgenesis. Birth Defects Res A Clin Mol Teratol 2010;88:722–7.
20. Kolon TF, Gray CL, Sutherland RW, et al. Upper urinary tract manifestations of the VACTERL association. J Urol 2000;163:1949–51.
21. Dursun H, Bayazit AK, Büyükçelik M, et al. Associated anomalies in children with congenital solitary functioning kidney. Pediatr Surg Int 2005;21(6):456–9.
22. Hoffman CK, Filly RA, Allen PW. The "lying down" adrenal sign: a sonographic indicator of renal agenesis or ectopia in fetuses and neonates. J Ultrasound Med 1992;11:533.
23. Cascio S, Paran S, Puri P. Associated urological anomalies in children with unilateral renal agenesis. J Urol 1999;162:1081–3.
24. Thompson DP, Lynn HB. Genital anomalies associated with solitary kidney. Mayo Clin Proc 1966;41:538.
25. Pereira BJ, Sousa L, Azinhais P, et al. Zinner's syndrome: an up-to-date review of the literature based on a clinical case. Andrologia 2009;41:322–30.
26. Heinonen PK. Unicornuate uterus and rudimentary horn. Fertil Steril 1997;68: 224–30.
27. Candiani GB, Fedele L, Candiani M. Double uterus, blind hemivagina, and ipsilateral renal agenesis: 36 cases and long-term followup. Obstet Gynecol 1997; 90:26.
28. D'Alberton A, Reschini E, Ferrari N, et al. Prevalence of urinary tract abnormalities in a large series of patients with uterovaginal atresia. J Urol 1981; 126:623.
29. Tong J, Zhu L, Lang J. Clinical characteristics of 70 patients with Herlyn–Werner–Wunderlich syndrome. Int J Gynaecol Obstet 2013;121(2):173–5.
30. Smith NA, Laufer MR. Obstructed hemivagina and ipsilateral renal anomaly (OHVIRA) syndrome: management and follow-up. Fertil Steril 2007;87: 918–22.
31. Oppelt PG, Lermann J, Strick R, et al. Malformations in a cohort of 284 women with Mayer-Rokitansky-Küster-Hauser syndrome (MRKH). Reprod Biol Endocrinol 2012;10:57.

32. Pizzo A, Laganà AS, Sturlese E, et al. Mayer-Rokitansky-Küster-Hauser syndrome: embryology, genetics and clinical and surgical treatment. ISRN Obstet Gynecol 2013;2013:628–717.

33. Guerrier D, Mouchel T, Pasquier L, et al. The Mayer-Rokitansky-Küster-Hauser syndrome (congenital absence of uterus and vagina)—phenotypic manifestations and genetic approaches. J Negat Results Biomed 2006;5:1.

34. Duncan PA, Shapiro LR, Stangel JJ, et al. The MURCS association: Müllerian duct aplasia, renal aplasia, and cervicothoracic somite dysplasia. J Pediatr 1979;95(3):399–402.

35. Van Vuuren SH, Van Der Doef R, Cohen-Overbeek TE, et al. Compensatory enlargement of a solitary functioning kidney during fetal development. Ultrasound Obstet Gynecol 2012;40:665–8.

36. Volkan B, Ceylan E, Kiratli PO. Radionuclide imaging of rare congenital renal fusion anomalies. Clin Nucl Med 2003;28(3):204–7.

37. Kaneyama K, Yamataka A, Satake S, et al. Associated urologic anomalies in children with solitary kidney. J Pediatr Surg 2004;39:85–7.

38. Westland R, Van Wijk JA, Schreuder MF, et al. The reason why mother nature provided us with two kidneys: the risks of a congenital solitary functioning kidney. Nephrol Dial Transplant 2012;27(6):2603–4.

39. Westland R, Schreuder MF, Ket JC, et al. Unilateral renal agenesis: a systematic review on associated anomalies and renal injury. Nephrol Dial Transplant 2013; 28:1844–55.

40. Chevalier RL. When is one kidney not enough? Kidney Int 2009;76:475–7.

41. Sanna-Cherchi S, Ravani P, Corbani V, et al. Renal outcome in patients with congenital anomalies of the kidney and urinary tract. Kidney Int 2009;76: 528–33.

42. Westland R, Schreuder MF, Bökenkamp A, et al. Renal injury in children with a solitary functioning kidney—the KIMONO study. Nephrol Dial Transplant 2011;5: 1533–41.

43. Hegde S, Coulthard MG. Renal agenesis and unilateral nephrectomy: what are the risks of living with a single kidney? Pediatr Nephrol 2009;24:439–46.

44. Westland R, Kurvers RA, Van Wijk JA, et al. Risk factors for renal injury in children with a solitary functioning kidney. Pediatrics 2013;131(2):e478–85.

45. Westland R, Schreuder MF, Van Goudoever JB, et al. Clinical implications of the solitary functioning kidney. Clin J Am Soc Nephrol 2014;9:978–86.

46. Puddu M, Fanos V, Podda F, et al. The kidney from prenatal to adult life: perinatal programming and reduction of number of nephrons during development. Am J Nephrol 2009;30(2):162–70.

47. Abeshouse BS, Bhisitkul I. Crossed renal ectopia with and without fusion. Urol Int 1959;9:63.

48. Stevens AR. Pelvic single kidneys. J Urol 1937;37:610.

49. Delson B. Ectopic kidney in obstetrics and gynecology. N Y State J Med 1975; 75:2522.

50. Malek RS, Kelalis PP, Burke EC. Ectopic kidney in children and frequency of association of other malformations. Mayo Clin Proc 1971;46:461.

51. Borer JG, Bauer SB, Peters CA, et al. Single system ectopic ureter draining an ectopic dysplastic kidney: delayed diagnosis in the young female with continuous urinary incontinence. Br J Urol 1998;81:474–8.

52. Gleason PE, Kelalis PP, Husmann DA, et al. Hydronephrosis in renal ectopia: incidence, etiology and significance. J Urol 1994;151:1660.

53. McCrea LE. Congenital solitary pelvic kidney. J Urol 1942;48:58.

54. Anson BJ, Riba LW. The anatomical and surgical features of ectopic kidney. Surg Gynecol Obstet 1939;68:37.
55. Benchekroun A, Kasmaoui EH, Jira H, et al. Pathological pelvic kidney. Ann Urol 2002;36:231–5.
56. McDonald JH, McClellan DS. Crossed renal ectopia. Am J Surg 1957;93:995.
57. Glodny B, Petersen J, Hofmann KJ, et al. Kidney fusion anomalies revisited: clinical and radiological analysis of 209 cases of crossed fused ectopia and horseshoe kidney. BJU Int 2008;103:224–38.
58. Gu L, Alton DJ. Crossed solitary renal ectopia. Urology 1991;38:556.
59. Kakei H, Kondo A, Ogisu BI, et al. Crossed ectopia of solitary kidney: a report of two cases and a review of the literature. Urol Int 1976;31:40.
60. Campbell MF. Anomalies of the kidney. In: Campbell MF, Harrison JH, editors. Urology, vol. 2, 3rd edition. Philadelphia: WB Saunders; 1970. p. 1447–52.
61. Kolln CP, Boatman DL, Schmidt JD, et al. Horseshoe kidney: a review of 105 patients. J Urol 1972;107:203.
62. Pitts WR, Muecke EC. Horseshoe kidneys: a 40-year experience. J Urol 1975; 113:743.
63. Natsis K, Piaghou M, Skotsimara A, et al. Horseshoe kidney: a review of anatomy and pathology. Surg Radiol Anat 2013. [Epub ahead of print].
64. Glenn JF. Analysis of 51 patients with horseshoe kidney. N Engl J Med 1959;261: 684.
65. Scott JE. Fetal, perinatal, and infant death with congenital renal anomaly. Arch Dis Child 2002;87:114–7.
66. Voisin M, Djernit A, Morin D, et al. Cardiopathies congenitales et malformations urinaires. Arch Mal Coeur Vaiss 1988;81:703.
67. Whitaker RH, Hunt GM. Incidence and distribution of renal anomalies in patients with neural tube defects. Eur Urol 1987;13:322.
68. Cascio S, Sweeney B, Granata C, et al. Vesicoureteral reflux and ureteropelvic junction obstruction in children with horseshoe kidney: treatment and outcome. J Urol 2002;167(6):2566–8.
69. Boatman DL, Kolln CP, Flocks RH. Congenital anomalies associated with horseshoe kidney. J Urol 1972;107:205.
70. Lippe B, Geffner ME, Dietrich RB, et al. Renal malformations in patients with turner syndrome: imaging in 141 patients. Pediatrics 1988;82:852.
71. Raj GV, Auge BK, Assimos D, et al. Metabolic abnormalities associated with renal calculi in patients with horseshoe kidneys. J Endourol 2004;18:157–61.
72. Stimac G, Dimanovski J, Ruzic B, et al. Tumors in kidney fusion anomalies. Scand J Urol Nephrol 2004;38:485–9.
73. Neville H, Ritchey ML, Shamberger RC, et al. The occurrence of Wilms tumor in horseshoe kidneys. J Pediatr Surg 2002;37:1134–7.
74. Mesrobian HG, Kelalis PP, Hrabovsky E, et al. Wilms' tumor in horseshoe kidneys: a report from the National Wilms' tumor study. J Urol 1985;133:1002.
75. Sanna-Cherchi S, Caridi G, Weng PL, et al. Genetic approaches to human renal agenesis/hypoplasia and dysplasia. Pediatr Nephrol 2007;22:1675–84.
76. Winyard P, Chitty LS. Dysplastic kidneys. Semin Fetal Neonatal Med 2008;13(3): 142–51.
77. Thompson PA, Chintagumpala M. Renal and hepatic tumors in the neonatal period. Semin Fetal Neonatal Med 2012;17(4):216–21.
78. Isaacs H Jr. Fetal and neonatal renal tumors. J Pediatr Surg 2008;43: 1587–95.
79. Powis M. Neonatal renal tumors. Early Hum Dev 2010;86:607–12.

80. Furtwaengler R, Reinhard H, Leuschner I, et al. Mesoblastic nephroma – a report from the Gesellschaft für Padiatrische Onkologie and Hamatologie (GPOH). Cancer 2006;106:2275–83.
81. Giulian BB. Prenatal ultrasonographic diagnosis of fetal renal tumors. Radiology 1984;152:69–70.
82. Fuchs IB, Henrich W, Brauer M, et al. Prenatal diagnosis of congenital mesoblastic nephroma in 2 siblings. J Ultrasound Med 2003;22:823.
83. Vujanic GM, Delemarre JF, Moeslichan S, et al. Mesoblastic nephroma metastatic to the lungs and heart – another face of this peculiar lesion: case report and review of the literature. Pediatr Pathol 1993;13:143–53.
84. van der Heuvel-Eibrink MM, Grundy P, Graf N, et al. Characteristics and survival of 750 children diagnosed with a renal tumor in the first seven months of life: a collaborative study by the SIOP/GPOH/SFOP, NWTSG, and UKCCSG Wilms tumor study groups. Pediatr Blood Cancer 2008;50:1130–4.
85. Perlman EJ, Grundy PE, Anderson JR, et al. WT1 mutation and 11P15 loss of heterozygosity predict relapse in very low-risk Wilms tumors treated with surgery alone: a children's oncology group study. J Clin Oncol 2011;29:698.
86. Shamberger RC, Anderson JR, Breslow NE, et al. Long-term outcomes for infants with very low risk Wilms tumor treated with surgery alone in National Wilms Tumor Study-5. Ann Surg 2010;251:555.
87. Frazier AL, Shamberger RC, Henderson TO, et al. Decision analysis to compare treatment strategies for Stage I/favorable histology Wilms tumor. Pediatr Blood Cancer 2010;54:879.
88. Metzger ML, Dome JS. Current therapy for Wilms' tumor. Oncologist 2005;10: 815.
89. Orbach D, Sarnacki S, Brisse HJ, et al. Neonatal cancer. Lancet Oncol 2013; 14(13):e609–20.
90. Weeks DA, Beckwith JB, Mierau GW, et al. Rhabdoid tumor of kidney. A report of 111 cases from the National Wilms' Tumor Study Pathology Center. Am J Surg Pathol 1989;13:439–58.
91. Biegel JA, Zhou JY, Rorke LB, et al. Germline and acquired mutations of INI1 in atypical teratoid and rhabdoid tumors. Cancer Res 1999;59:74–9.
92. Agrons GA, Kingsman KD, Wagner BJ, et al. Rhabdoid tumour of the kidney in children: a comparative study of 21 cases. Am J Roentgenol 1997;168:447–51.
93. Fisher JP, Tweddle DA. Neonatal neuroblastoma. Semin Fetal Neonatal Med 2012;17(4):207–15.
94. Garnier S, Maillet O, Haouy S, et al. Prenatal intrarenal neuroblastoma mimicking a mesoblastic nephroma: a case report. J Pediatr Surg 2012;47:E21–3.
95. Moore SW, Stage D, Sasco AJ, et al. The epidemiology of neonatal tumors. Report of an international working group. Pediatr Surg Int 2003;19:509–19.
96. Nuchtern JG. Perinatal neuroblastoma. Semin Pediatr Surg 2006;15:10–6.
97. Katzenstein HM, Bowman LC, Brodeur GM, et al. Prognostic significance of age, MYCN oncogene amplification, tumor cell ploidy, and histology in 110 infants with Stage D(S) neuroblastoma: the pediatric oncology group experience—a pediatric oncology group study. J Clin Oncol 1998;16:2007.
98. Nickerson HJ, Mattay KK, Seeger RC, et al. Favorable biology and outcome of stage IV-S neuroblastoma with supportive care and minimal therapy: a Children's Cancer Group study. J Clin Oncol 2000;18:477.
99. London WB, Castleberry RP, Mattay KK, et al. Evidence for an age cutoff great than 365 days for neuroblastoma risk group stratification in the Children's Oncology Group. J Clin Oncol 2005;23:6459.

Disorders of the Bladder and Cloacal Anomaly

Angela M. Arlen, MD[a],*, Edwin A. Smith, MD, FAAP, FACS[a,b]

KEYWORDS

- Urachal remnant • Patent urachus • Bladder exstrophy • Cloacal exstrophy
- Persistent cloaca

KEY POINTS

- Urachal anomalies are uncommon, rarely diagnosed prenatally, and most often suspected during the neonatal period when continuous or intermittent umbilical drainage is observed; they often are managed conservatively in children less than 6 months of age.
- Classic bladder exstrophy is a complex congenital anomaly with musculoskeletal abnormalities of the lower abdominal wall and pelvis and genitourinary abnormalities of the bladder, urethra, and external genitalia.
- Cloacal exstrophy is among the most severe congenital anomalies compatible with live birth, with features of bladder exstrophy present in combination with exstrophic bowel segments, imperforate anus, and, commonly, omphalocele and spina bifida.
- Persistent cloaca is a form of anorectal malformation that results in a confluence of rectum, vagina, and urethra into a common channel that extends to the perineum as a single opening.

INTRODUCTION

Interpretation of antenatal imaging consistent with urachal, bladder, and cloaca anomalies and optimal management of these problems are guided by an understanding of their embryologic origins.[1,2] The cloaca is an endoderm-lined primordial organ that is first apparent at the beginning of the second week of gestation. This structure represents a confluence of the primitive hindgut (dorsally) and the allantois (ventrally). Between the fourth and sixth weeks of gestation, the urorectal septum divides the endodermal cloaca into a ventral urogenital sinus and a dorsal rectum.[3,4] The cranial portion of the urogenital sinus is continuous with the allantois and develops into the bladder and pelvic urethra. During the second trimester, the allantoic duct and ventral cloaca involute as the bladder descends into the pelvis. This epithelialized

Conflict of Interest: The authors have nothing to disclose.
[a] Children's Healthcare of Atlanta, Emory University School of Medicine, 201 Dowman Drive, Atlanta, GA 30322, USA; [b] Georgia Urology, PA, 5445 Meridian Mark Road, Suite 420, Atlanta, GA 30342, USA
* Corresponding author.
E-mail address: angarlen@gmail.com

fibromuscular tube obliterates into a thick fibrous cord, the urachus, which becomes the median umbilical ligament connecting the apex of the bladder with the umbilicus. Failure of the lumen of the allantois to completely obliterate results in a urachal remnant.[5] Exstrophy is thought to be secondary to the failure of the cloacal membrane to be reinforced by ingrowth of mesoderm. The cloacal membrane is subject to premature rupture, and, depending on the extent of the infraumbilical defect and the stage of development during which the rupture occurs, bladder exstrophy, cloacal exstrophy, or epispadias results.[6] The inciting event for persistent cloaca remains unclear but is thought to be secondary to the arrest of cloacal division by mesenchymal growth.[4]

URACHAL ANOMALIES

The urachus is an embryonic remnant derived from involution of the allantois; it is located in the preperitoneal space and connects the dome of the bladder to the anterior abdominal wall at the level of the umbilicus. The urachus is accompanied by umbilical arteries on either side, which undergo fibrosis and become the medial umbilical ligaments. Failure of the lumen of the allantois to completely obliterate results in a urachal remnant. Congenital urachal anomalies include patent urachus, urachal cyst, umbilical-urachus sinus, and vesicourachal diverticulum.[5,7] Patent urachus and urachal cyst account for most urachal anomalies, with patent urachus diagnosed most commonly in the neonatal period.[5,7-9] Although most often diagnosed postnatally, patent urachus can be detected on prenatal ultrasound or fetal magnetic resonance imaging (MRI). It is visualized as a cystic mass located at the base of the umbilical cord that communicates with the bladder.[10,11] Urachal cysts are more likely to present with infection or abdominal pain in later childhood or adulthood.[9,12] Patent urachus results from failure of the epithelial-lined urachal canal to obliterate, whereas urachal cysts have no communication with the bladder or umbilicus, although they can intermittently drain into either.[5] Given its location, a urachal remnant may be confused with other umbilical complications (ie, omphalitis, granulation tissue of the healing umbilical stump, or an infected umbilical vessel).[5]

Patient History/Physical Examination

- Patent urachus is suspected with umbilical drainage and abnormal-appearing umbilicus in the neonatal period; additional presentations include edematous umbilicus, granuloma, and delayed healing of the cord stump[13-15]
- Most common organisms cultured from umbilical drainage include *Staphylococcus aureus*, *Escherichia coli*, *Enterococcus*, *Citrobacter*, *Klebsiella,* and *Proteus*[8,9]
- Patent urachus must be distinguished from omphalitis, which typically presents as a superficial cellulitis and a patent omphalomesenteric duct remnant, which can present with feculent umbilical drainage[16,17]
- Associated anomalies causing in utero bladder outlet obstruction (ie, posterior urethral valves, prune belly syndrome, and urethral atresia) must be excluded; up to 14% of patients with patent urachus have postnatal confirmation of lower urinary tract obstruction[5]

Imaging/Additional Testing

- Diagnosis is confirmed by demonstration of a fluid-filled cystic structure on ultrasound scan extending from the dome of bladder to the umbilicus
- Passage of contrast at the umbilicus is seen on voiding cystourethrogram (**Fig. 1**); this is not always demonstrable

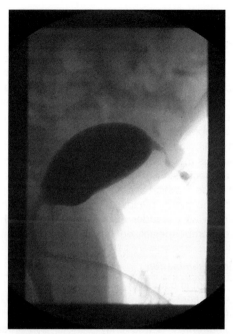

Fig. 1. Patent urachus. Voiding cystourethrogram image of a patent urachus in a newborn with umbilical drainage. Retrograde contrast filling of patent channel with pooling of contrast at the umbilicus is noted.

Management

- Urachal remnants in children younger than 6 months are likely to spontaneously resolve[8,9,18]
- Short-term urethral catheter drainage is reported to facilitate spontaneous closure of patent urachus[19]
- If symptoms persist or the urachal remnants fail to resolve, surgical excision is recommended to prevent recurrent infections[7,9]
- Management of infected urachus with abscess formation requires initial drainage and appropriate antibiotic therapy followed by complete surgical excision including a bladder cuff
- In infants, a small infraumbilical incision can be used, as the bladder dome is still high; urachal remnants can also be excised laparoscopically[5,20]

Summary

A small urachal remnant at birth may be viewed as physiologic. Patent urachus is most often diagnosed postnatally secondary to umbilical drainage, whereas other urachal anomalies (ie, urachal cyst) tend to present with abdominal pain or infection later in childhood or in adulthood. Observation in asymptomatic infants is reasonable; spontaneous resolution in children younger than 6 months is likely. Children with persistent urachal remnant or infection should undergo surgical excision.

BLADDER EXSTROPHY

The exstrophy-epispadias complex is a rare congenital malformation resulting in a lower abdominal wall defect exposing an open bladder and urethra, a wide diastasis of the pubic symphysis, and an epispadic urethral opening. The incidence of bladder exstrophy has been estimated between 1 in 10,000 and 1 in 50,000 and affects boys twice as often as girls.[6,21] The complex is more common in white infants.[22]

Bladder exstrophy can be diagnosed prenatally with fetal ultrasound scan between the 15th and 32nd weeks of pregnancy. Absence of bladder filling, a low-set umbilicus, widened pubic rami, small genitalia, and a lower abdominal mass that increases throughout pregnancy are characteristics of bladder exstrophy on prenatal imaging.[23–25] Despite ultrasound findings, accurate antenatal diagnosis of bladder exstrophy was recently reported to be just 25%.[26] Detection may be limited by habitus of the mother, oligohydramnios, and fetal position at the time of the scan.[27] In some cases, suspicious findings may be noted but not appropriately pursued with repeat ultrasound scan by a specialist.[26] More recently, fetal MRI was utilized to confirm bladder exstrophy in cases in which ultrasound findings are suspicious for exstrophy and also to evaluate the possibility of cloacal exstrophy.[28] Whether diagnosed prenatally or at birth, children with bladder exstrophy present a challenge to pediatric urologists and require prompt specialized care.

Patient History/Physical Examination

- Abdominal wall defect is caused by premature rupture of the abnormal cloacal membrane after descent of the urorectal septum; the exposed bladder and posterior urethra are situated on the anterior abdominal wall (**Fig. 2**)
- In girls, the vaginal orifice is frequently stenotic and anteriorly displaced, the clitoris is bifid, and the labia, mons pubis, and clitoris are divergent (**Fig. 3**A)
- In boys, epispadias is associated with prominent dorsal chordee and a short urethral plate (see **Fig. 3**B); the anterior corporal length of male patients with bladder exstrophy is approximately 50% shorter than that in normal age-matched controls[29]
- Distance between umbilicus and anus is foreshortened with anteriorly displaced anus
- Inguinal hernias are common (81.8% of boys and 10.5% of girls); attributed to a persistent processus vaginalis, large internal and external inguinal rings, and lack of obliquity of the inguinal canal[30,31]

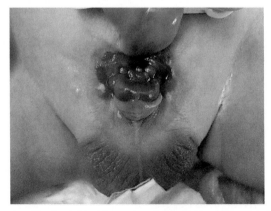

Fig. 2. Newborn male with classic bladder exstrophy and epispadias. Note the associated dorsal chordee, short urethral plate, and flattening of the scrotum. The umbilical clamp placed at the transferring facility was removed and the umbilical stump tied off with a silk suture.

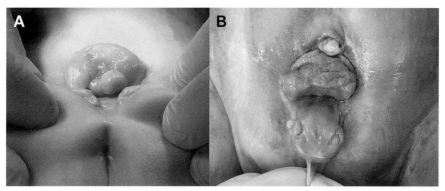

Fig. 3. (*A*) Newborn female with classic bladder exstrophy: note the bifid clitoral halves, divergent labia and mons pubis as well as anterior displacement of the anus. (*B*) Newborn male: note the short, exposed urethral plate.

- There is palpable diastasis of symphysis pubis with external rotation of the pelvis, retroversion of the acetabulum, and 30% shortening of pubic rami[32]

Imaging/Additional Testing

- Pelvic and hip plain films
- Renal-bladder ultrasound scan; although the upper urinary tract is usually normal, anomalous development does occur and horseshoe kidney, pelvic kidney, hypoplastic kidney, solitary kidney, and dysplasia with megaureter have been reported[6]

Management

- Children with bladder exstrophy should be treated at tertiary care centers with availability of experienced pediatric urology and pediatric orthopedic surgery teams
- Umbilical cord should be tied off with 2-0 silk close to the abdominal wall to prevent the umbilical clamp from traumatizing the delicate mucosa causing excoriation of the bladder surface
- Bladder should be covered with a nonadherent film of plastic wrap (ie, Saran Wrap) to prevent sticking of the bladder mucosa to clothing or diapers; each time the diaper is changed, the plastic wrap should be removed, the bladder surface irrigated with sterile saline, and clean plastic wrap placed over the bladder surface
- Infants should be placed on urinary tract infection prophylaxis secondary to vesicoureteral reflux
- A range of surgical techniques (complete vs staged repairs) have been used to achieve successful primary bladder closure with or without pelvic osteotomies[33,34]
- After osteotomy, 4 to 6 weeks of postoperative pelvic and lower extremity immobilization with either modified Buck's traction or spica casting (**Fig. 4**) is required[35]
- Early bladder closure within 72 hours was advocated in the past; more recently, delayed primary closure had comparable outcomes.[36,37]

Summary

The most important predictor of long-term bladder growth and continence is successful primary bladder closure.[38–40] Size and quality of bladder template, extent of pubic

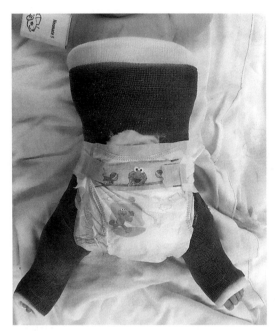

Fig. 4. Spica casting allows for immobilization of pelvis postoperatively without the use of external fixators or traction.

diastasis and urethral plate measurements affect timing and type of repair. Pelvic osteotomy and postoperative immobilization are found to decrease the rate of failed bladder closure (ie, wound dehiscence, bladder prolapsed or formation of vesicocutaneous fistula), highlighting the importance of a combined urologic and orthopedic repair.[41,42] After closure, children should be maintained on prophylactic antibiotics and require close urologic follow-up. Long-term outcome of classic bladder exstrophy is quite good, with preservation of renal and sexual function, achievement of normal-appearing abdominal wall and genitalia, and urinary continence rates approaching 80%.[6] Some children with small-capacity bladders and persistent incontinence may require adjunctive measures, including bladder augmentation.

CLOACAL EXSTROPHY

Cloacal exstrophy is a complex abdominal wall defect thought to result from a mesodermal abnormality with premature rupture of the cloacal membrane before complete descent of the urorectal septum.[6] It is commonly referred to as the omphalocele, exstrophy of the bladder, imperforate anus, and spinal abnormalities (OEIS) complex.[43] Cloacal exstrophy is accurately diagnosed with prenatal ultrasound scan in up to 50% of cases and can be confirmed with fetal MRI.[21,26,44] An incidence of 1 in 200,000 to 400,000 births makes cloacal exstrophy one of the rarest urologic anomalies, and it is one of the most severe congenital anomalies compatible with life.[45,46] Gastrointestinal abnormalities can be a source of significant morbidity.[47] Management of cloacal exstrophy requires a multidisciplinary team–based approach, with the principal goals of treatment focusing on patient function, psychosocial development, and overall quality of life.[48]

Patient History/Physical Examination

- Ileocecal and bladder exstrophy with associated omphalocele, hindgut remnant and imperforate anus is the most common presentation (**Fig. 5**)
- Omphaloceles may contain portions of the small bowel or liver (**Fig. 6**)
- Complete separation or absence of the phallic or clitoral halves may be observed; the scrotum or labia are also widely divided (see **Fig. 5**)
- In boys, the testes are frequently undescended and associated with bilateral inguinal hernias; in association with the diminutive phallus, boys often are declared to have ambiguous genitalia
- In girls, vaginal duplication and vaginal agenesis are common findings
- Pelvic deformity is characterized by widened pubic diastasis; scoliosis and kyphosis may also be noted[49]

Imaging/Additional Testing

- Baseline renal function and electrolyte and hematologic studies should be obtained
- Karyotyping can be performed if gender has not been determined previously or is not obvious on examination
- Plain films of the chest, spine, and pelvis; pelvic deformities are similar to those seen in classic bladder exstrophy, but are more pronounced in cloacal exstrophy[48]
- Renal ultrasound should be obtained; abnormalities of the upper urinary tract such as unilateral renal agenesis, pelvic kidney, hydronephrosis, horseshoe kidney and fusion anomalies have been reported in 41% to 66% of patients[45,50]
- Spinal ultrasound scan or MRI should be obtained to assess neurospinal defects; some form of spinal dysraphism is present in most patients[51,52]

Management

- Immediately after stabilization of the newborn, the exposed organs/mucosal surfaces should be protected by enclosing the infant's lower torso in a bowel bag or by applying saline followed by nonadherent plastic wrap; this aids in prevention of evaporative losses, trauma, and infection[53]
- Consultation should be obtained with pediatric urology, surgery, neurosurgery, and orthopedic surgery for operative planning

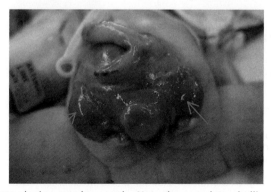

Fig. 5. Cloacal exstrophy in a newborn male. Note the complete phallic separation, exstrophy of the terminal ileum between the 2 halves of the bladder (bladder plates designated with *arrows*), rudimentary hindgut, imperforate anus, and the presence of an omphalocele.

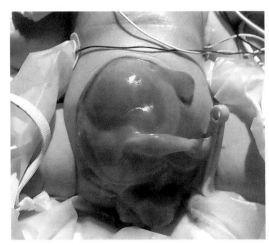

Fig. 6. Newborn female with cloacal exstrophy. Note the presence of the liver within the large omphalocele. This child also had a myelomeningocele, fulfilling criteria for OEIS complex (omphalocele, exstrophy, imperforate anus, spinal defects).

- Once the initial evaluation is complete, discussion should be had with the parents regarding gender assignment, surgical correction, possible functional deficits, and overall expected quality of life[48,53]
- Immediate closure of the omphalocele defect in the newborn period (within 48–72 hours) is advised to prevent subsequent rupture; the cecal plate is separated from the bladder plates and tubularized; a colostomy or ileostomy is created with preservation of the hindgut[48,51,54]
- Initial bladder management includes first stage approximation (**Fig. 7**) versus primary repair; dependent on multiple anatomic variables, including size of bladder plates and associated spinal defects[55,56]

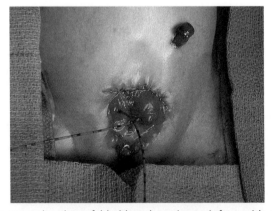

Fig. 7. First-stage approximation of bladder plates in an infant with cloacal exstrophy, essentially converting the bladder deformity to a classic bladder exstrophy. The ureteral orifices are cannulated with 3F feeding tubes bilaterally. Also note the ileostomy and closure of the omphalocele.

Summary

Cloacal exstrophy is a rare and challenging diagnosis that requires a multidisciplinary management team. Quality-of-life issues predominate in children born with cloacal exstrophy, as surgical and medical advances have led to a dramatic improvement in survival. Parents often require extensive counseling. Cloacal exstrophy patients generally require multiple surgical procedures and face a host of medical and psychosocial challenges.

PERSISTENT CLOACA

Persistent cloaca is along the spectrum of anorectal malformations and presents in girls as a single perineal orifice. The vagina, urethra, and rectum are fused together inside the pelvis, creating a single common channel that emerges where the urethra typically opens. Persistent cloaca is rare, with an incidence of 1 in 50,000 births and accounts for approximately 10% of anorectal malformations.[57] Cloacal anomalies can be diagnosed on prenatal ultrasonography and should be considered in any female fetus presenting with bilateral hydronephrosis, poorly visualized bladder, and a cystic mass secondary to hydrometrocolpos arising in the pelvis.[58] Potential confusion of the bladder with the hydrocolpos when the bladder is either empty or compressed by the mass can lead to misdiagnosis prenatally. Surgical reconstruction represents a significant technical challenge, with goals to achieve urinary control, bowel control, menstrual function, sexual function, and obstetric potential.[59]

Patient History/Physical Examination

- Single perineal orifice is seen in a girl with imperforate anus (**Fig. 8**)
- Appearance of the external genitalia can range from normal female appearance to ambiguous with a phallic urogenital sinus opening
- Abdominal distention may be severe secondary to hydrometrocolpos and bladder and intestinal distention; hydrometrocolpos is present in 50% of cases[60]
- Lower back should be carefully examined to identify any evidence of spinal cord abnormalities (ie, sacral dimple, hair patch, or area of abnormal pigmentation, bone abnormality), as this anomaly exists in the VACTERL spectrum (vertebral, anorectal, cardiac, tracheoesophageal, renal, and limb)

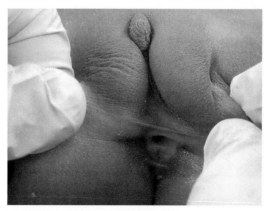

Fig. 8. Young female with persistent cloaca. Note the single perineal opening (representing confluence of the rectum, vagina, and urethra) and clitoromegaly and lack of labia minora.

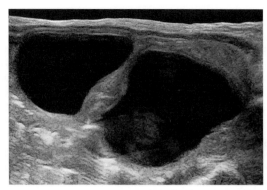

Fig. 9. Pelvic ultrasound scan of a newborn female with hydrometrocolpos. Note the bladder anteriorly, and the markedly distended vagina posteriorly. Principal ultrasound findings of hydrocolpos include an anechoic pelvic mass with or without a sagittal septum, located behind a normal bladder.

Imaging/Additional Testing

- Plain abdominal film should be obtained; pelvic mass may be obvious; retrograde flow of urine and meconium may result in the classic linear calcifications
- Abdominal ultrasonography is very important to visualize not only the pelvic anatomy but also the kidneys because hydronephrosis is common; hydronephrosis is usually related to hydrocolpos, with the distended vagina (**Fig. 9**) compressing the bladder neck and resulting in varying degrees of bladder outlet obstruction[61]
- Spinal ultrasound should be obtained
- Echocardiogram should be obtained to detect structural cardiac defects before general anesthesia; 13% of girls with cloacal anomalies have cardiovascular abnormalities[4,62]
- Genitography (filling the entire bladder, urethra, vagina, and sinus with contrast) provides anatomic detail[4]

Management

- Nasogastric tube should be used to decompress the bowel and rule out esophageal atresia[62]
- Diversion of gastrointestinal tract should be done by pediatric surgery (protective colostomy); definitive surgery is planned when the infant is older and the anatomy of the defect clearly defined
- At the time of colostomy formation, it is useful to perform endoscopy of the common channel to determine its length and to assess internal vaginal and urethral anatomy
- In some patients, it may be necessary to create more effective drainage of the urinary tract via a suprapubic catheter in the bladder or hydrocolpos; vesicostomy is considered in girls with impaired renal function[63–65]

Summary

Persistent cloaca remains a reconstructive challenge with the goal of future bladder and bowel continence and normal sexual function in adulthood. In the neonatal period, management includes a diverting colostomy, endoscopy to further delineate anatomy, and urinary tract drainage when necessary.

REFERENCES

1. Mandell J, Blyth BR, Peters CA, et al. Structural genitourinary defects detected in utero. Radiology 1991;178:193–6.
2. Carrera JM, Torrents M, Mortera C, et al. Routine prenatal ultrasound screening for fetal abnormalities: 22 years' experience. Ultrasound Obstet Gynecol 1995; 5:174–9.
3. Moore K, Persaud T. The developing human. 5th edition. Philadelphia: WB Saunders; 1995. p. 199–200.
4. Rink RC, Kaefer M. Surgical management of disorders of sexual differentiation, cloacal malformation, and other abnormalities of the genitalia in girls. In: Wein AJ, Kavoussi LR, Novick AC, et al, editors. Campbell-Walsh Urology. 10th edition. Philadelphia: Saunders; 2011. p. 3629–66.
5. Frimberger DC, Kropp BP. Bladder anomalies in children. In: Wein AJ, Kavoussi LR, Novick AC, et al, editors. Campbell-Walsh Urology. 10th edition. Philadelphia: Saunders; 2011. p. 3379–88.
6. Gearhart JP, Mathews RI. Exstrophy-epispadias complex. In: Wein AJ, Kavoussi LR, Novick AC, et al, editors. Campbell-Walsh Urology. 10th edition. Philadelphia: Saunders; 2011. p. 3325–84.
7. Galati V, Donovan B, Ramji F, et al. Management of urachal remnants in early childhood. J Urol 2008;180:1824–7.
8. Mesrobian HG, Zacharias A, Balcom AH, et al. Ten years of experience with isolated urachal anomalies in children. J Urol 1997;158:1316–8.
9. Ashley RA, Inman BA, Routh JC, et al. Urachal anomalies: a longitudinal study of urachal remnants in children and adults. J Urol 2007;178:1615–8.
10. Matsui F, Matsumoto F, Shimada K. Prenatally diagnosed patent urachus with bladder prolapse. J Pediatr Surg 2007;42:e7–10.
11. Fuchs F, Picone O, Levaillant JM, et al. Prenatal diagnosis of a patent urachus cyst with the use of 2D, 3D, 4D ultrasound and fetal magnetic resonance imaging. Fetal Diagn Ther 2008;24:444–7.
12. Cilento BG, Bauer SB, Retik AB, et al. Urachal anomalies: defining the best diagnostic modality. Urology 1998;52:120–2.
13. Razvi S, Murphy R, Shlasko E, et al. Delayed separation of the umbilical cord attributable to urachal anomalies. Pediatrics 2001;108:493–4.
14. Schiesser M, Lapaire O, Holzgraeve W, et al. Umbilical cord edema associated with patent urachus. Ultrasound Obstet Gynecol 2003;22:646–7.
15. Ozel SK, Kazez A, Akpolat N. An unusual presentation of a patent urachus: report of a case. Eur J Pediatr Surg 2004;14:206–8.
16. DiSantis DJ, Siegal MJ, Katz ME. Simplified approach to umbilical remnant abnormalities. Radiographics 1991;11:59–66.
17. Durakbasa CU, Okur H, Mutus HM, et al. Symptomatic omphalomesenteric duct remnants in children. Pediatr Int 2010;52:480–4.
18. Zieger B, Sokol B, Rohrscheider WK, et al. Sonomorphology and involution of the normal urachus in asymptomatic newborns. Pediatr Radiol 1998;28: 156–61.
19. Cuda SP, Vanasupa BP, Sutherland RS. Nonoperative management of a patent urachus. Urology 2005;66:1320.e7–9.
20. Khurana S, Borzi PA. Laparoscopic management of complicated urachal disease in children. J Urol 2002;168:1526–8.
21. Gambhir L, Holler T, Muller M, et al. Epidemiological survey of 214 families with bladder-exstrophy-epispadias complex. J Urol 2008;179:1539–43.

22. Nelson CP, Dunn RL, Wei JT. Contemporary epidemiology of bladder exstrophy in the United States. J Urol 2005;173:1728–31.

23. Gearhart JP, Ben-Chaim J, Jeffs RD, et al. Criteria for the prenatal diagnosis of classic bladder exstrophy. Obstet Gynecol 1995;85:961–4.

24. Mirk P, Calisti A, Fileni A. Prenatal sonographic diagnosis of bladder exstrophy. J Ultrasound Med 1986;5:291–3.

25. Clayton DB, Brock JW 3rd. Prenatal ultrasound and urologic anomalies. Pediatr Clin North Am 2012;59:739–56.

26. Goyal A, Fishwick J, Hurrell R, et al. Antenatal diagnosis of bladder/cloacal exstrophy: challenges and possible solutions. J Pediatr Urol 2012;8:140–4.

27. Hsieh K, O'Loughlin MT, Ferrer FA. Bladder exstrophy and phenotypic gender determination on fetal magnetic resolution imaging. Urology 2005; 65:998–9.

28. Goldman S, Szejnfeld PO, Rondon A. Prenatal diagnosis of bladder exstrophy by fetal MRI. J Pediatr Urol 2013;9:3–6.

29. Silver RI, Yang A, Ben-Chaim J, et al. Penile length in adulthood after exstrophy reconstruction. J Urol 1997;158:999–1003.

30. Connolly JA, Peppas DS, Jeffs RD, et al. Prevalence in repair of inguinal hernia in children with bladder exstrophy. J Urol 1995;154:1900–1.

31. Husmann DA, McLorie GA, Churchill BM, et al. Inguinal pathology and its association with classical bladder exstrophy. J Pediatr Surg 1990;25:332–4.

32. Sponseller PD, Bisson LJ, Gearhart JP, et al. The anatomy of the pelvis in the exstrophy complex. J Bone Joint Surg Am 1995;77:177–89.

33. Grady RW, Mitchell ME. Complete primary repair of exstrophy: surgical technique. Urol Clin North Am 2000;27:569–78.

34. Phillips TM, Gearhart JP. Primary closure of bladder exstrophy. BJU Int 2009; 104:1308–22.

35. Inouye BM, Massanyi EZ, Di Carlo H, et al. Modern management of bladder exstrophy repair. Curr Urol Rep 2013;14:359–65.

36. Baradaran N, Cervellione RM, Stec AA. Gearhart JPDelayed primary repair of bladder exstrophy: ultimate effect on growth. J Urol 2012;188:2336–41.

37. Ferrara F, Dickson AP, Fishwick J, et al. Delayed exstrophy repair (DER) does not compromise initial bladder development. J Pediatr Urol 2014;10:506–10. pii:S1477-5131(13) 00322-7.

38. Novak TE, Costello JP, Orosco R, et al. Failed exstrophy closure: management and outcome. J Pediatr Urol 2010;6:381–4.

39. Baradaran N, Cervellione RM, Orosco R, et al. Effect of failed initial closure on bladder growth in children with bladder exstrophy. J Urol 2011;186:1450–4.

40. Oesterling JE, Jeffs RD. The importance of a successful initial bladder closure in the surgical management of classical bladder exstrophy: analysis of 144 patients treated at the Johns Hopkins Hospital between 1975 and 1985. J Urol 1987;137:258–62.

41. Meldrum KK, Baird AD, Gearhart JP. Pelvic and extremity immobilization after bladder exstrophy closure: complications and impact on success. Urology 2003;62:1109–13.

42. Arlen AM, Cooper CS, Morcuende J, et al. Safety and efficacy of spica casts for immobilization following initial bladder closure in classic bladder exstrophy. J Pediatr Urol 2011;7:456–9.

43. Carey JC, Greenbaum B, Hall BD. The OEIS complex (omphalocele, exstrophy, imperforate anus, spinal defects). Birth Defects Orig Artic Ser 1978;15: 253–63.

44. Calvo-Garcia MA, Kline-Fath BM, Rubio EI, et al. Fetal MRI of cloacal exstrophy. Pediatr Radiol 2013;43:593–604.
45. Hurwitz RS, Manzoni GA, Ransley PG, et al. Cloacal exstrophy: a report of 34 cases. J Urol 1987;138:1060–4.
46. Martinez-Frias ML, Bermejo E, Rodriquez-Pinilla E, et al. Exstropy of the cloaca and exstrophy of the bladder: two different expressions of a primary developmental field defect. Am J Med Genet 2001;99:261–9.
47. Davidoff AM, Hebra A, Balmer D, et al. Management of the gastrointestinal tract and nutrition in patients with cloacal exstrophy. J Pediatr Surg 1996;31:768–70.
48. Phillips TM. Spectrum of cloacal exstrophy. Semin Pediatr Surg 2011;20:113–8.
49. Loder RT, Dayioglu MM. Association of congenital vertebral malformations with bladder and cloacal exstrophy. J Pediatr Orthop 1990;10:389–93.
50. Diamond DA, Jeffs RD. Cloacal exstrophy: a 22-year experience. J Urol 1985; 133:779–82.
51. Lund DP, Hendren WH. Cloacal exstrophy: a 25-year experience with 50 cases. J Pediatr Surg 2001;36:68–75.
52. McHoney M, Ransley PG, Duffy P, et al. Cloacal exstrophy: morbidity associated with abnormalities of the gastrointestinal tract and spine. J Pediatr Surg 2004; 39:1209–13.
53. Woo LL, Thomas JC, Borck JW 3rd. Cloacal exstrophy: a comprehensive review of an uncommon problem. J Pediatr Urol 2010;6:102–11.
54. Ricketts RR, Woodard JR, Zwiren GT, et al. Modern treatment of cloacal exstrophy. J Pediatr Surg 1991;26:444–8.
55. Smith EA, Woodard JR, Broecker BH, et al. Current urologic management of cloacal exstrophy: experience with 11 patients. J Pediatr Surg 1997;32:256–61.
56. Thomas JC, DeMarco RT, Pope JC 4th, et al. First stage approximation of the exstrophic bladder in patients with cloacal exstrophy-should this be the initial surgical approach in all patients? J Urol 2007;178:1632–6.
57. Brock WA, Pena A. Cloacal abnormalities and imperforate anus. In: Kelais PP, Belman AB, King L, editors. Clinical pediatric urology. 3rd edition. Philadelphia: Saunders; 1992. p. 920–42.
58. Winkler NS, Kennedy AM, Woodward PJ. Cloacal malformation: embryology, anatomy, and prenatal imaging features. J Ultrasound Med 2012;31:1843–55.
59. Levitt MA, Bischoff A, Pena A. Pitfalls and challenges of cloaca repair: how to reduce the need for reoperations. J Pediatr Surg 2011;46:1250–5.
60. Levitt MA, Pena A. Pitfalls in the management of new cloaca. Pediatr Surg Int 2005;21:264–9.
61. Hendren WH. Cloaca, the most severe degree of imperforate anus: experience with 195 cases. Ann Surg 1998;228:331–46.
62. Warne SA, Hiorns MP, Curry J, et al. Understanding cloacal anomalies. Arch Dis Child 2011;96:1072–6.
63. Warne SA, Wilcox DT, Ransley PG. Long-term urological outcomes of patients presenting with persistent cloaca. J Urol 2002;168:1859–62.
64. Hendren WH. Urological aspects of cloacal malformations. J Urol 1988;140: 1207–13.
65. Alexander F, Kay R. Cloacal anomalies: role of vesicostomy. J Pediatr Surg 1994;29:74–6.

Abnormalities of the External Genitalia

Lauren Baldinger, DO, MS, Abhijith Mudegowdar, MD, Aseem R. Shukla, MD*

KEYWORDS

- External genitalia • Genital malformations • Penile anomalies • Scrotal anomalies
- Inguinal hernia • Hydrocele

KEY POINTS

- Perinatologists and neonatologists should recognize common malformations of the foreskin that preclude a neonatal circumcision, including the webbed penis, concealed penis, chordee, and hypospadias.
- A presumed male infant with bilateral nonpalpable gonads should undergo an evaluation to rule out congenital adrenal hyperplasia.
- An undescended testis is not expected to descend spontaneously after 4 months of age, so pediatric urology consultation should be sought.
- Perinatologists and neonatologists should endeavor to differentiate an inguinal hernia from a communicating hydrocele and scrotal hydrocele by understanding the relevance of the processus vaginalis.

ABNORMALITIES OF THE EXTERNAL GENITALIA

Concealed Penis and Trapped Penis

The term inconspicuous penis was coined by Bergeson and colleagues[1] in 1993. It described conditions in which the penis appears undersized and small. A small penile shaft referred to as a micropenis can be a cause of the inconspicuous penis and is defined as being less than 2 standard deviations of the average size for a given age group or a stretched penile length of less than 2 cm in a term male neonate.[2] However, more commonly, inconspicuous penis is caused by a congenital condition of surrounding tissue. In the latter, the penis is normal in size but concealed by adjacent tissue, skin, or adipose. These conditions include webbed penis or scrotal webbing, buried penis, and trapped penis. The inconspicuous penis can become a great concern for parents, and, of immediate significance, may proscribe a standard

Disclosures: None.
Division of Pediatric Urology, The Children's Hospital of Philadelphia, Perelman School of Medicine, University of Pennsylvania, 34th Street and Civic Center Boulevard, 3rd Floor Wood Building, Philadelphia, PA 19104, USA
* Corresponding author.
E-mail address: shuklaa@email.chop.edu

newborn circumcision. It is important to be able to help distinguish which cases need referrals for surgical management and which require reassurance.[3]

Scrotal webbing or webbed penis (**Figs. 1** and **2**) refers to skin from the scrotum being tethered to the ventral surface of the penile shaft or the penoscrotal junction being too close to the dorsum of the penile skin. The typical anatomy is that the superficial fascia of the penis along with the skin makes a well-defined penoscrotal angle on the ventral aspect of the penis below which the dartos fascia begins incorporating with more smooth muscle fibers. This fascia, then, is closely adherent to the skin of the scrotal wall, and, hence, if the penoscrotal angle is distorted because dartos fascia anchors the penile skin to the scrotal wall, scrotal webbing ensues. Often this is associated with other external genital abnormalities, and the physician must look for hypospadias, chordee, and a micropenis. This condition is corrected with surgical intervention and a newborn circumcision should be avoided.

A concealed penis encompasses the buried and trapped penis: one is a congenital condition; the other is an acquired condition. Maizels and colleagues[4] defined the hidden penis as a penis that is hidden below the preputial skin. The penis is retracted in and beneath the suprapubic fat in the case of an excessively fat prepubic area coming off the abdominal wall. Concealment also occurs because of weak anchoring of the superficial fascia and penile skin to the deeper fascia at the penile base. As a child grows, the excessive fat pad could diminish and the penis will become unburied, whereas in other cases, the buried penis requires surgical intervention because of fascial laxity.[5] If the scrotum is swollen secondary to a hernia or hydrocele, the penis can also look buried; resolution or correction of the scrotal pathologic abnormality will resolve this cause of a buried penis.

The acquired trapped penis (**Fig. 3**) results after circumcision, when the penile skin forms a circumferential distal scar and traps the penis below this scar. The incidence of trapped penis following neonatal circumcision is estimated to be 2.9%.[6] An overzealous circumcision or a circumcision performed without addressing scrotal webbing or scrotal swelling can result in a secondary phimosis causing a trapped penis. This condition can be troublesome, presenting with urinary tract infections, painful phimosis, and ballooning of the penis during urination. Often this can be corrected with topical steroid cream, but may need surgical correction if conservative management fails.

Abnormalities of penile curvature are a commonly encountered concern in the newborn. The 2 most common causes of penile curvature in the male newborn are penile torsion and chordee. Penile torsion is a congenital rotational defect of the penile

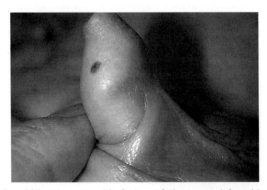

Fig. 1. Penoscrotal webbing is seen with fusion of the ventral foreskin with the scrotum causing a tethering effect.

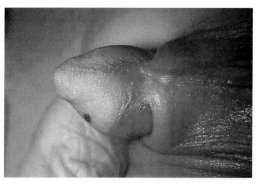

Fig. 2. Ventral view of penoscrotal webbing in same patient seen in **Fig. 1**.

shaft and it is almost always rotated in a counterclockwise fashion. It has been estimated to occur in isolation from other genital abnormalities in varying extents—ranging from 2% to 27% of newborns—but less than 1% of the time the penile is rotated more than 90°.[7,8] The rotation is often associated with other congenital abnormalities, such as hypospadias, and dorsal hooding with or without a urethral defect. If the rotation is less than 90°, no functional or physiologic significance has been reported. Correction is performed for cosmetic reasons.

Chordee

Up to 1 in 300 newborns are born with a hypospadias, and of those, up to one-fourth will have an associated penile curvature known as chordee (**Fig. 4**).[9] The true incidence is likely higher because chordee often occurs in the setting of a normal urethral meatus.[10] Surgical correction of penile curvature should take place within the first year of life. Chordee can result in psychosocial issues, painful intercourse, and difficulty with a straight urinary stream while standing.

When the foreskin is unable to be retracted over the glans due to a tight preputial ring, it is referred to as phimosis. Phimosis can be physiologic or acquired. At birth, approximately 96% of male newborns have a physiologic phimosis[11,12]; by 3 years of age, 90% of boys can retract their foreskin, and at age 17, less 1% of boys have difficulty retracting their foreskin. Preputial adhesions are common in younger boys,

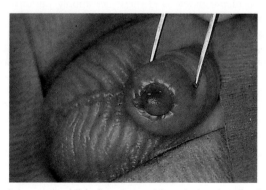

Fig. 3. Trapped penis is seen in child after circumcision. A cicatrix adhesion causes the glans to be trapped within the remaining shaft skin.

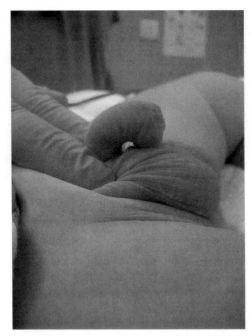

Fig. 4. Chordee of penis. Penis is noted to have a significant ventral curvature.

and this needs to be separated from true phimosis in which the foreskin is truly scarred or fibrotic in a concentric ring, known as a cicatrix. Phimosis may be the cause of urinary tract infections in young boys and this should be the first consideration to easily address in a boy presenting with a urinary tract infection. Poor hygiene may also result from phimosis and can lead to infections of the foreskin and glans, known as balanitis and balanoposthitis. Phimosis can be treated conservatively with topical steroids, and circumcision should be considered in rare situations where symptoms are recurrent, where phimosis is refractory, or there is strong family preference.

Circumcision

Circumcision is one of the oldest and most commonly performed surgical procedures.[13] It has been a ritual of religion and culture dating back to Biblical history.[14] Although the preponderance of circumcisions in the United States is completed due to family preference, clinical indications for performing a circumcision include phimosis refractory to medical therapy and recurrent urinary tract infections.[15–17] A recent meta-analysis by Morris and Wiswell[18] demonstrated a 23.3% lifetime chance of a urinary tract infection in uncircumcised men and boys. In addition, multiple reports and the American Academy of Pediatrics Task Force on Circumcision posit additional putative benefits of circumcision including protection from penile cancer and transmission of some sexually transmitted diseases, including the human immunodeficiency virus (see http://pediatrics.aappublications.org/content/130/3/585.full. html).[19,20] Despite all available clinical evidence, parents are empowered to make decisions regarding circumcision that is largely performed on an elective basis for cultural or cosmetic reasons. Like any other surgical procedure, circumcision carries identifiable risks, although profound disfigurement is exceedingly rare.

Multiple factors affect the complication rate, including medical comorbidities, patient age and size of the penis, surgical technique, and anatomic abnormalities. The perioperative rate of complications for in hospital circumcisions is reported at the low rate of 0.2% and can vary up toward more than 20% when performed outside of the hospital.[21] The most common complications are bleeding and local infection.[22] The timing of circumcision procedure can affect the complication rate. It has been shown that age and the rate of circumcision complications are directly proportional.[23] During the hormonal surge that begins around 4 weeks of life and lasts until 3 months of age, the risk of bleeding increases. The lower frequency of complications in neonates is likely related to the simpler nature of the procedure and the natural ability of the newborn to heal well.[22] Pain is also a factor to consider, and the first week of life is arguably a period of reduced pain sensitivity.[24] Still, the use of local anesthetic is recommended to be administered as a penile block injection in the penopubic space in all cases.

Complications can be divided into early and late complications and further subdivided into minor and serious adverse events. Early simple complications include local infection at the surgical site, bleeding, pain, and excess or inadequate amount of skin removal. Bleeding after a circumcision that is persistent is unusual, and when it occurs, is often a sentinel event leading to a clinical workup that may reveal a bleeding diathesis. Other early serious complications that injure the penis include creation of an iatrogenic hypospadias in the case where a ventral slit is performed rather than a dorsal slit, iatrogenic chordee if too much ventral skin is removed, and glanular necrosis or amputation depending of the method of circumcision performed. Pieretti and colleagues[25] reported on circumcision complications over a 5-year period at a single institution. They reported that 7.4% of all urology visits over a 1 year period were for concerns related to newborn circumcisions. Over the 5-year period, 424 procedures were performed to repair concerns related to newborn circumcisions. Late complications included thick skin bridges, preputial adhesions, buried penis, epidermal inclusion cysts, suture sinus, urethrocutaneous fistula (**Figs. 5** and **6**), meatal stenosis, chordee or penile torsion, and phimosis. Outpatient surgery can commonly correct all of these complications.

Proper patient selection and meticulous technique with attention to identifying certain anatomic variations and contraindications to circumcision are critical to avoiding many of the aforementioned complications. Circumcision should be delayed in any

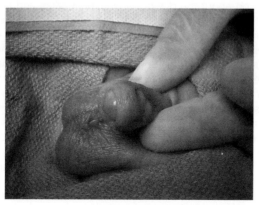

Fig. 5. A postcircumcision injury is seen with a visible urethrocutaneous fistula at the coronal incision line.

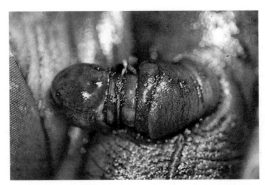

Fig. 6. A plastibell used for a newborn circumcision has created a tourniquet effect with necrosis of tissue visible under the plastic ring.

neonate that is premature with a small penis size or has a bleeding disorder, an abundant suprapubic fat pad, penoscrotal webbing, chordee, hypospadias, megameatus intact-prepuce, or any anatomic variation that may require the foreskin for reconstructive repair.

Labial Adhesions

In the prepubertal girl, labial adhesions are a common disorder of the external genitalia, usually occurring between 3 months and 6 years of age.[26] This finding is usually corrected by topical estrogen creams or by an in-office lysis of adhesions. The adhesions are usually asymptomatic and often detected by the parents or on physical examination. Although these adhesions are completely benign in the most cases, they can be a cause of skin rashes because of retained urine and urinary tract infections, emphasizing the importance of physical examination of the genitalia, including separating the labia minora in any female neonate with a urinary tract infection. Rarely, the labial adhesions can be associated with 21-hydroxylase deficiencies, and any case of persistent labial adhesions refractory to treatment should raise the question of ruling out a nonclassic case of congenital adrenal hyperplasia (CAH).

Hypospadias and CAH

A detailed discussion about the diagnosis of hypospadias and CAH is beyond the scope of this article, but recognizing the signs that should raise suspicion of further investigation is important.

Hypospadias refers to an abnormal development of the penis that leaves the urethral meatus proximal to its normal glanular position anywhere along the penile shaft, scrotum, or perineum. A spectrum of abnormalities, including ventral curvature of the penis (chordee), a hooded incomplete prepuce, and an abortive corpus spongiosum, are commonly associated with hypospadias (**Fig. 7**). A unifying cause of hypospadias remains elusive and is likely multifactorial. The hypospadiac anatomy appears consistent with incomplete embryologic development because of (1) abnormal androgen production by the fetal testis, (2) limited androgen sensitivity in target tissues of the developing genitalia, or (3) premature cessation of androgenic stimulation due to early atrophy of the Leydig cells of the testes.[27]

In 1997, 2 independent surveillance systems in United States, the nationwide Birth Defects Monitoring Program (BDMP) and the Metropolitan Atlanta Congenital Defects Program (MACDP), reported a nearly doubling of the rate of hypospadias when

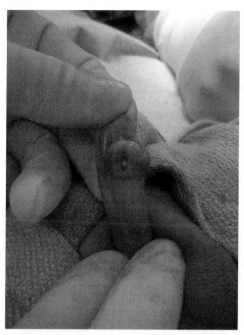

Fig. 7. Coronal hypospadias with the appearance of a coronal, stenotic meatus and dorsal hood prepuce.

compared with immediately preceding decades.[28] The incidence of all types of hypospadias increased from 20.2 to 39.7 per 10,000 live male births during the period from 1970 to 1993 (ie, 1 in every 250 live male births was a boy with hypospadias [measured by BDMP]). MACDP reported an increase in rate of severe hypospadia of between 3-fold and 5-fold. These rising trends, however, may reflect earlier diagnosis or an increase in reporting to registries of congenital defects. The increased reporting of more proximal than distal hypospadias cases, however, refutes the argument that these findings represent more frequent reporting of minor cases, and changes in the environment affecting maternal ingestion such as various endocrine disruptors may also play a role.[29]

Evaluation of hypospadias requires an understanding that the abnormal dorsal prepuce and ventral glans tilt often herald the presence of a hypospadias if close examination is performed. A proximally displaced urethral orifice that is often stenotic in appearance may be noted. In approximately 6% of all cases, the prepuce may be intact and diagnosis is rendered after the prepuce is retracted at time of neonatal circumcision. In such cases, the circumcision may be completed if the hypospadias is very mild and the meatus is located on the glans.[27] If there is any question of meatal location, stop after the dorsal slit has commenced to leave adequate prepucial skin for reconstructive surgery.

The location of the meatus and extent of ventral curvature, or chordee, should always be determined, realizing that often multiple pinpoint dimples may be present on the surface of the urethral plate in addition to the hypospadiac meatus. It is important to recognize that in such cases, the most proximal dimple represents the actual urethral meatus. Although 80% of hypospadias cases will be milder variants of distal hypospadias, the 20% of proximal hypospadias cases comprise the cohort of very challenging reconstructive cases for the pediatric urologist.[30,31]

For CAH, the classic presentation is that of a neonate with evidence of an enlarged clitoral structure with labial fusion and labioscrotal folds. In more extensively virilized forms, there may be the appearance of a normal penis with or without hypospadias (**Fig. 8**). The indication that workup should commence for a normal-appearing male infant is the absence of any palpable gonads, severe perineal hypospadias with an undescended testis, or when the phenotypic appearance fails to match a 46,XX karyotype based on amniocentesis obtained in some cases. For an assumed female neonate, workup should proceed based on the clitoral hypertrophy and labioscrotal fusion.

CAH occurs because of a deficiency in the enzyme 21-hydroxylase that is critical in the production of cortisol and aldosterone along the cholesterol biosynthesis pathway. With the deficient enzyme, 17-hydroxyprogesterone, one of the progenitors of cortisol is elevated. The adrenal cortex then fails to produce cortisol, forcing the pituitary to compensate by raising ACTH levels that cause skin pigmentation.

The serum 17-hydroxyprogesterone should be obtained immediately, while the serum electrolytes, blood glucose, and karyotype should be checked to rule out a salt-wasting form of CAH. The 21-hydroxylase deficiency affects approximately 1:14,000 live births and is the most common cause of CAH, affecting up to 95% of patients with CAH. A female neonate with 21-hydroxylase deficiency has a 75% chance of being a salt-waster and delayed diagnosis may be fatal in those cases after the first week of life as serum potassium increases, and a decrease in sodium drives down the blood pressure, consistent with an adrenal crisis.

The evaluation and management of a newborn with ambiguous genitalia must be tackled with great sensitivity and urgency. It requires a multidisciplinary team of specialists including pediatrics, urology, endocrinology, genetics, and psychiatry to care for the child with a disorder of sex development such as CAH.

CRYPTORCHIDISM

An undescended testis is a common disorder with an endocrine cause in boys.[32] Cryptorchidism is bilateral in one-third and unilateral in two-thirds of presenting infants.[33] Cryptorchidism is considered a significant neonatal morbidity because the

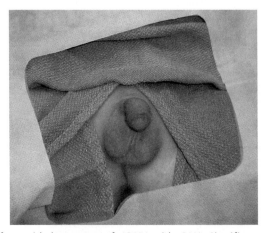

Fig. 8. Female infant with karyotype of 46,XX with CAH. Significant virilization of the clitoris is seen with fusion of labioscrotal folds.

long-term consequences on fertility and increased risk of testicular malignancy necessitate careful evaluation and prompt referral to a pediatric urologist.

Cryptorchidism is a developmental defect marked by the failure of the testes to descend into the scrotum, which is the normal anatomic location. The urologist will be faced with distinguishing whether a suspected nonpalpable testis is present at all or is what is termed a vanishing testis. The neonatologist will also be tasked with determining whether an undescended testis is truly absent from the scrotum or is palpable somewhere along the inguinal canal.

The incidence of cryptorchidism is estimated at 3% in full-term boys and up to 45% in preterm neonates. Because the testis will descend within the first few months of life, the 3% incidence decreases to 1% by 3 months of age.[34] According to the embryology of testis development and descent, testicular descent is known to occur after the 28th week of development. After birth, descent may continue for the first 3 months of life because of the normal gonadotropin surge that occurs around 60 to 90 days of life. For this reason, testicular descent in a child with cryptorchidism should not be expected after 4 months of age and surgical referral is recommended.

The pathogenesis of isolated cryptorchidism without other congenital abnormalities remains largely unknown, although it is likely multifactorial with genetic, hormonal, and environmental risk factors. Perinatal risk factors include prematurity, low birth weight, maternal diabetes, advanced maternal age, and breech presentation.[35,36] Schnack and colleagues[37] reviewed more than 1 million male births and demonstrated that risk ratios for cryptorchidism were 10.1 in twins, 3.5 in brothers, and 2.3 in offspring of fathers who have an undescended testis.[38] The presence of a hypospadias is associated with cryptorchidism in 12% to 24% of cases.[39]

In cases of a nonpalpable testis, the testis may be in a "peeping" or abdominal location 25% to 50% of the time; a "vanishing" testis, which is a completely atrophied testis, in 15% to 40% of cases; and an extra-abdominal location hidden by fat or examiner error in another 10% to 30% of boys.[40–42]

Testicular examination in infants and young children requires experience and should always use a 2-handed technique. Hrebinko and Bellinger[43] found that an experienced pediatric urologist may find a testis in 30% of cases where another practitioner was unable to render a diagnosis.[43] The child is placed in a supine position in a warm environment to minimize the cremasteric reflex, which will cause retraction of the testes. During the examination, it is important to note the ability to palpate a testis, the position, mobility, size, and any associated findings such as a hernia, hydrocele, penile size, and urethral meatus position. One hand starts with a stroke from the anterior iliac spine along the inguinal canal in the direction of the pubic bone, while the other hand attempts to palpate the testis. Wetting or lubricating the hand will help in identifying the testicle. Often the examiner will note an ability to locate the testicle and milk it down toward the direction of the scrotum. Differentiating between a retractile testis and an undescended testis occurs during the physical examination. A testis is retractile if the testis can be brought down to the scrotum and stays there without tension, but quickly retracts once the child moves. A gliding testis is one that can be brought down to the scrotum on palpation, but does not rest in the scrotum at all and feels attached to the inguinal canal. Finally, an ascending testis is one that was clearly felt within the scrotum at one point in time, but gradually ascended as the child experienced linear skeletal growth.

In boys with bilateral undescended testis or a boy with associated abnormalities including hypospadias, further testing is warranted. A chromosomal and endocrinologic evaluation may be performed after a multidisciplinary team discussion has been conducted with the family. When bilateral testes are noted and the male infant is less than 3 months of age, determining whether or not the testes or a testis is present can be done by checking serum luteinizing hormone (LH), follicle-stimulating hormone (FSH), and mullerian inhibiting substance (MIS) levels. Lee and colleagues[44] found that serum MIS correlates with the presence of testicular tissue; a measurable value of MIS is predictive of an undescended testis. The postnatal testosterone surge will be absent in a patient with anorchia. After 3 months of age, the human chorionic gonadotropin (hCG) stimulation test is used to determine the presence of an intra-abdominal testis. If testis tissue is present, an increase in testosterone will be seen after a weight-based single injection of hCG is administered. A failure to respond to the stimulation test and elevated FSH and LH levels are consistent with anorchia.[45–47] For the typical boy with a unilateral undescended testis, no further laboratory testing is necessary.

Imaging studies may aid in locating an undescended testis; however, studies have shown that they often do not affect treatment decisions, and a physical examination by an experienced physician is superior. A diagnostic laparoscopy has a higher yield for finding an intra-abdominally located testicle compared with imaging studies. Magnetic resonance imaging (MRI) is useful in identifying ectopic testes.[48] The cost of MRI and the need for sedation make it a less desirable test owing to the need for examination under anesthesia, and subsequent laparoscopy and inguinal exploration will still be required to confirm the presence of an undescended testicle.

Treatment of the undescended testis can be medical or surgical. The use of hormone therapy is more widely used in Europe than in the United States, where the mainstay of treatment is surgical. Hormonal treatment using gonadotropin-releasing hormone and hCG is most successful when the undescended testis is low in the distal inguinal region. Lala and colleagues[49] reported a success rate of 38% for testicular descent after combined treatment. Several meta-analyses of the published literature suggest that the effectiveness of hormonal therapy for the treatment of cryptorchidism is less than 20%.[50,51] A recent consensus statement discourages the use of hormonal therapy for cryptorchidism.[52]

Surgical therapy to bring the testicle into the scrotum is performed to achieve the prevention of ongoing thermal damage to the testis, treat the associated hernia, prevent testicular torsion, and allow easy palpation of the testicle for monthly examinations and for a good cosmetic result. The surgical steps are beyond the scope of this article, but it is important for the neonatologist and pediatrician to understand the different surgical options available. The standard inguinal orchidopexy is performed for the palpable testis. A primary scrotal approach can be offered to patients that have a palpable testicle close to the scrotum or one that is easily drawn into the scrotum. For the nonpalpable testis, surgical exploration can occur through an extended inguinal incision, an abdominal incision, or by diagnostic laparoscopy.

Parents are often concerned about future fertility. In patients who have an orchiopexy at an early age, abnormalities in semen quality is common; however, 90% of boys with unilateral cryptorchidism and 65% with bilateral cryptorchidism will achieve paternity.[53,54] Parents also must be counseled that every boy who has undergone an orchiopexy for an undescended testis must perform self-testicular examinations due to the elevated, although still overall low, risk of testicular cancer.

HERNIA AND HYDROCELE

The communicating hydrocele and inguinal hernia (**Fig. 9**) occur in neonates because of failure of the processus vaginalis to obliterate after the descent of the testis through it. In contrast to the direct inguinal hernias seen in adults, the infant hernia is directly

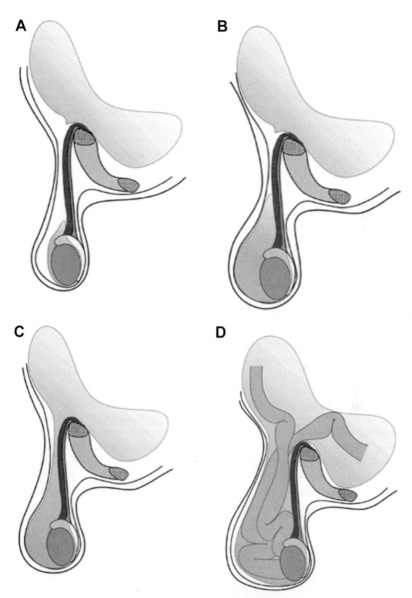

Fig. 9. Illustration depicts the normal inguinoscrotal anatomy along with variations of hydrocele and hernia that result from a patent processus vaginalis, which has failed to obliterate after the descent of testis through it. (*A*) Schematic representation of normal anatomy of spermatic cord and inguinal canal. (*B*) Collection of fluid around testis in tunica vaginalis without patency of processus vaginalis constitutes scrotal hydrocele. (*C*) Communicating hydrocele is seen with patency of processus vaginalis. (*D*) Herniation of bowel loops into scrotum in an inguinal hernia. (*Courtesy of* [*D*] P. Gleich, MD, Minneapolis, MN.)

linked to descent of the developing gonad. The processus vaginalis is first seen as an outpouching of the peritoneal cavity in the third month of gestation, but obliterates after the testis descends to the scrotum after the seventh month. Shortly after descent of testis, sometime in the first few months of life, most of the processus gradually obliterates except the terminal portion around the testis, which persists as the tunica vaginalis.[55] The tunica normally contains a small amount of fluid and invests the testis on almost all sides in the scrotum, forming an important covering and a protective layer for the testis. Hydrocele and hernia occur as a variation of this theme itself whereby a part of processus vaginalis remains behind. The caliber of the patent processus determines whether a hernia or a hydrocele will manifest. A small-caliber channel allows only peritoneal fluid to seep through, leading to a communicating hydrocele, while a larger defect allows intra-abdominal viscera to migrate, manifesting as an inguinal hernia.[56]

Inguinal hernia (**Fig. 10**) is documented to occur in close to 5% of all children; the incidence is higher in neonates and infants.[57] The incidence of pediatric inguinal hernia is highest during the first year of life and then gradually decreases thereafter. One-third of children undergoing surgery for hernia are less than 6 months of age and premature infants have an even higher risk of developing inguinal hernia with reports of incidence of up to 25%.[58] Incidence of hernia is 6 times more common in boys than in girls, and the sex ratio has been reported to vary from 3:1 to 10:1.[55] This increased ratio is possibly related to descent of testis through the inguinal canals in male infants.

The hernia or communicating hydrocele presents as a swelling in the inguinal or scrotal area. Neonatal hernias have a dramatic appearance and may be easily visible with peristaltic waves seen passing through the obvious inguinal swelling. The presentation may also be intermittent in nature, and a history will elicit increased swelling when the infant cries, coughs, grunts, or strains during bowel movements. At other times, the scrotum may even appear normal. Significant pain signifies onset of complications such as incarceration or strangulation.

Examination for hernia requires patience and involvement to keep the small child engaged. Hands are warmed as well as the ambient temperature in the room. Clinically, in a child with an evident hernia, a smooth soft mass would be seen emerging from external ring, which lies cephalad and lateral to pubic tubercle. This mass would be seen to enlarge when the child strains, cries, or coughs. In the case of an uncooperative child or in the preverbal age, straining can be induced by one of many techniques to elicit hernia. A communicating hydrocele will appear differently than an inguinal hernia to the extent that fluid will be felt and, transilluminated if necessary, within the scrotum. In a communicating hydrocele, compression of the scrotum will

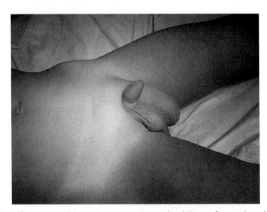

Fig. 10. Child with left inguinal hernia seen as a palpable, soft, and reducible mass within the left hemiscrotum.

result in the compression of fluid out of the scrotum, and retrograde flow of the hydrocele fluid through the processus vaginalis and back into the peritoneal cavity.

In cases of less apparent swelling or communicating hydroceles, a hernia may be suspected only on the basis of history but cannot be demonstrated on examination in the outpatient setting. If the history is classical and the referring pediatrician/physician has seen the swelling and confirmed it to be a hernia, then surgery can be recommended. In case of any doubt, it may be wise to call for a second visit or ask the pediatrician/physician to confirm whenever possible. With the widespread availability of digital photography, a parent may be asked to capture an image of the enlarged scrotum to confirm the intermittency of the inguinal or scrotal swelling.

Inguinal hernia predominantly occurs in boys, as girls comprise less than 10% of all reported cases.[59] Whenever a hernia is suspected in a girl, suspicion of the coexistence of a disorder of sexual differentiation must be considered. Up to 1% to 2% of all female children with hernia are found to have androgen insensitivity syndrome.[59,60] In such a circumstance, a testis may be palpable in the inguinal region. In a girl with inguinal hernia, investigations should be done to rule out androgen insensitivity syndrome if there is any suspicion. The various investigations include ultrasound and karyotype. Routine screening with karyotype, although most specific, may not be feasible for economic and technical reasons except when the hernia sac contains palpable gonads. In girls with only a hernia without a palpable gonad, ultrasound examination from a trained radiologist may be an adequate screening tool.

Once diagnosis is confirmed, referral to a pediatric urologist is recommended for surgical intervention. A surgeon may proceed immediately to the operating room in cases of a small infant with a large inguinal hernia that is at higher risk of incarceration and may delay intervention even up to 6 months of age in a less severe case. These decisions are rendered clinically guided by the risk and benefit scenario of surgical intervention in the small infant.

SUMMARY

This article aims to provide an understanding of commonly diagnosed abnormalities of the external genitalia. Variants of foreskin anatomy may preclude a newborn circumcision. Hypospadias is a profound abnormality that can be corrected, but must be recognized in its less severe presentations to ensure proper referral and evaluation. Cryptorchidism and the hernia and hydrocele comprise the most common abnormalities affecting the scrotum and inguinal examination and also require an astute physician to ascertain that these findings are not missed and ultimately neglected. This article provides a brief survey of these anomalies that can serve as the basis of further reading and investigation.

REFERENCES

1. Bergeson PS, Hopkin RJ, Bailey RB Jr, et al. The inconspicuous penis. Pediatrics 1993;92(6):794–9.
2. Aaronson IA. Micropenis: medical and surgical implications. J Urol 1994;152(1):4–14.
3. Srinivasan AK, Palmer LS, Palmer JS. Inconspicuous penis. ScientificWorldJournal 2011;11:2559–64.
4. Maizels M, Zaontz M, Donovan J, et al. Surgical correction of the buried penis: description of a classification system and a technique to correct the disorder. J Urol 1986;136(1 Pt 2):268–71.
5. Crawford BS. Buried penis. Br J Plast Surg 1977;30(1):96–9.

6. Blalock HJ, Vemulakonda V, Ritchey ML, et al. Outpatient management of phimosis following newborn circumcision. J Urol 2003;169(6):2332–4.

7. Sarkis PE, Sadasivam M. Incidence and predictive factors of isolated neonatal penile glanular torsion. J Pediatr Urol 2007;3(6):495–9.

8. Ben-Ari J, Merlob P, Mimouni F, et al. Characteristics of the male genitalia in the newborn: penis. J Urol 1985;134(3):521–2.

9. Baskin LS, Duckett JW, Lue TF. Penile curvature. Urology 1996;48(3):347–56.

10. Kramer SA, Aydin G, Kelalis PP. Chordee without hypospadias in children. J Urol 1982;128(3):559–61.

11. Gairdner D. The fate of the foreskin, a study of circumcision. Br Med J 1949; 2(4642):1433–7.

12. Oster J. Further fate of the foreskin. Incidence of preputial adhesions, phimosis, and smegma among Danish schoolboys. Arch Dis Child 1968;43(228): 200–3.

13. Hutcheson JC. Male neonatal circumcision: indications, controversies and complications. Urol Clin North Am 2004;31(3):461–7, viii.

14. Alanis MC, Lucidi RS. Neonatal circumcision: a review of the world's oldest and most controversial operation. Obstet Gynecol Surv 2004;59(5):379–95.

15. Ginsburg CM, McCracken GH Jr. Urinary tract infections in young infants. Pediatrics 1982;69(4):409–12.

16. Rushton HG, Majd M. Pyelonephritis in male infants: how important is the foreskin? J Urol 1992;148(2 Pt 2):733–6 [discussion: 737–8].

17. Schoen EJ, Colby CJ, Ray GT. Newborn circumcision decreases incidence and costs of urinary tract infections during the first year of life. Pediatrics 2000;105(4 Pt 1):789–93.

18. Morris BJ, Wiswell TE. Circumcision and lifetime risk of urinary tract infection: a systematic review and meta-analysis. J Urol 2013;189(6):2118–24.

19. Schoen EJ, Oehrli M, Colby CD, et al. The highly protective effect of newborn circumcision against invasive penile cancer. Pediatrics 2000;105(3):E36.

20. Bailey RC, Moses S, Parker CB, et al. Male circumcision for HIV prevention in young men in Kisumu, Kenya: a randomised controlled trial. Lancet 2007; 369(9562):643–56.

21. Okeke LI, Asinobi AA, Ikuerowo OS. Epidemiology of complications of male circumcision in Ibadan, Nigeria. BMC Urol 2006;6:21.

22. Weiss HA, Larke N, Halperin D, et al. Complications of circumcision in male neonates, infants and children: a systematic review. BMC Urol 2010;10:2.

23. Krill AJ, Palmer LS, Palmer JS. Complications of circumcision. ScientificWorldJournal 2011;11:2458–68.

24. Banieghbal B. Optimal time for neonatal circumcision: an observation-based study. J Pediatr Urol 2009;5(5):359–62.

25. Pieretti RV, Goldstein AM, Pieretti-Vanmarcke R. Late complications of newborn circumcision: a common and avoidable problem. Pediatr Surg Int 2010;26(5): 515–8.

26. Janus D, Wojcik M, Malunowicz E, et al. A case of recurrent labial adhesions in a 15-month-old child with asymptomatic non-classic congenital adrenal hyperplasia due to 21-hydroxylase deficiency. J Pediatr Endocrinol Metab 2012; 25(9–10):1017–21.

27. Kraft KH, Shukla AR, Canning DA. Hypospadias. Urol Clin North Am 2010;37(2): 167–81.

28. Paulozzi LJ, Erickson JD, Jackson RJ. Hypospadias trends in two US surveillance systems. Pediatrics 1997;100(5):831–4.

29. Dolk H. Rise in prevalence of hypospadias. Lancet 1998;351(9105):770.
30. Patel RP, Shukla AR, Snyder HM 3rd. The island tube and island onlay hypospadias repairs offer excellent long-term outcomes: a 14-year followup. J Urol 2004; 172(4 Pt 2):1717–9 [discussion: 1719].
31. Shukla AR, Patel RP, Canning DA. The 2-stage hypospadias repair. Is it a misnomer? J Urol 2004;172(4 Pt 2):1714–6 [discussion: 1716].
32. Berkowitz GS, Lapinski RH, Dolgin SE, et al. Prevalence and natural history of cryptorchidism. Pediatrics 1993;92(1):44–9.
33. Scorer CG. The descent of the testis. Arch Dis Child 1964;39:605–9.
34. Sijstermans K, Hack WW, Meijer RW, et al. The frequency of undescended testis from birth to adulthood: a review. Int J Androl 2008;31(1):1–11.
35. Damgaard IN, Jensen TK, Petersen JH, et al. Risk factors for congenital cryptorchidism in a prospective birth cohort study. PLoS One 2008;3(8):e3051.
36. Virtanen HE, Toppari J. Epidemiology and pathogenesis of cryptorchidism. Hum Reprod Update 2008;14(1):49–58.
37. Schnack TH, Zdravkovic S, Myrup C, et al. Familial aggregation of cryptorchidism–a nationwide cohort study. Am J Epidemiol 2008;167(12):1453–7.
38. Berkowitz GS, Lapinski RH. Risk factors for cryptorchidism: a nested case-control study. Paediatr Perinat Epidemiol 1996;10(1):39–51.
39. Cendron M, Huff DS, Keating MA, et al. Anatomical, morphological and volumetric analysis: a review of 759 cases of testicular maldescent. J Urol 1993; 149(3):570–3.
40. Cisek LJ, Peters CA, Atala A, et al. Current findings in diagnostic laparoscopic evaluation of the nonpalpable testis. J Urol 1998;160(3 Pt 2):1145–9 [discussion: 1150].
41. Kirsch AJ, Escala J, Duckett JW, et al. Surgical management of the nonpalpable testis: the Children's Hospital of Philadelphia experience. J Urol 1998;159(4): 1340–3.
42. Radmayr C, Oswald J, Schwentner C, et al. Long-term outcome of laparoscopically managed nonpalpable testes. J Urol 2003;170(6 Pt 1):2409–11.
43. Hrebinko RL, Bellinger MF. The limited role of imaging techniques in managing children with undescended testes. J Urol 1993;150(2 Pt 1):458–60.
44. Lee MM, Misra M, Donahoe PK, et al. MIS/AMH in the assessment of cryptorchidism and intersex conditions. Mol Cell Endocrinol 2003;211(1–2):91–8.
45. Kolon TF, Miller OF. Comparison of single versus multiple dose regimens for the human chorionic gonadotropin stimulatory test. J Urol 2001;166(4): 1451–4.
46. Davenport M, Brain C, Vandenberg C, et al. The use of the hCG stimulation test in the endocrine evaluation of cryptorchidism. Br J Urol 1995;76(6):790–4.
47. De Rosa M, Lupoli G, Mennitti M, et al. Congenital bilateral anorchia: clinical, hormonal and imaging study in 12 cases. Andrologia 1996;28(5):281–5.
48. Desireddi NV, Liu DB, Maizels M, et al. Magnetic resonance arteriography/venography is not accurate to structure management of the impalpable testis. J Urol 2008;180(Suppl 4):1805–8 [discussion: 1808–9].
49. Lala R, Matarazzo P, Chiabotto P, et al. Combined therapy with LHRH and HCG in cryptorchid infants. Eur J Pediatr 1993;152(Suppl 2):S31–3.
50. Henna MR, Del Nero RG, Sampaio CZ, et al. Hormonal cryptorchidism therapy: systematic review with metanalysis of randomized clinical trials. Pediatr Surg Int 2004;20(5):357–9.
51. Pyorala S, Huttunen NP, Uhari M. A review and meta-analysis of hormonal treatment of cryptorchidism. J Clin Endocrinol Metab 1995;80(9):2795–9.

52. Thorsson AV, Christiansen P, Ritzen M. Efficacy and safety of hormonal treatment of cryptorchidism: current state of the art. Acta Paediatr 2007;96(5): 628–30.

53. Chilvers C, Dudley NE, Gough MH, et al. Undescended testis: the effect of treatment on subsequent risk of subfertility and malignancy. J Pediatr Surg 1986; 21(8):691–6.

54. Cortes D, Thorup JM, Visfeldt J. Cryptorchidism: aspects of fertility and neoplasms. A study including data of 1,335 consecutive boys who underwent testicular biopsy simultaneously with surgery for cryptorchidism. Horm Res 2001;55(1):21–7.

55. Rowe MI, Copelson LW, Clatworthy HW. The patent processus vaginalis and the inguinal hernia. J Pediatr Surg 1969;4(1):102–7.

56. van Veen RN, van Wessem KJ, Halm JA, et al. Patent processus vaginalis in the adult as a risk factor for the occurrence of indirect inguinal hernia. Surg Endosc 2007;21(2):202–5.

57. van Wessem KJ, Simons MP, Plaisier PW, et al. The etiology of indirect inguinal hernias: congenital and/or acquired? Hernia 2003;7(2):76–9.

58. Boocock GR, Todd PJ. Inguinal hernias are common in preterm infants. Arch Dis Child 1985;60(7):669–70.

59. Sarpel U, Palmer SK, Dolgin SE. The incidence of complete androgen insensitivity in girls with inguinal hernias and assessment of screening by vaginal length measurement. J Pediatr Surg 2005;40(1):133–6 [discussion: 136–7].

60. Burge DM, Sugarman IS. Exclusion of androgen insensitivity syndrome in girls with inguinal hernias: current surgical practice. Pediatr Surg Int 2002;18(8): 701–3.

Neuropathic Bladder in the Neonate

Michael C. Carr, MD, PhD

KEYWORDS

- Myelomeningocele • Urodynamics • Spina bifida
- Detrusor external sphincter dyssynergy

KEY POINTS

- Newborn urodynamic evaluation can provide valuable information allowing appropriate evaluation of infants with spina bifida.
- The Management of Myelomeningocele Study trial demonstrated a reduced incidence of ventriculoperitoneal shunting and improvement in lower motor function in prenatally repaired myelomeningocele infants.
- Detrusor external sphincter dyssynergy can lead to progressive deterioration in bladder function and upper urinary tract drainage.
- Most patients with spina bifida ultimately require intermittent catheterization and pharmacologic therapy to improve storage and facilitate drainage of their bladders.

INTRODUCTION

Bladder function can be defined by two simple processes, storage and emptying. Children who are born with myelomeningocele (also known as spina bifida or myelodysplasia) can have significant effects on both of these processes, leading in some situations to upper tract deterioration unless it is recognized and treated in a timely fashion. Pioneering work by Lapides and coworkers[1] demonstrated that clean intermittent catheterization (CIC) could be used to empty the bladder, thus improving the situation for children with poor bladder emptying. Pharmacologic measures have been used to improve bladder storage and the combination of pharmacotherapy and CIC has become the mainstay in the management of children with myelomeningocele.

Myelomeningocele lesions are distributed among thoracic, lumbar, and sacral vertebrae (**Fig. 1**).[2] Most of the bony abnormalities occur in the lumbosacral region. The actual level of the meningocele may not correspond to the distribution of the

Disclosure: None.
Division of Urology, The Children's Hospital of Philadelphia, 3rd Flr Wood Center, 34th Street & Civic Center Boulevard, Philadelphia, PA 19104, USA
E-mail address: Carr@email.chop.edu

Clin Perinatol 41 (2014) 725–733
http://dx.doi.org/10.1016/j.clp.2014.05.017
0095-5108/14/$ – see front matter © 2014 Elsevier Inc. All rights reserved.

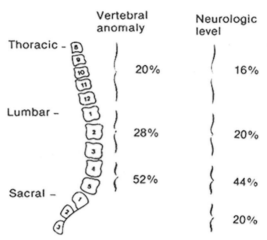

Fig. 1. Distribution of level of lesion in children with myelodysplasia. Most lesions involve the lumbosacral area.

injured nerve roots. In general, nerves opposite the level of the bony defect or more caudally positioned ones are affected. Occasionally the injury may affect more cranially positioned nerve roots and there may be differences on opposite sides of the spinal cord even at the same level.[3] Quite often, a lipoma of the filum terminala, or dura, is associated with the meningocele compressing or stretching the nerve roots. These patients, too, have an Arnold-Chiari malformation, which affects the brain and brainstem, so that most children require placement of a ventriculoperitoneal shunt. All of this leads to a considerable variation in the type and extent of neurologic injury. There remains ongoing debate concerning the appropriate evaluation, management, and treatment of patients with myelomeningocele.[4–6] Previously, urodynamic investigation, which is the best way of assessing the function of the bladder, was commonly not performed in children until after they reached school age. It was deemed important at that age to achieve social continence. Increasingly the evaluation of the bladder in the newborn period has been favored once the back has been closed and the child's neurosurgical condition stabilized.[7] The initial assessment provides a baseline so that subsequent studies can look for evidence of progressive deterioration that may occur.

The prenatal diagnosis of myelomeningocele is now more common, with a triple screen being performed to look for the presence of a neural tube defect.[8] Confirmation of the myelomeningocele occurs with ultrasonography so that appropriate prenatal counseling can occur and a thorough explanation of the various sequelae of spina bifida provided to expectant parents. Recently, the Eunice Kennedy Shriver National Institute of Child Health and Human Development sponsored a randomized prospective trial, The Management of Myelomeningocele Study (Clinicaltrials.gov NCT00060606), which provided a critical assessment of the outcome of infants who are born with myelomeningocele and are repaired in utero during midgestation versus those infants who had postnatal closure in the first 24 hours of life. This landmark study was published in the *New England Journal of Medicine* in March 2011.[9] This study demonstrated that the incidence of ventriculoperitoneal shunting was 80% in those who underwent postnatal closure versus 42% of those with prenatal repair. In addition, at 3 years, 42% of those who had prenatal repair walked independently versus 21% of those with postnatal closure. The urologic outcomes of those patients who underwent repair in utero is forthcoming, because the original studies had outcomes determined at only 12 months and 30 months. For this reason, additional funding was obtained to look at this unique cohort of patients at 6 to 10 years of age to provide an accurate reflection of bladder status and continence.

Prevention of spina bifida, with a reported incidence of 1 in 2500 live births and 1500 births per year in the United States, would have a dramatic effect and be the optimal public health goal. Folate deficiency was believed to be the primary cause of neural tube defects. Hence the US Food and Drug Administration mandated that enriched grain products be fortified with folic acid in 1998. Data collected as part of the Slone Defect study from 1998 to 2008 were used to identify 205 mothers of spina bifida cases. Interviews were conducted to discern pregnancy exposure, including details of diet and vitamin intake and comparison made to 6357 mothers of nonmalformed control subjects. Spina bifida was not associated with regular folic acid supplementation either around the time of conception or initiated in early pregnancy. Thus, in the setting of folic acid fortification of grains, folic acid supplementation does not seem to offer further benefit for reducing risk of spina bifida.[10]

BLADDER EVALUATION

The initial structural evaluation of the lower urinary tract can be accomplished by evaluating the kidneys and bladder ultrasonographically. Functional information about the bladder comes from urodynamic evaluation, which is able to assess bladder capacity, compliance (overall pressure in the bladder at a given time), and bladder emptying.[11] The use of urodynamics in infants with spina bifida allows the early detection of potentially injurious conditions so that the appropriate intervention can occur.

The external sphincter is designed to provide a resting tone that maintains urinary continence. Normal bladders have the unique property of maintaining a low pressure (low compliance) that is generally less than 10 cm H_2O over a variable volume. Once the bladder becomes full, the signal is transferred via the afferent sacral nerves to the pontine micturition center. These signals are then processed allowing for appropriate relaxation of the pelvic floor musculature and external sphincter, which are innervated by the pudendal nerve so that there is coordinated relaxation of these muscles before the time that the detrusor muscle begins to contract. Alteration of external sphincter function in children with spina bifida can contribute to persistent incontinence (low leak point pressure, external sphincter denervation) or detrusor sphincter dyssynergia that leads to detrusor hypertrophy of the bladder caused by a functional obstruction (**Fig. 2**). These changes alter the storage capability of the bladder, with progressive loss of bladder capacity and compliance. As long as the bladder stores urine at low pressure with coordination between the detrusor and the external sphincter, then effective emptying should occur and the kidneys remain normal. When this process is somehow circumvented, the compliance of the bladder may be altered, bladder emptying worsens, and the child is at greater risk for urinary tract infections and potentially kidney dysfunction. A urodynamic evaluation becomes critical in defining the activity of the external sphincter looking for evidence of synergy, dyssynergy, or the absence of activity. Bauer and colleagues[7] performed an evaluation of newborns with myelomeningocele and found that 55% of babies had detrusor sphincter dyssynergia, 18% had synergy, and 27% had absent activity.

Urodynamic studies have also been performed on healthy newborns that have demonstrated that the detrusor and external sphincter can function in a discoordinated fashion for as long as the first 12 to 15 months of life. There is a gradual neural maturation that occurs, which facilitates the synergic voiding pattern that should occur over time.[12]

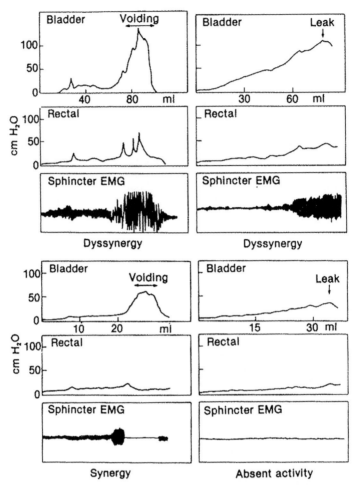

Fig. 2. Types of lower urinary tract function in children with myelodysplasia. The activity of the external urethral sphincter is classified as dyssynergic, synergic, or absent according to its response during a detrusor contraction or a sustained increase in intravesical pressure. Absent activity implies complete denervation of the sphincter. EMG, electromyogram.

Infants with detrusor sphincter dyssynergy are at higher risk for upper tract dysfunction than those with synergy or absent function. Further work in Bauer's cohort of newborns determined that 79% of children with detrusor sphincter dyssynergy had or developed deterioration of the upper urinary tract within the first 3 years of life. Children with synergic sphincter activity rarely show deterioration. Only those who converted to a dyssynergic pattern on subsequent studies did so and usually within a year of the alteration from synergic to dyssynergic.[13] Similarly, children with complete denervation of the sphincter were unlikely to show signs of upper urinary tract deterioration. Those children who did were presumed to develop increased outlet resistance caused by progressive fibrosis of the denervated skeletal muscle component of the external sphincter.[14]

Bauer[2] proposed a set of guidelines for the surveillance of infants and children who were born with myelomeningocele. These guidelines were based on the premise that those infants and children with dyssynergia are at greatest risk for upper tract deterioration and require the greatest amount of surveillance. Renal ultrasonography provides an assessment of the upper tracts, ureteral dilation, bladder wall changes, and bladder emptying. The dyssynergic group were monitored with a postvoid residual urine volume and urine culture every 3 months, renal ultrasonography every 6 months, and urodynamic studies annually to look for evidence of deterioration. Urodynamics that are done immediately following closure of the myelomeningocele need to be interpreted carefully because some infants manifest spinal shock and show evidence of a flaccid bladder that does not empty well. Generally, the spinal shock resolves within a period of several weeks so that it may be best to defer doing the initial urodynamic study until this resolves. In the interim infants are placed on intermittent catheterization. If the external sphincter is synergic, then annual renal ultrasound and urodynamic studies should be performed. Those patients who have complete denervation of the detrusor and external sphincter require annual renal ultrasounds to monitor the urinary tract (**Fig. 3**).

At The Children's Hospital of Philadelphia, we have further refined the guidelines and have devised an algorithm that is applied to those infants who have had either fetal repair or postnatal repair of their myelomeningocele (see **Fig. 3**). This provides consistent guidelines that can also be shared with parents who may have ongoing care provided at another institution.

THERAPEUTIC OPTIONS

Intervention is necessary when there are signs of outflow obstruction or elevated detrusor pressure on filling or both. High bladder filling and voiding pressures, particularly in the face of uncoordinated external sphincter activity, are worrisome signs suggesting that either bladder decompensation or upper urinary tract deterioration

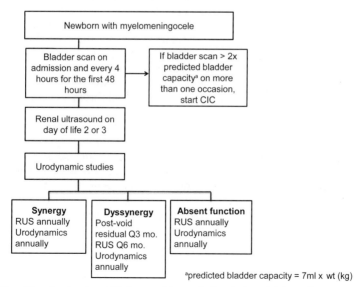

Fig. 3. Algorithm for testing of infants with myelodysplasia. Initial urodynamic studies are done after 4 weeks of age to avoid potential spinal shock that can occur after closure of the myelomeningocele. CIC, clean intermittent catheterization; Q, every; RUS, renal ultrasound.

will occur. Thus, newborn infants who demonstrate these worrisome features traditionally have been started on intermittent catheterization.[15] Additionally, they are placed on anticholinergic therapy to potentially decrease intravesical pressures and also to minimize the occurrence of uninhibited bladder contractions.[16] In situations in which children develop recurrent urinary tract infections or have changes in their continence patterns, then urodynamic studies can be used to look for changes in overall bladder compliance and external sphincter activity.

Newer methods of dealing with detrusor sphincter dyssynergy include the use of urethral dilation of the external sphincter[17] or the injection of onabotulinumtoxinA (Botox) directly into the external sphincter. Park and colleagues[18] have shown that urethral dilation can be effective in altering the guarding reflex so that infants or children with evidence of detrusor sphincter dyssynergy empty their bladders more effectively and lessen the chance of upper tract deterioration. Urethral dilation is easily accomplished in female patients, because the urethra is short and able to accommodate progressively larger urethral sounds (8–32F catheter). The male infant urethra cannot accommodate such large sounds, so the University of Michigan group recommended a temporary perineal urethrostomy to allow access to the posterior urethra. Alternatively, the external sphincter can be approached via an infant cystoscope and onabotulinumtoxinA injected directly into the external sphincter. Credé voiding, which involves applying pressure to the suprapubic region to facilitate bladder emptying, is contraindicated in those infants or children with an intact sacral reflex function. Such children have a reflexive increase in external urethral sphincter electromyographic activity during a Credé maneuver. Failure of such conservative approaches may lead to a cutaneous vesicostomy as an alternative option.

Video urodynamic studies that combine the use of fluoroscopic imaging and monitoring of intravesical, intra-abdominal, and electromyographic activity of the external sphincter have become the ideal way of assessing infants and children with a neuropathic bladder. Such studies are particularly helpful in the evaluation of a child with persistent urinary incontinence with a neurogenic bladder. Such a child with persistent incontinence may have uninhibited detrusor contractions, elevated intravesical pressures, a low urethral resistance, or excessive urine volume. The institution of anticholinergic therapy (Oxybutynin, Detrol, Ditropan) may lower detrusor tone and contractility. Newer agents that are long acting improve overall patient compliance for the medication and increase the likelihood that this will be successful. Patients who have a diminished leak point pressure may benefit from α-sympathomimetic agents, such as ephedrine.[19]

The child with denervation of the external sphincter may not empty well because of a fixed urethral resistance caused by fibrosis. Such a patient would benefit from intermittent catheterization to facilitate bladder emptying. That same patient may only be plagued with stress incontinence because of the fixed nature of the external sphincter.

The use of onabotulinumtoxinA has become more popular by treating the external urethral sphincter and the detrusor muscle.[20] First described for use in spinal cord injury patents with detrusor external sphincter dyssynergy, the technique was applied for male infants with detrusor external sphincter dyssynergy, in which 100 IU of onabotulinumtoxinA is injected at the 12-, 3-, 6-, and 9-o'clock positions, 25 IU per quadrant. The effects of the injections last anywhere from 6 to 9 months and obviate the need to begin CIC and anticholinergic therapy. For some families, delaying the process of CIC can be very beneficial because the logistics of CIC being conducted in a daycare situation is not always easy to accomplish. What is not known is the likelihood of futurè success following a single injection into either the detrusor or the external sphincter.[21,22]

The final option in the management of patients who have persistent urinary incontinence despite maximal pharmacotherapy and an intermittent catheterization regimen involves reconstructive surgery. Such surgery ultimately represents a failure of medical management and the hope is that early and aggressive management of such patients limits the need for reconstructive surgery in the future. These patients require an increase in bladder capacity and improvement in overall bladder compliance that can be accomplished by augmenting the bladder with a segment of intestine.[23] For those patients with persistent incontinence, this alone does not render the patient dry because many have a diminished leak point pressure. Several surgical procedures have been devised to increase the outlet resistance but none seems to have universal applicability and overall success.

Female patients can be managed by injecting a bulking agent at the bladder neck, trying to co-opt the tissues more effectively as urethral resistance is increased.[24] If reconstructive surgery is needed to increase bladder capacity, then a combination of a urethral sling and a catheterizable channel is necessary to maximize the success of the surgery.[25]

Male patients with decreased urethral resistance pose an even greater surgical challenge, because there is no surgical procedure that proved to be uniformly successful. Attempts at bladder neck reconstruction include such procedures as the Kropp procedure,[26] Pippi Salle,[27] bladder neck suspensions and slings, and artificial urinary sphincters.[28] Each procedure has advantages and disadvantages that need to be carefully explored with the patient and family.[29]

A concept used in the past but modified today is the use of an indwelling Foley catheter. Typically, the catheter is left in place only at nighttime, so that the patient resumes CIC during the daytime. The use of a catheter for anywhere from 8 to 12 hours can decrease the postobstructive diuresis that occurs in some patients who have not been catheterized overnight. Their urine output is not as great during the day, increasing the likelihood that they will remain dry with their CIC regimen during the day.[30]

Patients who are born with myelomeningocele need a coordinated team approach to maximize their management. The success that is achieved in the newborn, toddler, school-aged, and adolescent years needs to be tailored to that age group and closely monitored. The successes that are achieved in the pediatric population contribute to a new dilemma because this population is maturing into adulthood and bringing with them a unique set of ongoing challenges.[31]

REFERENCES

1. Lapides J, Diokno AC, Silber SJ, et al. Clean intermittent self-catheterization in the treatment of urinary tract disease. J Urol 1971;107:458.
2. Bauer SB. Pediatric neurology. In: Krane RJ, Siroky MB, editors. Clinical neurourology. Boston: Little, Brown; 1979. p. 279.
3. Barson AJ. The vertebral level of termination of the spinal cord during normal and abnormal development. J Anat 1970;106:489.
4. Johnston JH, Farkas A. Congenital neuropathic bladder: practicalities and possibilities of conservative management. Urology 1975;5:729.
5. McGuire EJ, Woodside JR, Bordon TA, et al. Prognostic value of urodynamic testing in myelodysplasia patients. J Urol 1981;126:205.
6. Webster GD, el-Mahrouky A, Stone AR, et al. The urological evaluation and management of patients with myelodysplasia. Br J Urol 1986;58:261.
7. Bauer SB, Hallett M, Khoshbin S, et al. Predictive value of urodynamic evaluation in newborns with myelodysplasia. JAMA 1984;252:650.

8. Adzick NS, Walsh DS. Myelomeningocele: prenatal diagnosis, pathophysiology and management. Semin Pediatr Surg 2003;12(3):168.

9. Adzick NS, Thom E, Spong C, et al. A randomized trial of prenatal versus postnatal repair of myelomeningocele. N Engl J Med 2011;346:993–1004.

10. Ahrens K, Yazdy MM, Mitchell AA, et al. Folic acid intake and spina bifida in the era of dietary folic acid fortification. Epidemiology 2011;22(5):731–7.

11. Ghoniem GM, Bloom DA, McGuire EJ, et al. Bladder compliance in myelomeningocele children. J Urol 1989;141:1404.

12. Sillen U. Bladder function in infants. Scand J Urol Nephrol Suppl 2004;215:69–74.

13. Van Gool JD, et al. Vesico-ureteral reflux in children with spina bifida and detrusor-sphincter dyssynergia. Contrib Nephrol 1994;39:221–37.

14. Bauer SB, Spindel MR. The changing neurological lesion in myelodysplasia. JAMA 1987;258:1630.

15. Hopps CV, Kropp KA. Preservation of renal function in children with myelomeningocele managed with basic newborn evaluation and close follow-up. J Urol 2003; 169(1):305.

16. Goessl C, Knispel HH, Fiedler U, et al. Urodynamic effects of oral oxybutynin chloride in children with myelomeningocele and detrusor hyperreflexia. Urol 1998;51:94.

17. Bloom DA, Knechtel JM, McGuire EJ. Urethral dilation improves bladder compliance in children with myelomeningocele and high leak point pressures. J Urol 1990;144:430.

18. Park JM, McGuire EJ, Koo HP, et al. External urethral sphincter dilation for the management of high risk myelomeningocele: 15-year experience. J Urol 2001; 165:2383.

19. Diokno AC, Taub M. Ephedrine in treatment of urinary incontinence. Urology 1975;5(5):624–5.

20. Marte A. Onabotulinumtoxin A for treating overactive/poor compliant bladders in children and adolescents with neurogenic bladder secondary to myelomeningocele. Toxins (Basel) 2012;5(1):16–24.

21. Chancellor MB, Elovic E, Esquenazi A, et al. Evidence-based review and assessment of botulinum neurotoxin for the treatment of urologic conditions. Toxicon 2013;67:129–40.

22. Riccabona M, Koen M, Schindler M, et al. Botulinum-a toxin injection into the detrusor: a safe alternative in the treatment of children with myelomeningocele with detrusor hyperreflexia. J Urol 2004;171(2 Pt 1):845–8.

23. Kass EJ, Koff SA. Bladder augmentation in the pediatric neuropathic bladder. J Urol 1983;129:552.

24. Misseri R, Casale AJ, Cain MP, et al. Alternative uses of dextranomer/hyaluronic acid copolymer: the efficacy of bladder neck injection for urinary incontinence. J Urol 2005;174(4 Pt 2):1691.

25. Dik P, Klijn AJ, van Gool JD, et al. Transvaginal sling suspension of bladder neck in female patients with neurogenic sphincter incontinence. J Urol 2003; 170(2 Pt 1):580 [discussion: 581].

26. Kropp KA. Bladder neck reconstruction in children. Urol Clin North Am 1999; 26(3):661.

27. Pippi Salle JL. Surgical management of urinary incontinence in children with neurogenic sphincteric incompetence. J Urol 2000;164(5):1668.

28. Gonzalez R, Merino FG, Vaughn M. Long-term results of the artificial urinary sphincter in male patients with neurogenic bladder. J Urol 1995;154(2 Pt 2): 769.

29. Cole EE, Adams MC, Brock JW 3rd, et al. Outcome of continence procedures in the pediatric patient: a single institutional experience. J Urol 2003;170(2 Pt 1): 560–3 [discussion: 563].
30. Koff SA, Gigax MR, Jayanthi VR. Nocturnal bladder emptying: a simple technique for reversing urinary tract deterioration in children with neurogenic bladder. J Urol 2005;174(4 Pt 2):1629.
31. Burke R, Liptak GS. Council on children with disabilities: providing a primary care medical home for children and youth with spina bifida. Pediatrics 2011;128(6): e1645–57.

Index

Note: Page numbers of article titles are in **boldface** type.

Clin Perinatol 41 (2014) 735–747
http://dx.doi.org/10.1016/S0095-5108(14)00068-2
0095-5108/14/$ – see front matter © 2014 Elsevier Inc. All rights reserved.
perinatology.theclinics.com

Moving?

Make sure your subscription moves with you!

To notify us of your new address, find your **Clinics Account Number** (located on your mailing label above your name), and contact customer service at:

Email: journalscustomerservice-usa@elsevier.com

800-654-2452 (subscribers in the U.S. & Canada)
314-447-8871 (subscribers outside of the U.S. & Canada)

Fax number: 314-447-8029

Elsevier Health Sciences Division
Subscription Customer Service
3251 Riverport Lane
Maryland Heights, MO 63043

*To ensure uninterrupted delivery of your subscription, please notify us at least 4 weeks in advance of move.